Here's what readers are saying about The Body Sculpting Bible for Women

The best book on weight training for women...period!

—*A reader from New York, N.Y.*

I have been following the advanced 14-day workout and diet for one week and plan to continue indefinitely. I love your book—I love the plan. Thank you!

—*Ellen*

I received my copy of the *Body Sculpting Bible for Women* not even a week ago and I was so impressed that I read it from cover to cover in less than three days. It answered all of my questions and I found the information extremely helpful. I was a little concerned about the instructions to workout with weights five to six days straight; I was always told that muscles need a day or so of recovery time—but I'm no expert. . . I've recommended this book to all of my friends interested in resculpting their bodies. On a scale of 1 to 10, I'd definitely give this book a 10!

—*A reader from Phoenix, Ariz.*

My husband starting using the *Body Sculpting Bible for Men* and loved it, so I decided to see if it would work for me. Thank you guys—I feel great and look great! The 14-day workout program is a great motivational start and I realized that even if I don't want to go to the gym seven days a week I can do a lot of the exercises at home. It has also brought my husband and I closer together. Thank you Hugo and James!

—*A reader from Ft. Meyers, Fla.*

I'm a 22-year-old who used to hate working out. This book has changed all that...It was fun, and the best part is I saw results! I never thought I'd be writing a review for a "fitness" book or that a program would actually work for me. Thank you authors of the *Body Sculpting Bible for Women*, for my new body and new outlook on life!

—*Nicole (N.Y.)*

I am almost 41 years old and have been weight training for years. This is the first book that covers everything! It truly is a bible for women's fitness. I plan to smoke most every 25-year-old on the beach this summer!

—*Linda (Radford, Va.)*

I have worked out and dieted on and off for years, but this is the first routine that produced immediate results. All I did was follow the workout routines, not even the eating plan or the meditation exercises. After each two-week cycle, I had lost inches!

—*A reader from Reno, Nev.*

I would recommend this to anyone who wants to add resistance training to her workout, or just get more proficient at designing a good, effective workout for herself. I would also recommend it to anyone who has been working out for some time and "eating healthy," but has not gotten the results she was expecting—this book will deliver them to you!

—A reader from Switzerland

This book is awesome! If you follow the nutrition plan and do the workouts everyday, you will see results. I am heavy and need to lose weight and tone down, and this book is the key...Results come; with dedication and heart, you will do it with this book. In a matter of a few weeks you start to see changes, physically, nutritionally, mentally. Thanks James and Hugo. A+. Ladies, this is our book.

—A reader from Hawaii

After looking at a variety of books on the subject of weight loss, nutrition, and weight lifting (for tone and shape) I finally settled on this one. It's geared toward females who are ready to take control of their bodies. I found the book to be very accessible and I liked the informal language...This book is like having a personal health and fitness instructor right there with you. I highly recommend it!

—A reader from Thousand Oaks, Calf.

If you are going to buy one book on women's body sculpting, this is the one. James Villepigue clearly knows bodybuilding, and understands female anatomy and physiology. His subject is covered thoroughly, and the individual exercises are precisely explained in comprehensible language. Follow the program, and you will see results in no time!

—Kristen M. (Belmont, Mass.)

This book is wonderful! If you are willing to change your eating habits and follow their exercise plan, you will see results. I really enjoy having a structured plan to follow. They have great explanations for the exercises, as well as pictures. The supplement and nutrition sections are very informative. I use this book as a reference almost every day. I can't say enough good things about this book!

—Jenell B. (Ottawa, Ohio)

With so many so called fitness authorities out there, it is refreshing to read a book that offers both fundamental information that must be included in order to successfully educate, coupled with a plethora of innovative and exciting material that actually works. The books are without question an essential tool for helping every woman achieve a fabulous body! Great work James and Hugo!

—Barbara M. (Bethesda, Md.)

Thank you so much for the great book. I started your routine about five weeks ago and wow, what a difference! Normally I get bored when I work out...so I stop. With the "bible" I find myself looking forward to my work-outs. I finally feel good about myself. I have better stamina, more energy, and a body that I'm not ashamed of. Thank you again so much for helping me see that working out and getting into shape doesn't have to be dull. Try the body sculpting bible...you'll love it. Five stars!

—A reader from Encino, Calif.

THE BODY SCULPTING BIBLE FOR WOMEN

PLATINUM EDITION

FEATURING THE 14-DAY BODY SCULPTING WORKOUT

JAMES VILLEPIGUE
HUGO RIVERA

FOREWORD BY NICOLE ROLLOLAZO

Library of Congress Cataloging-in-Publication Data is available.

ISBN: 978-1-57826-613-5

Disclaimer:
Before beginning any exercise program, consult your physician. The author and the publisher disclaim any liability, personal or professional, resulting from the application or misapplication of any of the information in this publication.

THE BODY SCULPTING BIBLE FOR WOMEN is available for bulk purchase, special promotions and premiums. For more information on reselling and special purchase opportunities, please call us at 1-800-528-2550 and ask for the Special Sales Manager.

Cover Design by Angel Harleycat, Deborah Miller, and Heather Daugherty
Interior Design by Fatema Tarzi, Deborah Miller, Allison Furrer, Jasmine Cordoza, and Nick Macagnone

10 9 8 7 6 5 4 3 2 1
Printed in the United States

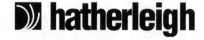

Dedications

This book is dedicated to my Twin Flame Cecile who has been my constant source of inspiration since the moment we met and who made me come alive. You are my air, the better part of me, and words cannot express the love that I feel for you. Thank you so much for being in my life.

This book is also dedicated to my son Chad who makes me proud on a daily basis, who has achieved Body Sculpting perfection much quicker than I did, and who is also on his way to beating me by achieving business success quicker than me as well!

I also dedicate this book to my parents and grandparents for always believing in me and who always ensured that I would get the best education possible as I was growing up, to my brother Raul whose superior computer knowledge made it possible for me to go online, and to my brother Javier who has pursued his dreams and achieved success regardless of obstacles. A special thanks to Alvaro and Edith who have always been there to help me and have provided me with support in time of need.

This book is also dedicated to my close friends who are also like family to me...you all know who you are. Words cannot express the gratitude I have.

Also, to every single person who has crossed my path and has helped me in one way or the other in my journey. And of course, to James Villepigue who was instrumental to getting this great piece of work done (James, you are awesome), as well as to everyone else involved in its publishing and distribution.

Last but not least, to all of the wonderful people who have ever gotten a copy of this book (many of you who have also served as our wonderful spokespeople to others) as without you there would not be any reason for what we do. Thank you!

And finally, to God, for giving me the talent to put this work together.

Hugo A. Rivera

Dedicated to my Lord and My Savior, Jesus Christ.

My Lord, I thank You, and am just so thankful for my life, my beautiful wife, my amazing children, my wonderful parents, my very talented sister, all my family, my friends, and for all of the blessed success that you have bestowed upon Hugo and myself, over the years. For *all* of these mighty blessings, I am eternally grateful!

"I can do all things through Christ who strengthens me."
—*Philippians 4:13*

James Villepigue

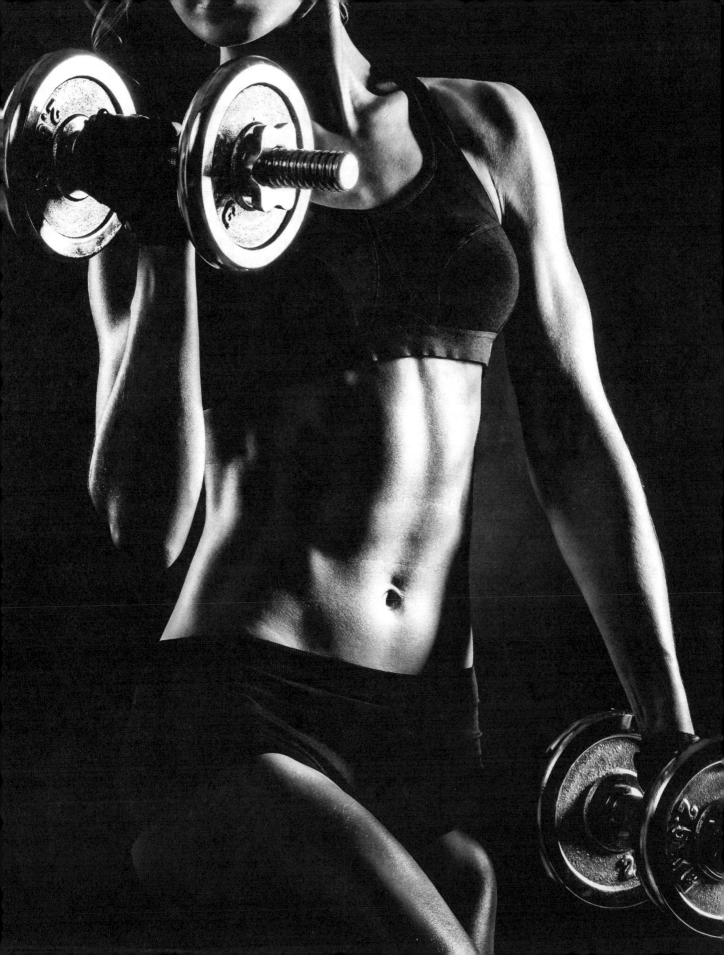

Foreword to the Original Edition

Finally, a book that dispels the myths about getting into shape! I started working out ten years ago and have been participating in fitness competitions for four years. Unfortunately, it has taken me all this time to gain even half of the knowledge you can learn just by reading *The Body Sculpting Bible for Women!*

This book is not filled with empty promises for a "quick fix" or a "miracle diet." Instead, it gives you priceless information on how to achieve your fitness goals. If you are really serious about changing your body for the better, the best thing you can do for yourself is to follow the advice on these pages. Don't give up or get discouraged! The 14-Day Body Sculpting Workout is a serious fitness plan, and if you use it seriously, you will get serious results.

As women, we generally have different nutritional and physical goals and needs than men. That is what is so great about this book! Inside you will find information on James and Hugo's 14-Day Body Sculpting Program, the Zone-Tone concept, nutritional programs and much more. The best part about it is that these programs are all designed specifically for women. When it comes to fitness and bodybuilding, women's needs often get lost in the shuffle. Sometimes it feels like every fitness magazine, workout program, and nutritional product out there is designed just for men! With this book, however, each and every point of information is targeted to a woman's fitness needs.

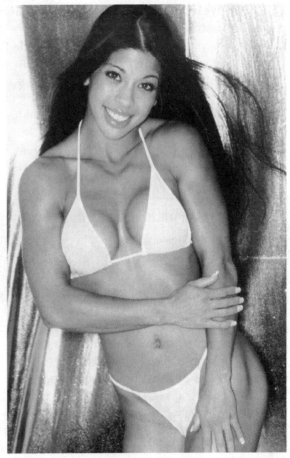

The Body Sculpting Bible for Women is not only filled with invaluable information, it is also easily accessible. The presentation is simple to understand and use. Whether you are a beginner or a professional athlete, you will definitely find this book to be rewarding and inspirational. You won't just change your body, you'll change your mind!

Nicole Rollolazo
Fitness America Pageant Champion 2000

Preface

Hi Folks! Welcome to the Platinum Edition of our *Body Sculpting Bibles!*

If you have already purchased our previous *Body Sculpting Bible* editions in the past, then we want to extend to you our most sincere gratitude for giving us the support you have since the beginning. If you are a new reader, then we want to personally congratulate you for taking your first step towards achieving the leaner, firmer, and stronger body that you are looking for.

The *Body Sculpting Bible* series has been around for over 11 years now. That's an extraordinary length of time for a fitness book series. Most fitness books only last a year or two in the market-place, if they even last that long.

So why have our books survived the test of time, and even flourished, when others seem to just disappear? Here are a few reasons why the *Body Sculpting Bible* series has differed from other fitness books:

THE WHO, WHAT, WHEN, WHERE, WHY & HOW

- **Who are the Creators:** James Villepigue and Hugo Rivera have been in the fitness industry and lifted in the trenches for a combined amount of over 40 years. They walk the talk and play the part.
- **What are They Most Recognized For:** The essence of the *Body Sculpting Bible* books is the underlying original 14-Day Body Sculpting Program—one of the very first periodized weight training programs for the mainstream fitness enthusiast. These systems utilize a logically arranged `muscle confusion' approach that yields the fastest and most consistent long-term body composition results possible.
- **When Were the Books First Created:** Back in 1998, the authors just happened to meet in Florida while working out separately. They started talking and two years later, they had developed this best-selling fitness book series.
- **Where:** *The Body Sculpting Bible for Women* is now in its 4th Edition. The 1st Edition was written by James and Hugo over 18 years ago, and so, it only made sense that each edition be updated with the latest and greatest information. James and Hugo spent over one year writing the 1st Edition and accomplished the collaborative work by way of phone and Internet.
- **Why:** The authors had discovered that average people needed top-tier fitness information and more guidance to help them achieve their dream physiques.
- **How:** James and Hugo created step-by-step guidelines and a direct plan of action that any-one could follow, all based on scientific analysis. Much like a business plan, where every-thing is laid out for success, the *Body Sculpting Bible* books equip people with the means to achieve body sculpting perfection.

Why is it that the *Body Sculpting Bibles* have sold well over one million copies and are revered as one of the most successful fitness book franchises in history? Well, they're solid books and provide a comprehensive, yet solid, plan of specific action steps to help you on your way. When we first set out, we offered one of the very first mainstream periodization programs called "The 14 Day Body Sculpting Program". Many of our innovative training principles were initially considered radical, but they were quickly embraced by our readers and fans because they worked (and worked very well).

So, yes, the *Body Sculpting Bible* books have had wild success, but we are not sitting pretty. Yes, we've managed to help millions of average people just like you to shape up, gain confidence, preserve their youth, and improve many areas of their lives. But still, there are millions of people we still need to help.

We came to the realization that we needed to come back and refresh some of the material within the book. As time passes, things naturally change as new research is conducted and new science comes about. It is up to us, as fitness experts, to take the science, decipher it, and pass it on in a way that makes sense and is easy for you to understand.

So, with that said, we're on a mission to help millions more people get up and get out of their own way. Get up off that couch, rid yourself of the fast food, do what most people won't take the time to do, and let's get you to a place of total body transformation and life empowerment.

Over the years, we have had to rely mostly on the books and e-mail to stay in communication with our fans. No longer do we each exist in a place where we are isolated in our homeland or limited to our own cities and close surroundings. The internet has allowed us to reach out and digitally shake hands with our global friends.

The new global approach of this latest edition was developed for two reasons. First, we want you to be an ambassador for fitness in your hometown. We want you to stand proud and represent where you're from. Gather your local friends, family, co-workers, and anyone else and create a fitness force. With this book, we want you to lead your clan and build them up to extraordinary health and fitness levels. Together, we can combat fat, obliterate obesity, do-in diabetes, kill many cardiac problems, and take more control over our lives than ever before.

The second reason for this global approach is that, even though we have greater reach to the world than ever before, many of us still hide behind our computers. It's time to reach out and tell the world who you are. We know the world is facing a lot of difficulties right now, and there is no better time to take a stand and refuse to give in to adversity. Today we are battling wars, a bullied economy, and the fight against obesity. The grim reality is that most people have not gotten healthier over the last decade. In fact, they have gotten even unhealthier! Perhaps this is partly a result of the negative things that are going on in the world at this time. Maybe the stress from everything that is happening has affected people and thus, they take comfort in food.

However, here is our advice to you: there is too much going on in the world that we have little or absolutely no control over. But here's the great news: there are some things that we can control. We can control our ability to do our very best in building ourselves up, both inside and out, so that we create better outcomes for ourselves and for the people around us. When we build ourselves up both physically and emotionally, we empower ourselves and we place ourselves in a rare position that allows us to have more control over many different things in our lives.

It is our hope that you will take advantage of

this powerful opportunity by following our lead, and we promise to help you achieve many truly remarkable and life-altering changes.

WHAT'S NEW

In this new edition we have updated our nutritional supplements section in order to make it current. We have also added the new highly effective 21-minute Express Body Sculpting Workouts. These time management masterpieces were developed to help those of you who are limited with the time they can spend working out. We've also made two options available; workouts you can do in the privacy of your home and in a commercial gym.

In addition, we have added an incredible section on healthy and delicious Body Sculpting recipes, which were created by renowned French Chef, Marie-Annick Courtier. These recipes will help you beat the boredom of tasteless diet food by introducing some incredible flavor into your healthy eating plan. Who says following a healthy diet has to be tasteless? Finally, you can truly enjoy the food you eat while blasting body fat and adding lean muscle. As if that wasn't enough, we have also added a section that expands on the revolutionary Zone-Tone method, which can be used to achieve virtually anything you want out of life, including the development of your dream physique!

We then added a section on training over 40. In these sections, we equip you with everything you need to know about becoming your very best at the best stage of your life!

Finally, we are in the final stages of developing a new Body Sculpting Bible website. This will be the official website of the Body Sculpting Bibles and the place to visit for personal coaching from your authors, James and Hugo. We aptly named this new membership program Body Sculpting Base Camp, as it will become the go-to spot for building and maintaining your physical masterpiece. Please visit us at www.BodySculptingBibles.com and add your name to our waiting list.

Since the beginning of the series, over 18 years ago, our goal has been to help people achieve the physique that they desire without having to deal with the pitfalls and the challenges that we experienced ourselves. A decade later, our commitment to help others is larger than ever! And thanks to the internet and to social networks like Facebook, we can now reach millions of more people with just one click!

Before you put this book down today, go to your computer and visit us here: www.facebook.com/bodysculptingbibles. This will now become the new *Body Sculpting Bible* home base and it's a place where you will find accountability from us and your fellow readers, where you will maintain motivation to keep going, and where you can communicate with us directly.

By frequenting our Facebook Fan Page, you will always be on top of your game and you can count on it. Whether you have questions, need support, motivation, or information on training, nutrition, or supplementations, we are here to help you succeed in achieving your physique goals. We want to turn this page into a massive community of like-minded people whose goal is to not only improve their physiques but also their lives and the lives of many others!

Over the years, we have been blessed with the great opportunity to touch the lives of well over 1 million people and now that we have Facebook, we feel that we can reach more people than we ever thought possible. And now, we are not alone, since we have you to help us spread the word and finally get people off the couch and into shape!

With that said, we're calling on you to help us make great change. We need you to help us touch the lives of many other people. The way to do this is simple:

1. **Become a fan of our Facebook Fan Page:** www.facebook.com/bodysculptingbibles.
2. **Share this page with your friends:** In this manner, you can help us reach out to others who are looking to get in shape but may not know how to do it.
3. **Share your expertise:** Don't be shy. Many of you are very talented and can help others by sharing your expertise. If you have read the books and used the information to transform your own life, this puts you in a position of power to help others achieve the same.

In fact, we have thousands of readers who, after reading the *Body Sculpting Bible*, decided to make a career out of fitness! While that may not be your goal, definitely don't be shy in sharing your expertise as just a simple word of encouragement can make a huge difference in the life of someone who could use a helping hand.

We look forward to working with all of you as we continue to improve our bodies (and lives). We are so excited to be connecting with new people throughout the world and together we can have a huge impact on global health!

See you soon on Facebook!

Best Always,
James & Hugo

Quick Start

To get started with the *14-Day Body Sculpting Workout* as quickly as possible, follow the reading outline below. It will take you approximately 60 minutes at the most to go through this outline. We feel you'll need this basic understanding of the *14-Day Body Sculpting Workout* principles in order to harness the maximum benefits of the program.

Depending on your knowledge of how to perform the exercises, read the exercise descriptions that pertain to the routine that you choose.

We do recommend that you read through the entire book progressively to obtain the full benefits of the program (there is much more than just training information). This book will not only teach you how to change your physique, but also how to change your life!

Table of Contents

Precautions

READ THIS SECTION THOROUGHLY BEFORE GOING ANY FURTHER!

You should always consult a physician before starting any fat reduction and training program.

If you are unfamiliar with any of the exercises, ask an experienced trainer to instruct you on the proper form and execution of the unfamiliar exercise.

The instructions and advice presented herein are not intended as a substitute for medical or other professional personal counseling.

The editors and authors disclaim any liability or loss in connection with the use of this system, its programs and advice herein.

Introduction

THE **BODY**
SCULPTING
BIBLE
FOR **WOMEN**

Every time we turn on the TV we are bombarded with the latest way to lose fat and achieve the body of our dreams. With so many diets, gadgets, and magic pills available it is no wonder that the public is confused about how to lose weight. This is why we decided to write this book. We are tired of seeing people getting taken advantage of by gimmick "solutions" that don't provide results. In addition, having dealt with weight problems throughout our youth, we can relate to people who desperately want to change the way they look but don't know how.

In this book you will learn how to lose weight without starving yourself. In fact, you may end up eating more than you ever have before and still achieve the shape you are looking for! We will also show you how to create lean muscle without having to exercise for hours a day—and you don't even need to join a health club. Our goal is to share the knowledge that we have accumulated in our combined 20 years of bodybuilding experience in training both ourselves and women just like you. With this newfound knowledge you will soon be in control of how you look and how much you weigh. No longer will it be a dreadful experience to step on the scale. No longer will you be at the mercy of an infomercial—you'll know exactly what to do in order to achieve the look you desire.

Now that we've laid out our goals, let's examine how you can reach yours.

THE WEIGHT LOSS OBSESSION

Have you noticed how many people are obsessed with losing weight? There is increasing evidence that the American fixation with diet and weight loss is hazardous. Concerns about weight can lead to obsessions about diet and weight control, dysfunctional lifestyles, abnormally high patterns of exercise, disordered eating patterns, metabolic depression, and inadequate nutrition. Study after study has proven the ineffectiveness of dieting. There is a misconception that losing "weight" is the best way to look and feel good, an idea that weight-loss companies promote. What exactly does losing weight entail? Traditionally, losing weight includes losing muscle, bone density, water, and even organ tissue. These vital components of your body are compromised severely during weight-loss stages. Is this healthy? Certainly not! But the diet and weight-loss industry will have you believe it is. Could this be a reason why people are unhealthy, become sick, and sometimes die? Indeed it is.

Conventional weight-loss programs focus on caloric reduction, often without providing proper nutrition. These programs are not concerned with how you feel, exercise, or the reasons why you are losing weight. Reducing your caloric intake so you burn many more calories than you are consuming is fine. But without exercise to help build and sustain lean muscle tissue, your body will be forced to cannibalize itself. Yes, commercial weight loss programs can help you lose "weight," but along with that, there is a good chance that you'll also feel terrible, weaken your immune system, and in most cases gain all of your weight back. In contrast, exercising will build muscle, which in turn will help neutralize your fat loss. Your body will keep what you need for health maintenance, and burn the rest off. Nutrients you consume must be in balanced ratios that provide sufficient protein, carbohydrate, and fat intake for optimal health. Consider these factors carefully before beginning any weight-loss program.

The first hurdle in your weight-loss journey is to stop obsessing about your body weight. Instead, focus on bodily measurements, fat composition and the way you look in the mirror.

Why? Because weight is not a good indicator of how much fat you are carrying. Remember, body weight is a combination of the weight of your bones, organs, muscles, water, and fat. If you lose five pounds in one week, how can you be sure that those five pounds were from fat? Think about it. It could have been two pounds of muscle, two pounds of water and one pound of fat. If this is the case, you are now in a worse situation than you were before. Why? Because your metabolism will be slower and you will have lost body shape (muscle is what increases your metabolism and also gives shape to your body). This is why crash diets don't work; you lose muscle and water, while simultaneously creating fat storage. These diets trick the body into thinking that it is starving. When the body thinks that this is the case, it begins storing fat for future use and eating away at valuable muscle. So while you may achieve your ideal weight, you'll look very different than what you envisioned.

In order to achieve the look you desire, forget about ideal weights—with so many varying frames and sizes, such a thing is impossible to determine. Follow the guidelines in the Nutrition chapter and let the tape measure and the mirror tell you when you have arrived at your destination.

A BOOK DESIGNED ONLY FOR WOMEN

Women generally have different goals than men. While most men want bulging biceps and a powerful chest and back, women are more often concerned with attaining a slim and toned figure—lean and cellulite-free legs, a defined midsection, and toned arms. With these goals in mind, we have created a program that will help any woman achieve the body of her dreams.

THE 14-DAY BODY SCULPTING WORKOUT

The 14-Day Body Sculpting Workout takes a safe and holistic approach to fat loss and muscle toning that enables you to reach your goals in a minimum amount of time. What is so unique about 14 days? Fourteen days is typically the amount of time that it takes us to get used to a new habit. Also, 14 days is the amount of time it takes the body to begin adjusting to a new training and nutrition regimen. Now, while it is good for us to get used to a new habit (like waking up early in the morning to work out), it is not good for the body to get used to our workout and nutrition program. Results will cease once your body adjusts to your workout routine and calorie intake. In other words, while you are dieting and working out in earnest, your body will maintain the same fat percentage and your muscles will not develop. This is why after you start a new exercise and nutrition program, you stop getting results after a few weeks.

Why does this happen? The body likes to remain in a state of homeostasis (balance). When you reduce calories in order to lose fat, eventually your metabolism slows down and fat loss comes to a standstill. You see, our prehistoric ancestors sometimes endured periods of famine with only the fat in their bodies to sustain them. As a result, the body adapted by conserving energy (in the form of fat) in order to ensure preparedness for periods of low food consumption.

When you start a weight training program, muscle mass comes quickly. However, after a period of time your body grows accustomed to the routine and remains at the same fitness level. It does this to conserve energy; when you have more muscle, you burn more calories.

So, how does the 14-Day Body Sculpting Workout solve these problems?

This regimen:

- Changes the parameters (sets, reps, rest in between sets) of weight training routines every 14 days in a logical and periodized manner to ensure maximum workout efficiency (more on this later).
- Adjusts the duration of cardiovascular activities every 14 days.
- Varies caloric intake every 14 days.

Also included in the 14-Day Body Sculpting Workout are: mind and visualization techniques to help you get the most out of your workouts, the Zone-Tone, a technique that dramatically increases the mind to muscle connection, and award-winning exercise descriptions. With all these unique features, you can easily see how this workout is designed to help you successfully reach all your fitness goals!

MORE ON THE 14-DAY BODY SCULPTING WORKOUT

You may wonder how a 14-Day Body Sculpting Workout can exist, right? We at Custom Physiques, Inc. have created the most powerful, dynamic, and simple system for creating lean muscle tissue and eliminating unwanted body-fat for good! We do not believe in starvation diets or long, exhaustive workouts in order to achieve results. We believe in a healthy, systematic, and scientific approach to fitness, offering a complete fat loss/muscle-building program providing fast and consistent results. Fast results? Yes, you heard it right! Did you think we were just going to leave the "14 day" part out? No way! Although it is physically impossible for you to completely change your body shape within 14 days (Unless you have a referral to a good plastic surgeon!), you can still make some very respectable changes within that time frame. Not just some changes to your physical body, but also some major

changes to your whole self. This book contains the finest fat loss and muscle building information available. How can we be so confident? We realized that we would have to take a different approach to fitness in order to make this program work best. Our strategy was to combine our own breakthrough knowledge with some of the traditional methods of fitness and health, to create the most thorough and complete fitness program ever produced. What you get is a complete and balanced approach to losing fat, building muscle and sculpting the body of your dreams.

We are about to introduce you to a new fitness training philosophy widely accepted by athletes ranging from the Olympic elite to

---

FAQ:
Is your 14-Day Body Sculpting program just a marketing gimmick?

ANSWER:
We are proud to say that the Body Sculpting Bibles are among the very first books to bring the very powerful principles of periodization training to the commercial market. Back in 2000, periodization training was known only to Olympic and elite athletes. Since 2000, with the release of the first Body Sculpting Bibles, periodization training has become widely known and regarded as the #1 type of training for eliciting remarkable and consistent results.

---

weekend warriors and college athletes. It is called periodization training, which is defined as "a training regimen done a specific way for a specific period of time and then modified and done a different way for a specific period of time." What would be the significance of changing a fitness routine from time to time?

Have you ever started a weight training routine, hoping to lose some fat while simultaneously putting on some muscle and found that it was much easier to do so in the very beginning? Do you remember how motivated you were at first and how easy it was to make immediate progress? What happened next? All of a sudden you stopped gaining muscle, you still had those last five pounds of fat attached to your body and because of that, you probably lost your motivation and desire to train. You hit a plateau and no matter how hard you trained or how much you dieted, you just couldn't make any more progress, right? What happened? Your body simply adapted! That's right, your body, in an attempt to neutralize and protect your system from further breakdown (tearing down muscle and losing fat), suddenly stopped responding to the catalyst (resistance training and diet).

Periodization training prevents this adaptation. It helps to avoid plateaus, thus increasing and continually creating results. This version of the 14-Day Body Sculpting Workout was completely designed for the woman whose goal is to create a more muscular and lean physique. Up until now, you have probably tried every fitness routine, gadget and/or supplement under the sun and still not reached your goals. Well don't lose hope! You will discover shortly just how powerful this program truly is.

We want to help the average woman attain her goal of sculpting a lean and muscular physique. We quickly realized that this would require certain criteria within the traditional periodization program to be customized. We knew that key components of the traditional periodization model such as sports specific training would not be necessary since the program would not be used for sports conditioning. At the same time, we realized that there had to be many specialized additions to help customize the program according to our female readers' objectives. Our main objective is to provide a direct plan of action for expediting the development of the ideal female physique (a lean and muscular body). We balanced this unique and complete revolutionary training program with the nutrition plan and a healthy mind-set method. The 14-Day Body Sculpting Workout's mind/muscle approach will help you to realize your potential!

We cannot and will not promise you unachievable results. Unrealistic promises can both sabotage your motivation to get in shape or, even worse, jeopardize your health. Companies that make such far-fetched claims are not concerned with your well-being. They only care about what they can get from you—your money. We, on the other hand, are concerned about your health. We are here to help you achieve amazing results, and to explain exactly what you should do to become and stay fit and healthy forever.

Both of us have been in situations where our health and self-esteems were in jeopardy. I (James) can remember when I was 14 years old. I was very heavy and very depressed. One day while watching television, I was drawn to a commercial advertisement for a new type of diet pill called the grapefruit diet. The ad guaranteed tremendous results within a very short time period. I was young and vulnerable to such claims. I also felt desperate and immediately decided, without conducting any type of research on the company or product, to rob my piggy bank. That very same day, I sent them my money through the mail. Do you see where this is leading? I received those pills, no questions asked! They had no concern for my health, my age, or my overall wellbeing. I took those pills and luckily, I didn't die. I see kids and adults all the time who make very similar mistakes. They have been struggling for some time, listening to this claim and that claim, promising to instantly and miraculously change their physical appearance. Do these companies ever stop to think that some people are just so frustrated, that they are blinded by the wonderful claims and left playing Russian roulette with their lives? Do these companies realize that a good portion of these frustrated people happen to be young kids, who from being abused and ridiculed about their physical appearance, become even more frustrated and are even more willing to take any product promising to change their appearance? These kids most likely will not stop to think about the major health implications involved with taking some of these potentially life threatening products. Although there are some great companies out there who pride themselves on creating safety for their customers, many have very little or no concern for their customers. They fulfill any order they receive, without screening or qualifying one person. We would never and could never hurt or deceive anyone. We have both come from painful childhoods and can both empathize completely with anyone who has a weight problem or any problem that relates to the body and can affect one's self-esteem. Either too heavy or too thin, we have both been through each scenario and because of that, our primary goal is to help anyone who needs or could benefit from our guidance and support. From now on, your new motto must be, "If the product or business has even a trace of uncertainty, move on!" If you don't learn to follow this motto, you will either get taken for your money and/or jeopardize your own health.

Our 14-Day Body Sculpting Workout contains only the safest, top-notch health and fitness information and techniques you need to become fit and healthy. Our program takes into account the importance of physical and mental health, and how they must be combined, in order to reach the pinnacle of good health and fitness. Our program was derived from our over 40 years of combined knowledge base of health, fitness and nutrition. What we can do for you in 14 days is to totally supply you with everything you need to reach and surpass your weight loss goals. In two weeks not only will you know exactly what to do, you will actually begin to see remarkable results. Even more exciting is the fact that the results you make during that very short time period will be permanent (provided you stick to the program) and only the beginning of your body sculpting success. Our one-of-a-kind program integrates the body and mind, offering you a completely fit body. A body that looks and feels great! Finally, we are most excited to let you know that this will be the last weight reduction and fitness book or program that you will ever need to buy. If your goal is to lose weight and get in amazing shape, welcome to results country: This is the place where you'll find both and then some! So now it's time to get excited, as you begin the 14-Day Body Sculpting Workout, for the body of your dreams. Enjoy!

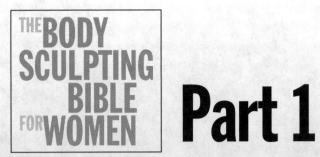

Part 1

The Foundations of Physical Perfection

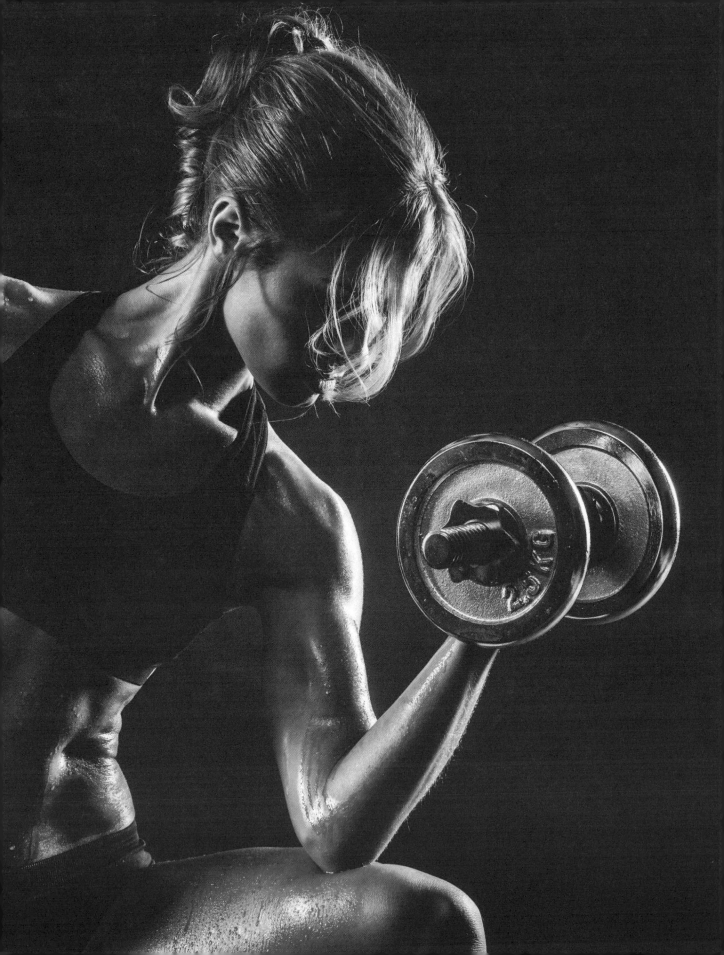

Chapter 1
Common Myths & Misconceptions

THE BODY SCULPTING BIBLE FOR WOMEN

1

In this chapter we will cover several topics that cause confusion in the fitness industry.

COMMON MYTHS DEBUNKED

Myth #1: Weight training makes you bulky. Due to the fact that women do not produce as much testosterone (the hormone responsible for increasing muscle size) as males do, it is impossible for a woman to gain huge amounts of muscle mass. The image that may come to your mind is of professional female body-builders. Many of those women unfortunately use anabolic steroids (synthetic testosterone) along with other drugs in order to achieve that high degree of muscularity. In addition, most also have good genetics that enable them to gain muscle quickly when they spend hours in the gym lifting very heavy weights. Believe us when we say that they do not look like that by accident. Women who conduct weight training without the use of steroids get the firm and fit cellulite-free looking body that you see in most fitness shows these days.

Myth #2: Exercise increases your chest size. Women's breasts are composed mostly of fatty tissue. Therefore, it is impossible to increase their size through weight training. As a matter of fact, if you go below 12 percent body fat (which we don't recommend as you'll see later), your breast size will decrease. Weight training does increase the size of the back, so this misconception probably comes from confusing an increase in back size with an increase in cup size. The only way to increase your breast size is by gaining fat or getting breast implants.

Myth #3: Weight training makes you stiff. If you perform all exercises through their full range of motion, flexibility will increase. Exercises like flys, stiff-legged deadlifts, dumbbell presses, and chin-ups stretch the muscle in the bottom range of the movement. Therefore,

by performing these exercises correctly, your stretching capabilities will increase.

Myth #4: If you stop weight training your muscles turn into fat. This is like saying that gold can turn into brass. Muscle and fat are two totally different types of tissue. What happens many times is that when people decide to go off their weight training programs they start losing muscle due to inactivity (use it or lose it) and they also usually drop the diet as well. Therefore bad eating habits, combined with the fact that metabolism is lower due to inactivity and lower degrees of muscle mass, give the impression that the subject's muscle is being turned into fat while in reality what is happening is that muscle is being lost and fat is being accumulated.

Myth #5: Weight training turns fat into muscle. More alchemy. This is the equivalent of saying that you can turn any metal into gold. The way a body transformation occurs is by gaining muscle through weight training and losing fat through aerobics simultaneously. Again, muscle and fat are very different types of tissue. We cannot turn one into the other.

Myth #6: As long as you exercise you can eat anything that you want. How we wish this were true! However, this could not be further from the truth. Our individual metabolism determines how many calories we burn at rest and while we exercise. If we eat more calories than we burn on a consistent basis, our bodies will accumulate these extra calories as fat regardless of the amount that we exercise. This myth may have been created by people with such high metabolic rates (lucky them) that no matter how much they eat or what they eat, they never meet or exceed the amount of calories that they burn in one day. Therefore, their weight either remains stable or goes down.

Myth #7: Once you lose motivation, it's impossible to get back to a healthy routine. It's true that it's difficult to get back on track after losing motivation, but it's not impossible!

When you get bored, it's easier for you to get depressed and your productivity can come to a screeching halt. Your body reacts similarly and stops producing results when you do the same exact activities day in and day out. How do you create results consistently? Change your action plan! In the following chapters, we will show you exactly how to constantly evolve your training and nutrition plan in order to keep getting results.

Myth #8: Exercising makes you tired and exhausts your body. If you're feeling too tired to exercise, it's most likely because you're just bored. Get up and start moving and you'll be surprised when you feel a surge of energy!

Myth #9: You don't need to work out if you're already in great shape or if you're still young. Despite fitness level and age, you can always manage to take care of yourself, and there's always room for improvement. Think of it as an insurance policy of sorts!

Myth #10: There's not enough time to exercise if you're working full-time. Even if you're feeling like your work schedule leaves you with no time to exercise, keep in mind that exercising can actually improve your work performance. Incorporating 30 minutes into your daily schedule for working out will be well worth it as exercise has been proven to elevate mood, which naturally leads to far better results and more productivity in the work place. Take a look at our 14-Day Rapid Body Sculpting Workout.

Myth #11: The gym is intimidating! The gym actually intimidates more people than you think. Even those so-called "gym rats" don't always feel confident. Any time you're feeling nervous about being in the gym, remember that you're in there to do a job and you owe it to yourself to conquer your fears by facing them head on! Motivate yourself by thinking about the fact that you're doing what most people won't do or don't think they have time to do. It's all about getting in great shape by doing what you gotta do!

Myth #12: The gym is crowded, dirty, and it's just not for me! If you really don't like the gym, build one in your own home—it's not as difficult as you would think. All you need is a pair of adjustable dumbbells. This is all the equipment that many of our Body Sculpting Programs require. If you want to get more fancy, you can get a weight bench as well. Remember: It's quality, not quantity that matters. You can still get a great workout with very little equipment.

Myth #13: If you've failed once, you're doomed to fail again. The first step in conquering past failures is to stop blaming yourself. Chances are, if you didn't stick to the plan, it's likely because the plan just wasn't right for you. Be sure to set realistic goals & outcomes for yourself and write down your short-term, mid-term & long-term goals. This will make a world of difference! Take a look at our Goal Setting Section on page 22 for help with this.

Myth #14: You need to give all of your attention to your family, which leaves no time for working out. If you don't start taking care of yourself, you won't be able to care for your family and they may even end up having to take care of you! Giving yourself the time to exercise and stay healthy doesn't mean you're being selfish. In fact, the healthier you are, the better equipped you will be to care for the people you love.

Myth #15: It's impossible to find the time to work out if you have a baby. Consider bringing your baby with you–many gyms and health clubs now have child-care services. If your gym doesn't offer this service, find a friend or family member to baby-sit for an hour or so while you work out. You can make it work if you really want to.

Myth #16: You need to stretch before training with weights. Not necessarily. You should not do any static stretching (also known as isometric stretching, in which you hold the stretch for a certain amount of time) before weight training. This actually sends a signal to the muscles that they should relax, which is the last thing you want your muscles doing before a set of exercises. You should instead be using dynamic stretches, which warm and ready the muscles for the upcoming workload by performing active stretches with no holding point. You can also prepare the muscles for the lifting activity by performing the actual weight training movement that you are about to perform, using either light weight or no weight.

UNNECESSARY GADGETS

Let's talk about all of the exercise contraptions we see on TV. First of all, why do we need to pay over $80 to perform an abdominal crunch? The abdominal crunch is perhaps the most inexpensive and simple exercise there is to target the abdominal muscles. Do we need a machine to help us do it? We think not!

Ads for such gadgets promise abs in minutes a day. But did you ever read the fine print on the TV screen? It usually reads that the statements are true as long as you combine the exercise with a sensible diet—which brings us to the next point. You do not need to enslave yourself everyday to hours of abdominal work—only 5 to 10 minutes of ab work is sufficient. What really brings out the definition in your midsection is a sensible nutritional program and aerobic exercise. Combined, these components burn fat in order for your definition to appear. The abdominal work only builds the muscle covered by the fat. Besides, there is no way in which you can only reduce

the fat in one section (spot reduction) without reducing it in the rest of your body.

Once again why do we need to purchase an ab machine? To avoid neck strain? If you don't know what you are doing you can strain your neck with or without the machine.

Unless you are recovering from a back injury and are not yet strong enough to do a crunch by yourself, save your hard-earned dollars for more meaningful things. All you need to perform an abdominal crunch is the floor and the proper instruction on how to execute the exercise correctly.

CELLULITE CREAMS

We have all seen commercials that promise to eliminate cellulite by rubbing the latest cream discovered in some secret tree in God-knows-where. At Custom Physiques we have talked with many women who have used such products with no results. Good luck finding any real scientific research that proves these products work. Again, save your hard-earned money.

The only thing that eliminates cellulite from your body is a systematic approach to eliminating fat through the nutritional practices we describe along with a training routine that is designed to tone and eliminate body fat from all angles. That is the only way that the battle against cellulite can be won. Don't let anybody mislead you.

WEIGHT LOSS CLINICS

Why pay others every month to tell you what to do when you are fully capable of figuring out what to do yourself after reading this book? We have seen what most weight loss clinics offer and we are not impressed! Not only do you have to pay an unbelievable fee (sometimes on a monthly basis) to get a diet that may not be as efficient as it could be (most of these programs are low protein diets); some require you to buy special foods (provided by them, of course, on top of the initial fee). Others charge you by the pounds you lose. Hey, what a concept! You do the work and you get to pay someone else for your success!

DRUGS FOR WEIGHT LOSS

If what you want is health and permanent weight loss, don't touch any kind of weight loss drugs. Many are very dangerous (remember Phen-Fen?) and can cause serious side effects such as heart problems and possibly death. Besides, once you stop using them you begin to gain all of the weight back. So what's the use? People criticize bodybuilders for using steroids and everybody preaches about their dangers. Well, using weight loss drugs (and this includes those formulas that claim to be natural but contain ephedrine) is exactly the same thing! There is nothing different here; it's using dangerous drugs in order to achieve a pleasing cosmetic effect.

When Phen-Fen came out people flocked to their doctors in order to get a prescription. Unfortunately, many were given the drug despite the fact that research indicated that this drug combination had some serious side effects. So after a few people got rich off it, the drug was pulled from the market. However, the damage was already done.

The only solid and safe solution that takes the weight off permanently is the correct combination of diet, exercise and rest. Anyone who tries to convince you otherwise is full of it! Therefore, once again, save your money, but more importantly, save your health. Stay off the drugs.

For more information on hormonal balance, see the "Fitastic at and after 40" section on page 481.

see the "Fitastic at and after 40" section on page 481.

> **FAQ:**
> What if one of these weight loss clinics actually motivates me to lose weight and keep me on track to meet my goals?
>
> **ANSWER:**
> By all means, if you find that you just can't stick to the program and need an outside source to keep you afloat, do what you need to do. We would like to think that anyone can stick to this program and motivate themselves to excel. However, life can sometimes get the best of us. If you find yourself needing additional support, do what you need to keep on your journey. Your health is with the extra money, don't you agree?

THE MOST COMMON DIETER'S MISTAKE: LESS IS BETTER

When people think of a diet they think of pain, hunger, and food deprivation. At first, most dieters reduce their food intake dramatically and see that in the first week they lose around ten pounds of weight. They say, "Great! In order to lose more weight I need to eat less." After a few weeks they notice that they are not losing as fast as they had hoped. Frustrated, they start to starve themselves even more. Before we continue, let's stop right here and explain what is going on inside the body.

The first week the person will lose weight as the metabolism gets shocked by the lessened food intake. However, most of the weight lost is derived from water with only three to four pounds coming from fat. The second week the body, still not adjusted to the shock, continues to lose weight (though not as fast as the first week). By the third week the body begins to take counter measures in order to adjust to the lowered caloric intake. Think about it, what do you do when your light bill goes up? You probably begin to save electricity in order

FAQ:
Isn't bulimia a problem that only females can get?

ANSWER:
Whenever I tell someone that I was bulimic, they are shocked and say that they never knew that a man could have such a disorder. The truth of the matter is that there are many men who are bulimic. You'd be surprised if you knew how many athletes--and average men--binge and purge. Men are very good at keeping to themselves. We are also not as likely to ask for help as our female counterparts.

Bulimia is not a gender specific disease; it is a problem that exists for us all. Please be advised that bulimia is a deadly eating disorder, and if you are bulimic or have ever considered binging and purging, your life is at serious risk. There is no part-time bulimia; if you think that binging and purging once in a while is okay, you're dead wrong. The effects of disturbing your digestive and nervous systems in such a way will add up and inevitably will catch up with you in ways that you'd rather not experience. Please educate yourself on its perils, and please feel free to email me, James Villepigue, for support: info@fitnessbusinesscoach.com. I've been there.

to save money. The body is just like you. When it sees that its metabolic costs are too high (in other words, losing fat because the metabolism is too high), then it decides to save energy and lowers the metabolism in an attempt to keep the fat on. Therefore, the person experiences a slowdown in weight loss or just comes to a standstill. The way you save electricity is by turning appliances off, etc. The way your body

saves energy is by losing muscle, because muscle is the most expensive tissue to maintain.

So by looking at the scenario above, let's see what may happen to someone (we'll call her Denise) who is determined to lose weight but does not know how to go about doing so.

As Denise notices that her weight loss comes to a sudden halt, she decides to reduce her caloric intake further. For the first few weeks this in fact works, but afterwards the weight loss comes to a standstill again. After a few cycles of the same thing, Denise continues to spiral downward. At this point most people (99 percent) just forget about the diet and start eating everything in sight. They gain back all of the weight and then some (remember it will be easier for them to gain weight now because they lowered their metabolism by using the wrong dieting practices). However, there is a very determined one percent of dieters who will not give up.

These people continue the cycle described above. They begin to look pale and feel cold. They are hungry all the time but deny it. Sometimes they go without food or water for the whole day. They look at themselves in the mirror and they still see themselves fat, even though everyone tells them that they are already skinny (very skinny). They are afraid to drink water because they think water will make them gain weight. This condition is called anorexia nervosa, a condition that I (Hugo) suffered from in my early teens.

People with this condition are not totally crazy in seeing themselves as fat. Even though they look very skinny in clothes, if you take their fat percentage you will probably see that it is around 20-30 percent. Anorexics had an original ideal physique in mind that was toned, hard and firm. In the hopes of attaining this physique they continue on their downward spiral. However, they never seem to achieve what they want so they figure that the answer is fewer calories. See how the cycle is created?

The only cure for conditions like this is education. We remember that when we used to be overweight everybody used to tease us, poke fun at us and tell us to stop eating. People treated us as if we were diseased. Therefore, we decided to take action and started doing what people told us to: "Stop eating!"

However, the only solution for losing weight (fat) and keeping it off, while at the same time building a lean and hard physique, is eating the correct combinations of food, along with doing weight training and aerobic exercise. So please, never fall into the trap of thinking that eating less will get you good results!

BULIMIA

Another eating disorder, bulimia (characterized by bingeing and purging) is somewhat of a difficult subject for me (James) to write about because I personally battled with it for a period of time in my life. When I was young, my physique was the last thing on my mind. I did not care about how I looked or what I ate. Being served seconds for lunch and dinner was not enticing for me; it was more like thirds and fourths that got my attention. My mother, who is a registered nurse and an amazing one at that, was not aware of the health implications and effects that too much food would cause to my body. As a matter of fact, most health practitioners, including medical doctors, are not always aware even today, of some of the implications food can have on a person's body. As I grew older and larger I was forced into realization of my obesity. One day, while in Junior High School, a gym teacher pulled me aside and made me step onto the scale. I weighed about 200 pounds at age 12/13. He thought that his way of revealing my weight problem to

me was a productive one. He was wrong! The only thing he did was embarrass and anger me.

From that point on, I began to gain more and more weight until finally I was at my all time high of 255 pounds. I was fat and depressed and had no idea what to do about my problem. I resorted to weight loss pills and liquid diets, which only frustrated me more. One of my family members, who was also quite heavy, began suddenly to lose weight. I was shocked at how she shed pounds of weight, yet didn't diet or exercise. It was odd, but I started to notice that her once beautiful olive complexion began turning pale. In addition, I would constantly see her falling into a deep depression accompanied by anxiety. I, like most people with eating disorders, paid no attention to the terrible things that she was going through. I just wanted to know how the heck she was losing that weight. Well I found out!

Staying up late and having good ears made it obvious. I could hear her throwing up in the bathroom and knew that this was the way she was losing weight. While initially I was afraid to try such a harsh thing, I went ahead and tried it. At first, I hurt the back of my throat by gagging. I then tried other ways to purge myself, all of which were ways of causing a gag reflex. That was when my terrible eating disorder began. In the beginning I lost some weight and actually felt good because I could eat junk food while getting the results I wanted. That was until I noticed some odd behavior in myself, such as an obsessive need to exercise and ongoing bouts of low self-esteem. I felt like my self-worth required that I be skinny. I continued until one day, while living with my parents, I heard my sister scream from the bathroom. I ran upstairs and tried to open the door, but it was locked! I screamed for my sister to unlock the door, but she didn't. I had to break open the door and found my sister on the floor naked, lying in a pool of water. She had fallen out of the shower due to her body becoming weakened by the abuse of bulimia. She was purple and looked as if she was having a seizure. I screamed to my mother and she immediately called the police. It was discovered that she had developed seven bleeding ulcers, among many other problems that were all the side effects of bulimia. I was never so scared in my life as when I saw what my sister had done to herself and realized that I was on the same exact path.

Since that time, my sister and I have both stopped abusing our bodies and have educated ourselves about eating disorders. With strong will and persistence, we conquered this eating disorder and I must say that my sister has become a beautifully strong and confident woman. We discovered through reading and from our personal dealings, that even though a person with any eating disorder may look happy and cheerful, that person is often depressed, lonely, ashamed and empty inside. Friends of bulimics may describe them as people who are competent and fun to be with. But underneath all of that, where they hide their guilty secrets, they are actually hurting real badly. They may feel unworthy and have great difficulty talking about their feelings. These feelings are often accompanied with anxiety, depression, self-doubt, and deeply buried anger.

So you see, bulimia is a very dangerous eating disorder that will never meet your expectations of acquiring a great looking physique. Bulimia is a disease and one that needs to be taken care of with the help of someone knowledgeable. Please remember that bingeing and purging is not the way to get in or stay in shape. *If you feel that you may have this terrible disease, please seek professional counseling.*

LOW CARB/HIGH PROTEIN/HIGH FAT DIETS

Low carb (less than 50 or even 30 grams a day), high protein, high fat diets might at first work. The reason? After the initial adaptation period of two weeks, in the absence of carbohydrates, the body has no choice but to go into a state of ketosis (carbohydrate deprivation) and start burning fats for fuel. This is assuming that more than 50% of your calories are coming from good essential fatty acids like olive oil and flaxseed oil. Basically, your body shifts its carbohydrate metabolism into an exclusively fat burning metabolism. Now, like any diet, the same basic principles apply. Even though you will be burning fats exclusively this does not mean that you will be able to eat everything and anything without getting fat. Remember if you take in more calories than you burn, you will get fat.

We have tried such diets for as long as a year at a time. The following are the drawbacks:

- If you are only allowed 30-50 grams of carbohydrates a day, your life will not be very tasty. You will only be limited to a small selection of foods.

- Even though at the beginning you lose incredible amounts of weight, it is mostly water weight. We also did not find a big difference between losing fat on a low carb diet and losing fat on a moderate carbohydrate diet. Both diets provide similar benefits.

- While on a low carbohydrate diet, the muscles feel flat (shrink in size) due to the fact that the glycogen (the carbohydrates that are stored inside the muscle cell and make the muscles look firm) gets depleted. On a moderate carbohydrate diet, your muscles always feel firm and tight.

- We experienced joint pains after the ninth month on the diet. We were drinking 2 gallons of water a day so lack of fluids was not the problem. We wonder if it was the lack of carbs that caused the fluid in the joints to diminish but this is mere speculation. Once we switched back to a moderate carb diet, the joint pains disappeared.
- You have to pay close attention to your cholesterol levels and to nutritional deficiencies caused by the lack of variety in the diet.

In order to get all the good fats in the diet, we had to take them in liquid form; not very tasty.

Even though this type of diet might work, we don't believe it can be maintained for a lifetime. If you feel like trying it, then please remember to pay close attention to cholesterol levels and nutritional deficiencies. We, however, believe that to get in shape the best approach is a more balanced one.

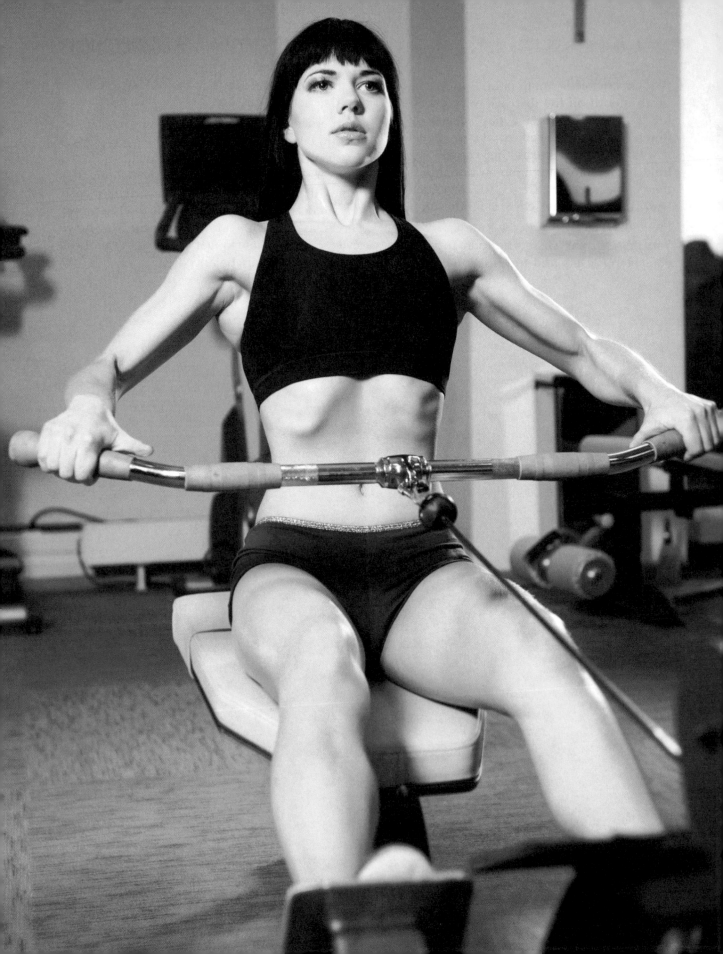

Chapter 2
The Power of
the Mind

Powerful Methods for Achieving Success

For immediate Body Sculpting Bible support &
coaching directly from James & Hugo, please visit
www.BodySculptingBibles.com

2

THE **BODY
SCULPTING
BIBLE
FOR WOMEN**

THINGS DON'T HAVE TO BE SO COMPLICATED; NOT WHEN YOU HAVE AN ARSENAL OF RESULTS AMMO!

What you have in your hands right now is a straightforward and logical formula that we have broken down and simplified, making the information easy to comprehend and follow. This manual gives you the most effective sure-fire plan to attain a better-looking body, in the shortest amount of time humanly and naturally possible.

The reason this book is called the 14-Day Body Sculpting Workout is because if you follow the guidelines we present, you will start to notice some amazing changes in your body within a couple of weeks. Please understand that this is not a magic program. We are not claiming that your body will miraculously change overnight. However, by applying these methods to your lifestyle, along with applying yourself to the program, you will achieve results and then "magic" may just be the word you'll use to describe our program. Often, people who have seen us train ask, "How do you guys make such noticeable physique changes with such a short workout?" That's just it! That's the underlying formula, the key to your success! Remember more is not necessarily better and in the case of this book, definitely not. If you understand how the body works, you will be successful in the shortest time possible. We live in a fast paced world, where time is a precious asset (time is money!). We don't have the time to spend long hours in the gym—even a short time in the gym can be a major commitment. Having extra time can greatly enhance your life, allowing you to do some of the things you've otherwise neglected. A basic, yet scientific approach to fitness training is what's needed, and is exactly what you're about to discover with the 14-Day Body Sculpting Workout!

FAQ:
You write about how important it is to make your workout short. Why is this better than longer workouts, where I can really work my body harder with the extra time?

ANSWER:
Your body is not meant to endure long periods of stress. The more stress you put your body through, The more it will break down and won't have the ability to recuperate. The best strategy for the best workout and results is to train as hard as you can as quickly as you can. Think of it this way: you have a certain amount of energy that you will use during your weight training session and it's not going to last forever. You begin to use this energy the moment you start to exercise. Thus, your objective should be to direct your energy towards lifting as intensely as possible.

Your ability to exercise intensely will vary from person to person, but for most people, you have a specific amount of time that allows you to get the best workout. Powerful muscle building and fat burning hormones are released, and your body is ready for results. When you go beyond this time block, you get diminishing returns, or your energy levels deplete and your focus wanders. When this happens, your muscle glycogen has been spent and toxins begin to release into your bloodstream. Have you ever seen a boxing match, where both opponents are fresh and ready to do battle at the very beginning of the fight? They come out and they are strong, powerful, and fierce! The second round comes around and they still have that fuel to sustain their attack, but when the third round arrives, their drive is restrained and conserved. What has happened?

They have blown their power energy. At the beginning of the round, their muscle glycogen is at peak evels, adrenaline is spilling over, and focus is sharp. It's these beginning rounds that are the most valuable. The same principles apply to weight training. Come out fierce, give it all you've got, and get it done before you run out of steam.

DIFFERENT ROUTINES: SOME WORK, MOST DON'T!

"What kind of workout routine should I choose?" This is probably one of the most frequently asked questions when it comes to exercise. With so many different routines and so-called "guru philosophies" out there, it would surprise us if only a few people were confused about this issue. Deciding what program to choose can be extremely difficult. Even professional trainers and elite athletes frequently have problems choosing a quality program. There are many different programs—some good, some bad, some terrible. The fact of the matter is that some of these programs may in fact work somewhat, if you dedicate yourself to them. That is the key word, "dedication." The dedication we're talking about isn't just committing or devoting yourself to something, for that alone is just not enough. The dedication we mean is the dedication to devoting yourself and your time (remember you are not in the gym to waste time!) to something, to get as much out of it as is humanly possible. To do this, you must define exactly what your training objectives are before and during a fitness session. Without this mindset, you will undeniably fail to achieve optimum results. You must realize that when you're not prepared you cannot expect to receive the maximum response from your actions, and therefore you will not see results. You must know what tools (exercise and technique) to use and what to expect at each workout session in order to receive your desired effect (more muscle tone and less fat). You must also make sure that your response or reactions to the stimulus are as accurate as you expected them to be.

The basic guidelines and training principles of your fitness program must always be based on information that is backed up by scientific fact. Please understand that the routine alone is not enough to make your dream body appear. You must follow the proper training methods and initial preparation techniques included in this manual to help make the program work optimally. Using correct exercise form alone is very important for steady results. If you follow the proper, often neglected, training techniques, form, and principles we describe, this program can be the program that changes your life forever! We do realize that there are currently several schools of thought concerning the best types of weight reduction and body sculpting workouts. We also realize that most of these so-called, state-of-the-art programs lack useful information and will not live up to their claimed benefits.

The 14-Day Body Sculpting Workout is based only on concepts that truly work. We include some traditional principles, which supply the building blocks of all reputable fitness programs, as well as new and exciting principles and techniques that are considered breakthroughs in the field.

EXPECTATIONS AND DESIRE; EXPECT AND YOU SHALL RECEIVE

Where would we be without our expectations? Expectations are a driving force in our ability to plan effectively. If you want to be a success, whether in the gym or in the office, you must set goals for yourself. But setting goals is not enough. In order to reach those goals as smoothly and as quickly as possible, you must think about what it is that you expect to receive.

When you begin the 14-Day Body Sculpting Plan, expect optimal results. Expect to receive what you bought this manual for. By doing this you are creating a positive mindset, a vital component of this wonderful program. Once you commit yourself to anything, do not question its power or validity (unless of course it's dangerous, which should be evident from research on both the seller's and readers' parts). Instead, dedicate yourself to it until you've accomplished your objective. Many of the fitness programs available today could work somewhat if a positive mindset was followed. Now imagine what you will accomplish by creating a positive mindset with this program. You are almost ready to begin on your journey to success. Why a journey? Because all of the following techniques can be applied to all aspects of your life! Now let's move on to our first powerful tool for success.

MIND SCULPTING: VISUALIZATION AND MENTAL IMAGERY (THINK AND BECOME!)

Although the information below seems difficult to comprehend and follow, it is not! The techniques can help you achieve fitness goals and affect virtually all aspects of your soon to be (if not already) amazing life!

Before you can sculpt your body into a piece of art you must first sculpt your mind into a powerful tool. How would you like to guarantee success and accelerate your results exponentially? Well, this next portion of the 14-Day Body Sculpting Workout addresses a very powerful technique that is virtually non-existent in the fitness realm. The special tool we speak of is known as visualization or mental-imagery. In the next few minutes you are going to learn how to develop and use some fantastic possibilities that lay dormant within each one of us. They will allow you to perform remarkable feats that you would have never believed possible. By thinking powerfully about what it is you want and repeating your thoughts long enough, these thoughts will turn into solid realities.

You may ask how such influences occur. Do you know that medical doctors consider many illnesses psychosomatic, that is, caused or provoked in part by the patient's own thoughts? Even diseases such as cancer may have psychosomatic origins, since the power of our minds over our bodies is so strong.

Right now, you are going to learn how to cultivate a talent for visualization that you already possess. This power is more or less developed from one person to the next. But, with the right training anyone can achieve excellent results. Just as exercise develops the muscles, the appropriate physical and mental training will make you a master of visualization. The balance of body and mind exercise is too often neglected, but is the key to astonishing success individual possesses a strong and confident attraction to her goals. The disciplined!

There are three conditions that you must have in balance for optimum results. The first is desire, as we already discussed. How can you expect to obtain anything, if you don't want it badly enough? Desire is that fire you feel in your belly when you so badly want something, creating the drive and **determination** to achieve. The stronger your **desire**, and

FAQ:
Why do you talk so much about the mind when it's my body I'm concerned with?

ANSWER:
The mind is without question your most powerful asset. Every action you take begins with a thought. Your mind helps control your body and your muscles. When you lift a weight and simply put yourself through the motions, moving it from point A to point B, you will stimulate your muscles, but not to the degree you could if you put your mind to work. When you really think about and focus on the muscles you intend to stimulate, something much more powerful begins to happen: The mind begins to help further stimulate your muscles, helping them respond at their highest degree possible. When you mentally visualize yourself in great shape and what it would feel like to be in great shape, your subconscious cannot tell the difference between this visualization and reality. In other words, your mind starts to act as if this is reality and begins to adjust to make it a solid truth. This is not science fiction; it is hard science. Training and utilizing the power of the mind can help you achieve more than you ever knew was possible.

the more sustained it is, the more certainty you add to reaching your goals quickly. In order for your desires to become powerful, you have to feed them with the intense fire of your will and imagination. How? By thinking about them on a daily basis and imagining that your goal has already come true.

By doing this, you will be in the optimum mental state to make your goal a reality. Your

mind will attract the events that are capable of producing the results you seek.

The next component in the model is **discipline,** the essential condition for all personal development and accomplishment. Without this component, you cannot expect to achieve or accomplish great things. In order to become fulfilled, your mind needs discipline. In fact, how can you expect to accomplish or receive anything at all if you're not able to fix your attention on the goal you have set out to achieve? Do you really want to lose weight and get into great shape? The disciplined individual possesses a strong and confident attraction to her goals. The disciplined individual succeeds where most fail, and always ends by conquering the obstacles blocking her path. The person who could care less about creating discipline constantly falls prey to failure. Success is the exception rather than the rule for this person, despite the many other great qualities she may possess. Most of the time she ends up where she is by chance, certainly not by choice. So how do you learn and practice discipline? By tirelessly repeating exactly what it is you want to achieve in your life. You must constantly remind yourself of what it is you are out to achieve (more muscle? less fat? better tone? more definition? all of the above?) from your fitness plan. Discipline your mind, apply the principles we've outlined here, and you will realize wonderful results.

The last of the components in the model, is **action!** Even if you possess **desire** and **discipline,** without **action** you will never obtain what you want. Combining action with desire and discipline creates the three musketeers of achievement. Many people have great ideas, foolproof plans and creative knowledge, yet everything falls apart for them. Why? Because they never act or they never act persistently enough. ***The difference between a person***

APPLYING THE VISUALIZATION TECHNIQUE: AN INTRODUCTION TO SELF-HYPNOSIS FOR UNPRECEDENTED RESULTS

Before beginning a visualization session, you must be fully rested. As the body needs adequate rest for exercise and activity, so does the mind for concentration and focus. Have you ever noticed that when you are tired you can't keep your concentration and things don't seem to work? When you feel like this, don't continue trying; take a nap! This allows for optimum concentration, the most important subcomponent of the visualization technique.

You should try to set aside a time allotment for practicing the method. It will only take about 15 minutes a day to put the technique into action. But without a set time, procrastination can and will set in, making it impossible to find the time needed. By setting a specified time each day (i.e. right before sleep or upon rising) you will condition your mind to be ready and effective every day at the same time. Also, try not to eat prior to the session because it will divert your needed energy (just as you should not eat prior to a workout for circulatory and digestive reasons). Be enthusiastic about your sessions too. Take pleasure in knowing that you are on your way to your personal best physique.

When practicing visualization you don't have to force it like exercise. Take it easy and relax! We are not doing bodybuilding exercise, yet the results achieved will blow your mind! The more relaxed you are, the clearer your image will be, thus allowing for more powerful results.

The first step in practicing visualization is to become entirely relaxed and calm. If you have already had some practice with relaxation or self-hypnosis techniques, you should be able to relax very quickly. We will assume that you have no experience with relaxation techniques.

First, direct all of your energies toward obtaining a state of very deep physical and mental relaxation. Your mindset will be that you feel remarkably calm and relaxed. We will now cover in detail a self-hypnosis session to rid your body of tensions and help you relax completely.

Stretch out comfortably on your favorite recliner or lay in your bed. Next, concentrate on one single point: either directly in front of you or above you (the ceiling, for example). Begin by saying the following sentences either out loud or to yourself, consciously focusing on feeling the physical effects they produce.

"My mind is fully concentrating on my focal point and the harder I concentrate on this point the more my mind and body are relaxed." (Note: Take as much time as necessary to feel the intended effect of total relaxation.)

"My eyes are getting more tired and my eyelids are getting heavier with every passing second." (Focus on your heavy eyelids as you fall deeper into your desired state.)

"I want to close my eyes, and I close my eyes."

"I feel totally calm and relaxed. My body is getting heavier and heavier, sinking into my bed (or seat). I can feel myself so, so relaxed. My eyes are now completely closed and I am so, so relaxed, yet focused on my body." (Do not fall asleep; you are relaxed, not sleepy!) "I will now begin to consciously relax my body." (Always begin with your feet, focusing first on your toes and moving body part by body part up towards your head. Proceed as outlined below with the following suggestions.)

"I am concentrating all of my attention on my feet, which are growing heavier and becoming so, so relaxed." (You may start to feel a tingling sensation as if very slight pins and needles were in your feet and toes.)

"A very comfortable and warm feeling is vibrating throughout my entire body."

"I will now focus on my legs, which are beginning to sink deeply into themselves." (Concentrate on this feeling but do not force it. This should be fun, not work! When you practice regularly, you will automatically fall into the desired state quickly.)

"My stomach is now beginning to feel very heavy, sinking deeper and deeper into itself." (Allow relaxed and easy breathing to occur. As you progress and move on to each body part, simply allow that part to lazily relax while you concentrate on the amazing feelings of relaxing your body. What you are doing right now may very well change your life forever!)

"My hands and fingers are growing heavier and heavier. They are totally relaxed."

"My chest is now sinking deeper and deeper into itself. With each breath I fall deeper and deeper into relaxation. I feel so, so calm and relaxed; I feel a warm vibration throughout my whole body."

"My neck is growing heavy and feels so relaxed as I allow it to sink deeply into itself. My head is relaxing more and more. I feel no pressure, only the heaviness allowing my head to sink deeply into itself. All of my thoughts are calming and relaxed. I feel as if I am in a dream floating."

"In this mind state, every thought that I wish to focus on is so powerful, so very powerful that nothing can stop it from becoming reality, whatever the obstacles in my way." (Repeat this last sentence mentally three times.)

Now form a mental image of exactly what it is that you want to achieve (a totally ripped or defined physique, more muscle, smaller dress size, entering and winning a competition, losing ten pounds of fat, gaining ten pounds of muscle), visualizing the object or goal towards which your message will be transmitted. The image must be as vivid and real as possible. Keep it in your mind's eye for about ten to fifteen minutes, without going over fifteen minutes.

Think about your message strongly. Do this for ten to fifteen minutes depending on the state of relaxation you have achieved. If you start getting tired or tense, stop, rest and begin in a few minutes. Think about your message by concentrating all of your attention on it. The more you are absorbed by it, the stronger the effect, thereby creating better success. The more the message is present in your mind during the session, the greater your success. Act with conviction that your message will come true. Don't forget that everything that you believe to be true will come true. This is the universal rule. Act with desire, discipline and faith to achieve. These actions cannot fail to produce the desired results.

What you have just read and experienced is a technique that really does work. We passionately believe in the power of the technique for attaining an abundance of success and achievement in your life. You can apply this powerful visualization technique to any and all aspects of your life. It is universal. Enjoy!

You may find relaxation and visualization foreign; you may not be comfortable with it. However, in order to change your life and make your desires reality, you must be willing to do what may initially be uncomfortable or different. The visualization technique can change your life, but only if you open your mind for change. Don't be afraid of change. You have the power to open up and accept new challenges. Are you capable of letting go and willing to try new things? If you want to dramatically change your physique and create a more exciting life for yourself, then take some chances, move out of your comfort zone and open your mind and life to new possibilities. These mind powering techniques are not commonplace or commercialized. Most teachers, whether it be fitness or academics, are afraid to teach what is not ordinarily taught. They are scared to cross the threshold of beliefs in fear that they will be the first to teach a method and possibly fail. We are not afraid to teach you our methods because we are confident that what we teach works: it has worked for us and thousands of others as well. We are not trying to be different by any means, nor are we trying to put down other traditional methodologies. We are simply revealing what may be the single most powerful life-changing tool in existence. Open your mind and begin to make changes where you never thought possible.

who knows and one who succeeds resides in the individual's ability to act.

Everything that you read in this book is the fruit of experience born of practice. If you apply the techniques and principles that we have discussed and you put action into the equation, you will meet your goals with astonishing success. To put action into use, we should reiterate something we discussed earlier, the premise of application and putting knowledge into practice. Many people wrongly believe that anything that doesn't fit their way of thinking must be false. Unfortunately, these people limit themselves by thinking that they are always correct. They never question their own beliefs. Whatever you do, never allow yourself to become this type of person. Always question others and follow your own instincts; but most importantly, **act as often as possible!**

ZONE-TONE CONCEPT

Obviously, one of your goals is to get in great shape as quickly as possible, right? If you don't know already, you will soon discover that the mind-to-muscle connection coupled with proper exercise technique and form are crucial if you want to stimulate the necessary muscle fibers needed to create a dynamite physique. While one may think this knowledge to be obvious and common sense, strangely enough, most people neglect the mental aspect behind exercise execution. It is not unusual to go to a gym and see people that are just "going through the motions;" in other words, moving

FAQ:
Isn't this mind-training material really unscientific and "New Age"?

ANSWER:
I can understand how things like meditation and visualization can get a bad rap but this material is based on science. The act of taking time to really go within yourself to think and focus your goals will have a profound effect. It is one thing to read about meditation and visualization; it's another thing to take the time to really let go and focus on your target. It's not easy to lie back and focus for any length of time on one vision, and it's very easy to be distracted. Wouldn't it be fair to say that if things were easy to achieve, everybody would be doing them? Your goals are not going to be simple to accomplish, but if you put your due diligence into practicing these methods on a consistent basis, you will inevitably be successful.

Make sure you know the difference between being attracted and being distracted. When you are attracted, your focus can be redirected and you will be drawn to outside influences. In other words, if you find yourself being easily attracted to socializing, perusing the environment and all its beauty or towards the things you need to get done outside of working out, distract yourself from the clutter and regain focus immediately!

a weight from point A to point B with little stimulation being directed towards the working muscles.

In this section you will soon learn yet another very powerful technique that will immediately provide astonishing performance and enhanced results to your physique by teaching you how to enhance your mind-to-muscle connection!

We have decided to name this very unique concept the "Zone-Tone" technique. It is the art of mentally zoning in and pre-isolating specific muscles just before an exercise is to be executed while at the same time maintaining that zone throughout the execution of the movement. This wonderful technique is very easy to grasp and will deliver enormous benefits to your fitness program. Combining proper form and technique (covered in the upcoming sections) with the Zone-Tone method will help you reach all of your fitness program. Combining proper form and technique (covered in the upcoming sections) with the Zone-Tone method will help you reach all of your fitness goals much faster than conventional practices. The level of isolation and stimulation you will get every time you perform an exercise using this method will increase tenfold.

There are several reasons why people fail to create a successful mind-to-muscle connection:

- Lack of knowledge about anatomy combined with lack of information available on how to successfully create a mind-to-muscle connection.

- Misinformation on the part of our teachers or books regarding exercise execution.

- Humans have a difficult time with change since they get accustomed to doing the same old thing and feel more comfortable and less at risk by doing so. As a result, they refuse to change the way in which they conduct their exercises.

- Lifting gargantuan weights without any concern for proper exercise form in order to satisfy our ego.

Of all of these possibilities, perhaps the biggest reason is the lack of information available on how to successfully create a mind-to-muscle connection coupled with a lack of knowledge on basic anatomy. If I asked you where your biceps were, would you be able to point to their exact location on your body? Are you aware that there are actually two biceps muscles, hence the prefix "bi"? Now, the next question is, if I asked you to flex your biceps muscle, could you do it effectively? How about your hamstring muscles located behind your thigh. Could you make that muscle contract really hard? Let's talk triceps; those three relatively small muscles located on the back of the upper arms. If I asked you to squeeze those muscles hard so that they tensed up intensely, could you do so immediately? The answers to these simple questions will soon lead to perhaps the most profound, beneficial, and eye opening mental exercise technique the fitness industry has ever experienced. (Note: Please do not feel bad if you do not know where these muscles are located. Our job is to teach you where they are and how to use them. As a matter of fact, in Appendix I, you will see a simple anatomical chart that contains the location of each muscle group.)

Now, when you're getting ready to do an exercise, do you ever stop to think about exactly what muscles you are about to train? Some of you will say yes and mean it. Some of you will say yes and not tell the whole truth. Most of you will say NO! This is the amazing reality that we are dealing with. I must admit to you though, that we truly love this fact too. We love it, of course, because we are the ones who will teach the world how to correctly and effectively transform their physiques ten

THE 10 COMMANDMENTS OF BODY SCULPTING PERFECTION

Commandment #1: Believe in Yourself! If not, you won't be able to achieve your desired results!

Commandment #2: Write down your goals. How can you get somewhere if you don't know where you are heading?

Commandment #3: Set new goals every six weeks. After six weeks, compare your results against your original goals.

Commandment #4: Place a calendar on your fridge. Mark a back slash on the days that you followed your diet without cheating. Make a forward slash on the days that you trained. If you trained and followed a good diet on a given day, you should have an X marked on that day.

Commandment #5: Place a picture of how you currently look somewhere that you will be able to see on a daily basis. This picture should provide you with additional motivation to follow this program.

Commandment #6: Take pictures of yourself every 4 weeks and place them on the refrigerator next to your "before" picture. That way, whenever you have a craving and go to the refrigerator you will remember the reason that you are doing this and also get motivated by seeing what you're achieving.

Commandment #7: Write down the reasons why you are following this program and put them on your refrigerator. Same benefit as item 6.

Commandment #8: Keep your house free from any foods that are not good for your program. Only on Sundays can you bring these foods in the house.

Commandment #9: Remember to prepare all your meals the day before, so that when you are at work, you already have all of the food that you will need for the day with you. That way you limit the amount of times you'll be tempted.

Commandment #10: Remember that only you control what goes in your mouth. Food does not control you!

FAQ:

I've read your techniques concerning Zone-Tone and I'm having difficulty actually making it work for me.

ANSWER:

Harnessing the power of your mind can sometimes be challenging. Just like exercising the body, you must practice your mental form and technique in order to truly harness the power of your mind. When you have perfected form and technique for both mind and body, the exercise begins to feel effortless and fluid. Then, you can trust that every movement you make is doing exactly what it should, and you are getting the most out of your training. It may take some time to get the hang of this, but with practice and dedication, your mind can quickly become your biggest and most valuable asset.

times quicker. We love it even more because of the fact that neglecting the mind-to-muscle connection while performing an exercise means that you all have a tremendous window of opportunity for major improvements to be made in your physique!

The key to improving the mind-to-muscle connection is to become attuned to our bodies before and throughout the movement. This means knowing what muscles you are targeting before you start the exercise and moving the muscle from its fully extended position to its fully contracted position while feeling the muscles (and only the intended muscles) contract and extend throughout the movement. Carelessly going through the motions of exercise is a complete waste of time and a great way to get nowhere quickly.

SO HOW DO WE USE THE ZONE-TONE?

While at the beginning the Zone-Tone concept might seem difficult to learn, it really is not! You might think that you won't be able to do it effectively but we know you can! We have taught it successfully to many others and now we will do the same for you.

There are only two simple steps to the Zone-Tone method:

Step #1: Focus and zone in on the individual muscle/s you intend to train before you begin the exercise. Knowledge of where each muscle is located is crucial; look at the anatomical chart in Appendix I of this book. Tense and flex the muscle to be trained as hard as comfortably possible before you even start to execute the exercise. This way you will be sending a message to that muscle, preparing it by completely isolating it even before the exercise begins. By doing so you have successfully created a mind-to-muscle connection.

Step #2: Maintain your mind-to-muscle connection during the execution of the exercise. Throughout the execution of the exercise feel the muscle extend and contract as you move from point A to point B. What we really want you to do while you are performing the exercise is to flex the muscle as hard as you can in the same way you did on Step 1, but this time with the exception that now you have a weight in your hand. This is crucial as it is of no benefit to activate the muscles before the exercise begins if the mind-to-muscle connection is lost as the movement starts. Many people waste their time by exercising without thinking about what they're doing. They exercise on a physical plane rather than on both the mental and physical planes. This is fine if you are content with average results, but who really wants to be average? On the other hand, if you want to compound your efforts exponentially and undeniably create the body you've always dreamed about having, then you must effectively develop the mind-to-muscle connection that we have been describing.

When you effectively call out to that muscle and prepare it for the following set, you create a mind-to-muscle connection. By maintaining this connection throughout the execution of the exercise that one set will produce the results of five sets! Did you read that? Do you realize what this can mean for you? If you implement these principles into your training regimen, you can create unbelievably toned and incredibly defined muscles in half the time. Imagine then the type of results you will get by combining the Zone-Tone method with the 14-Day Body Sculpting Workout and the exercise execution techniques that are presented later in this book. We guarantee that by combining all of these concepts you will achieve the most astounding and unbelievable physical transformation in the minimum amount of time.

FURTHER ENHANCING ZONE-TONE'S EFFECT

How would you like to multiply the effects of the Zone-Tone method? Here is a way to compound your efforts with little or no additional time expenditure.

Remember what you did during your meditation and visualization sessions as you focused on relaxing each and every muscle in your body starting with the feet? Well, at this time you have an invaluable opportunity to implement the Zone-Tone method.

IMPLEMENTATION

Starting with the feet, as you begin to relax and focus upon your toes, slightly wiggle each toe and concentrate on feeling the slightest movement in each individual toe.

You might feel a strange tingling sensation as you may never have stopped to pay attention to the feeling of these individual parts of your body. You might wonder why we would

waste time focusing on the feet first, right? We want to do this so that you become completely familiar and in sync with each and every part of your body. This will eventually give you the ability to isolate any muscle you desire at will. It is very important to remember and focus upon each and every part of your body without neglecting any specific part! As you move on from the feet towards your knees and up, zone in on every body part along the way. *Now here's where it can get tricky, so pay attention.* Simply focusing on the individual muscles of the body is not enough. When you simply think about them you cannot truly get a feel for how they feel when they are in action. To help you hone in and experience the feel for each of these muscles you should do the following:

- As you get to each individual body part, stop and contract the muscle as best as you know how. Do this three to five times and then relax.

- Remember the exact area where you felt that muscle contract and now focus all of your attention and energy on relaxing that same area. Do you realize what you will be accomplishing here? You are giving yourself an amazing ability to become in complete control of your entire superficial muscular system and will have the opportunity to call upon their action for maximum muscular efficiency.

Here is yet another technique you should use to further enhance the effects of the Zone-Tone method:

After you complete each set of an exercise, stand in the mirror and flex the muscles that you were exercising as hard as you can and hold for a count of 3-5 seconds. What will this do for you? It will help you to create a stronger mind-to-muscle connection and help you to accurately identify and call upon those individual muscles during exercise.

We can't tell you enough how important it is to practice the Zone-Tone method both when you're working out and also while at rest. As with anything, the more you practice the Zone-Tone method the quicker and more powerful the method will become. Soon you will realize, firsthand, the astonishing results gained from this powerful concept. Good luck!

For more information on the Zone-Tone, plus some amazing updates for this 4th Edition, check out Appendix K: The Zone-Tone.

LIFE'S DILEMMAS, SIMPLE SOLUTIONS; SOME PEOPLE MAKE EXCUSES, OTHERS FIND SOLUTIONS

In life we are bound to face adversity or dilemmas at one time or another. When this happens the key is to not freeze up. This is the problem many people have. Instead of doing something about their problems, they dwell upon them, feel sorry for themselves, and let the problems overtake them. In order to be successful at anything in life, instead of accepting adversity, **combat it!** Instead of finding a reason to be sad about a problem, **find solutions for the problem!** By finding solutions, you never give in to failure. You never admit defeat, and therefore are never defeated. It is only when you admit and give in to failure that you become a failure. The most successful people in the world have learned this philosophy and adapt it to their lives on a daily basis. Finding a solution to a problem is not as hard as it seems. You must use your imagination in order to achieve solutions. You must be willing to do what most people are not willing to do. Namely, you must create solutions by using your God-given talents. Brainstorming is one such talent, in which you write down any and all ideas to help solve your problem. It might be a quick fix,

such as changing an exercise. It might be a long-term solution, such as the one you discovered by applying these new principles into your life. Whatever solution or strategy you choose to apply, just make sure it is realistic and based on sound knowledge.

In the next section, you will learn why it is important for you to understand that your subconscious mind cannot tell the difference between a real experience and one that you imagine.

THE BLUEPRINT FOR A PERFECT BODY

The method below is an extremely powerful tool that can help you accomplish any of your goals (both in and outside the gym). If you're as skeptical as we once were, try to let go of your inhibitions and open up your mind to endless possibilities. People don't realize how incredibly happy and successful they can be with just this one technique. So we hope that you make good use of it.

The conscious mind has the ability to conjure up fantastic dreamlike images of the things you most desire. However, it is the subconscious mind (that feeds from the information you program into it with your conscious mind) that can turn your imagined visions into realities. Your subconscious mind reacts not only to what is true, but also to what you imagine. Your subconscious mind will store your emotional fantasies or dreams as reality. For instance, if you see yourself with a perfectly lean and muscular body, and if you truly believe this is possible, you are programming your subconscious mind with your imagination to bring this dream into reality.

Creating a mental blueprint of your dream body with your conscious mind is the first step. But when you program these mental blueprints into your subconscious mind believing that you can have them, or better yet, believing that you already have them, your subconscious mind will go to work for you to devise the methods that will make your fantasy come true. The value in creating mental pictures is enormous in that it gives the mind a constructive course of action to follow. It can and will help guide and motivate the practitioner into doing what is necessary in order to emerge with the desire. How would you like to see yourself, say in the next two months? Would you like to lose five inches around your waist? Would you like to gain five pounds of muscle for an unbelievably attractive body? Would you like to make a complete metamorphosis of your body type? If you said yes to any one of these, or perhaps have other desires which you'd like to attain, it is to your utmost advantage to incorporate the "mental-blueprint" method into your life. This same technique can be applied to any other aspect of your life as well.

In order to receive the best results from your visualization and mental blueprint principles, you must learn to create the proper mindset. Creation of the proper mindset is not a "think positive and everything will be great" type of method. This powerful weapon is fantastic for wiping out any negative thoughts, helping to keep you on the right track to success! Combining the right attitude with the proper training (visualization and blueprint imaging) is the surest way to reach your goals in no time. When training our clients we explain the importance of paying attention to their thoughts and mindset at all times. The attitudes that you project during your daily life can play a significant role in determining future occurrences. In other words, paying attention to your thoughts and changing them if necessary into positive thoughts is important for an optimal life and the creation of wonderful things.

Too many people have little faith in themselves. They have no belief that they can actually create better things or a better life for themselves. If you believe in yourself, have strong desires and act upon them with faith, desire and diligence, then that dream body, that beautiful house, that nice car, that wonderful life can all be yours. Your subconscious mind will react automatically to give you whatever you program into it, either real or imagined. Haven't you noticed that when we have a bad dream, the body reacts as if it were a reality; heart rate, adrenaline and blood pressure go up. The mind cannot distinguish the difference! However, your subconscious mind will not take the trouble to work for you unless you truly believe what you program into it. You must visualize or see yourself the way you want to look. It is also highly important that while transmitting your intended message to your subconscious mind, that you do so in the spirit that you already possess your dream body (or possess whatever it might be that you wish for). Have confidence in yourself and your goals, making sure that nothing or no one gets in the way of reaching them. You must realize, unfortunately, that many people will not want you to reach your objectives, not always by fault and sometimes because of insecurities of their own. You must learn to stay clear of these people and, even more, to stay strong in your convictions. If someone says that you cannot do or achieve certain things, use that negative energy as a way to fuel your determination in order to get there. By doing this, you will conquer any and all obstacles in your way and reach your goals.

Having said this, realize that you must use these mental images in order to fuel your determination to actually do what you have to in order to get there (e.g. train, eat right and rest). Just believing that it is possible to reach your goals is not enough; we need to take **action** in order to get there.

So in conclusion, the secret to achieving success is to program what you want into your subconscious mind by believing in yourself and seeing yourself as you would ultimately like to look or live. Such mental programming will then motivate you to set a plan (in this case a sound workout and nutrition program), follow through with the plan, and persevere. By programming yourself for success, everything you desire can and will be yours.

THE MANY BENEFITS OF EXERCISE AND CORRECT EATING: YOU WILL GET MUCH MORE THAN YOU HOPED FOR!

Exercise provides many benefits:

- **Increased energy:** When you exercise and eat right your energy levels go through the roof as the body is working at peak efficiency. This is due to the fact that the correct combination of diet and exercise produces a hormonal environment that leads to increased energy, fat loss and increased muscle tone.

- **Increased mental focus:** Did you know that exercise actually boosts brainpower? That's right; in fact, the latest research indicates that exercise can help keep the brain sharp well into old age, and might prevent many diseases, such as Alzheimer's disease, along with other mental disorders that accompany aging. If the brain is able to operate in peak condition, imagine the improvements that could be attained with business, decision-making, brainstorming, and every aspect of your life.

- **Increased self-esteem:** Since you are feeling good about the way that you look, your self-esteem goes up. This leads to self-confidence, something that empowers you with feelings of control and the

ability to make critical decisions under pressure with the certainty that you are making the correct one.

- **Increased sense of control over your life:** Once you are able to change the way you look and feel with exercise you'll notice that you can change anything else that you want in life using the same basic principles that allowed you to make the initial transformation (e.g. Desire, Discipline, & Action). No longer will you be afraid of setting a goal and not meeting it. If you are able to change yourself, you can change anything else that surrounds you.

- **Reduced chances of a heart attack:** By exercising and dieting you lower your cholesterol and your blood pressure, greatly reducing your chances of a heart attack.

- **Reduced chances of osteoporosis:** Correct exercise and diet increase bone density, reducing your risk of osteoporosis.

- **Reduced chances of breast cancer by 60%:** Exercise lowers the body's production of two ovarian hormones linked to breast tumor production: estradiol and progesterone.

According to Deborah Kallen, M.S., "the body's susceptibility to exposure to these hormones is greatest between ovulation and the beginning of menstruation. Habitual exercise postpones ovulation until later in a woman's monthly cycle, reducing the number of days her body must combat these potentially harmful hormones.

Medical researchers have long been aware that exercise burns fat, a known catalyst in the production of estrogen. So, if a woman has a regular exercise regimen, she gets an automatic two-for-one breast cancer prevention ticket. One ticket reduces the amount of time the body must protect itself against unwanted estrogen, and the other burns the fat that helps to manufacture the unwanted estrogen. For more information on hormonal balance, see the "Fitastic at and after 40" section on page 481.

- **Increased strength and stamina:** Naturally, exercise provides you with more strength and stamina which becomes useful in your daily activities.

- **Less Depression:** Exercise increases your production of endorphins (hormones that make us feel good and happy). Due to increased endorphin production, your chances of getting depressed are greatly reduced.

- **Exercise helps control stress level:** Note that with exercise, worries dissolve while mood rises. Say you had a bad day—the traffic was horrendous, the boss was in a foul mood, the phones wouldn't stop ringing, and you were late for an important meeting. Could you imagine going to bed with all of that accumulated stress? I certainly couldn't. Exercising right after work (for those of you that like late afternoon training sessions) is a great natural therapy that lets you forget about all of that and puts you in a great mood at the same time. After a good night's sleep you'll be refreshed and ready to tackle anything the next day throws at you.

When you exercise, you improve your whole lifestyle. By knowing the most intelligent, scientific way to train for optimal results you will be able to get so much out of life.

THE FORMULA FOR SUCCESS

Since we are engineers it is hard for us to write a book that has no formulas. Consider the following formula for success in changing your appearance; it is based on determination.

$$S = D \times (T+N+R)$$

S is the success that you achieve in your program, D is your determination to succeed, T is your training, N your nutritional program, and R stands for rest.

Each component in the formula above can only have two values. A value of 1 is given to a component if it is followed completely. A value of 0 is given to any component that is not followed or just followed halfway. Therefore, if every single component is followed, you get a maximum value of 3. In this case you would get the fastest results possible from your program. If you stop following one of the components inside of the parenthesis then you get a lesser value and sub-optimal results. However, note that if you don't have any determination you get a value of 0 and then your whole program fails and you don't get any results. The reason? ***Determination is by far the most important factor in determining the amount of success you will achieve in your Body Sculpting workout.***

After examining the formula above, it is easy to see why just purchasing a sophisticated gadget or a couple of magic pills at the health food store is not going to cut it. In order to achieve permanent weight loss all of the factors described above have to be present and in perfect harmony. Follow one but not the other and your success will be negatively affected.

Now that you have an idea of what it will take to get the body of your dreams, let's learn how to apply this knowledge. After all, only **applied knowledge** is power.

THE FIRST COMPONENT: DETERMINATION

Determination is the first component of the formula for good reason. Of all of the four components that make up the formula this is the most important. If you are not determined enough to make the sacrifices necessary to get in shape, then nothing is going to happen. You can have all the knowledge that we have on how to get in superb shape, but if you don't apply it then all you have is wasted knowledge. You need to want to change your appearance as badly as you would need to breathe if you were drowning. You also have to believe in yourself and know that you can do it. You must not doubt your ability to change. If you have doubts, you will fail! You will also need tunnel vision; in other words focus goal and, no matter how much adversity you encounter, stick to your plan, follow through, and get there. It is not an easy path. In a day and age where skepticism and negativity rule, roadblocks will appear (such as people telling you that you will not succeed or putting your program down, etc.). Every time you encounter a negative situation like that, use it to your own advantage. Use it to fuel your desire to achieve your goal. Don't let anybody put you down! This is important stuff. This not only applies to changing your appearance; this applies to every aspect of your life! If you want something, and you want it badly enough, you will be able to get it no matter what. Set a goal, develop an action plan and follow through—no matter what happens—until you reach that goal. In this book we give you a proven plan to change the way you look. Whether you want to lose a few pounds and firm up or lose 100 pounds, we provide you with a road map on how to get there. Use your desire and put the plan to work for you.

THE OTHER COMPONENTS OF THE FORMULA FOR SUCCESS

In the next few chapters we will cover the topics of training, nutrition, and recuperation. Due to the enormous amount of information necessary to thoroughly cover these topics, we have decided to dedicate a full chapter to each one of them.

Chapter 3 covers training, **Chapter 4** discusses nutrition and delves into the importance of supplements, and **Chapter 5** is dedicated to the often neglected components of rest and recovery.

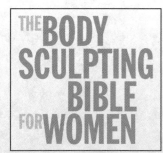

Part 2

The Building Blocks of Body Sculpting

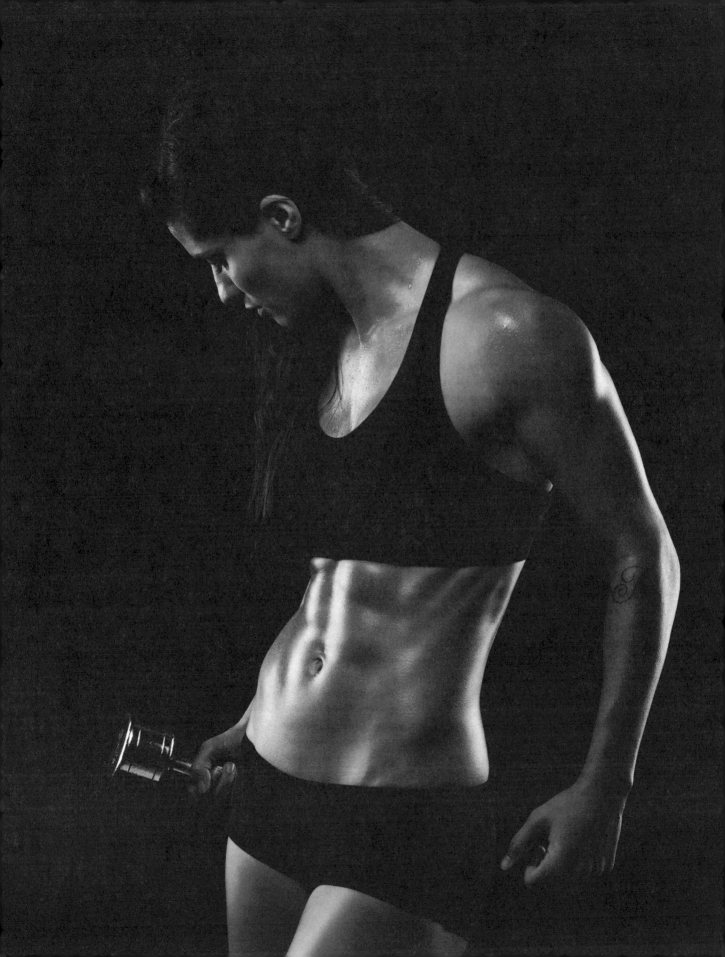

FIRST THINGS FIRST

Before you move any further in this book, you should first ask yourself what has brought you here. This may seem like a silly question, but it's not. In order for this program to help you achieve your body sculpting goals, you first need to identify your exact reasons for wanting to create a perfect physique.

A seemingly crazier question may be: are you *really* ready to get your body in amazing shape? We have always believed that there is a time and a place for everything. Have you ever wondered what makes the difference when someone finally quits smoking after so many failed attempts? Or how a person can finally lose 200 pounds after trying for years without success? The answer is surprisingly simple: **Those people were ready!**

Being ready is just as important as being able. Once you are truly ready to begin, you'll find that your fitness goals will finally become a reality. Sound familiar? We've watched people shovel in a five-course meal on Tuesday night and then wake up on Wednesday morning and eat healthy for the rest of the year, dropping dozens of pounds in the process and enjoying a life they never thought possible before. How? Simple: they'd had enough; they were finally ready. I've watched people slouch past the gym every day for years before they finally came inside; but once they did, they all had one thing in common: they were ready for action!

Creating your ultimate body is not as simple as just wanting to create your ultimate body. It requires a time commitment, sacrificing some of your favorite foods, rearranging your schedule, embracing a new philosophy and, let's face it, a lot of blood, sweat, and tears. We are not going to lie to you. To make such a commitment, to draw that proverbial line in the sand between your old life and your new, you simply have to be ready. Otherwise, it's all just pomp and circumstance.

Call it intuition, but we can always tell which of our clients will succeed and which won't. This judgment doesn't have anything to do with how they look, how much money they have, how old they are, how close they live to the gym, what kind of sneakers they wear, or what they do for a living. It all boils down to whether or not they're ready.

Don't just take our word for it, though; let's turn to science for evidence. According to a study done by Sarah Whitehead, and reported in the February 2005 *Journal of Sport Sciences*, research has shown that the enjoyment of exercise and the willingness to go it alone (e.g. without a friend) are both related to our level of physical activity and participation in sports. The research revealed that the more a person finds pleasure in exercise and the more his desire to exercise comes from within, the more likely he is going to engage in physical activity.

Another study, done by Amanda Daley and Gaynor Parfitt, and reported in the June 1996 *Journal of Occupational and Organizational Psychology*, found that exercise improves both mood and job performance.

Both studies support our theory that when you embrace health, fitness, and nutrition you don't just look better; you feel better! You don't just lose weight; you gain confidence. These are scientific studies delving into the matters of sports and fitness and yet they have both revealed that your physical and mental realities are interdependent.

Mind and body are not mutually exclusive; where one benefits, the other benefits. The better you feel, the better you perform; the better you perform, the better you feel. Like a snowball rolling downhill, the benefits just keep increasing until one day you look up to find the best looking you that you can be staring back in the mirror. If you haven't yet felt this, stick with us and we guarantee that you soon will!

READY, SET, GO! DISCOVERING YOUR READINESS!

We all think that strong muscles and proper nutrition are the backbone upon which your perfect body is built. Yes, they're absolutely important, but your intentions and attitude toward your fitness lifestyle are two of the most important factors when it comes to your decisions about finally being ready to get in great shape.

In order to achieve success you must first decide exactly what you want to attain from it, verbalizing your goal and visualizing it, picturing what you want in your mind, and keeping that image firmly before you, every moment, until your goals are brought to fruition.

Naturally, in order to receive you must give something, so it's necessary to decide what you are going to give. Fair enough? First and foremost, be willing to invest a feasible amount of time, as there are no shortcuts in achieving a beautiful physique. When you are an all-natural athlete, one of the most rewarding gifts is the empowerment in knowing that you and you alone are fully responsible for all of your wonderful body sculpting results! Therefore, results cannot be expected to appear in five minutes.

However, by investing your time equally between the most important elements of your fitness lifestyle—weight training, cardiovascular, nutrition, rest and recuperation, supplementation, and mindset—nothing short of miraculous results are quite achievable.

Your intention guides all of these pieces to help them work together. Clearly, intent is critical to success. So, what exactly is intention? According to Princeton University, it is "an anticipated outcome that is intended or that guides your planned actions". Your intention for this book is likely to look better than you ever have, right? Yes, that's certainly a broad way of looking at it, but we want you to have a more specific and direct intention. Perhaps your intention is to lose 20 pounds of fat and to add 2-5 pounds of muscle to your frame in 1½ months. That's a specific intention; a very direct and realistic goal, combined with an exact time frame.

In order to define your intention, we have discovered an exercise that is most effective and should always be used when focusing your intention. While many of us confuse intention with purpose, it is important to note that intention and purpose are not the same. So first we need to make the distinction between intention and purpose.

The difference between the two is that purpose is achieved through reflexes, and intention is achieved through planning.

It might be helpful to look at it this way: If I were to tap you on the knee with a hammer, your leg would automatically move; this is the same as purpose. Purpose revolves around seeing a stimulus and reacting to the stimulus. Intention would be similar to asking why the hammer is hitting the knee and discovering why your leg moves when hit. Intention is a much deeper conflict and will, in fact, help you in your quest for a fulfilling fitness regimen.

Exercise involves concentration on the goal at hand. For instance, if you are beginning an exercise such as a bench press, you should look at the weights and grow intent on using them to build your muscles. Think to yourself, "If I do this bench press I will work my upper body and will further develop it by breaking down and rebuilding the muscle tissue." Do not use purpose, which would be saying, "If I do this bench press my chest muscles will start burning and I'll be sore when I am done."

The distinction in this case may be accurate,

but recognizing the short-term nature of purpose will help you focus on the bigger picture. Use intention exercises to understand the underlying goal of the exercise, not just the reaction to the exercise.

So, how does one go about creating this point of finally being "ready"?

You must begin by recognizing that right now is the most important point of your life!

Get up off the couch, get your kids up off the couch, get your brothers, sisters, cousins, friends, and foes off that couch! Our country depends on this, folks!

Now, let's hit the fast forward button...

FAILING FORWARD

Most of you reading this book may have already attempted to follow a workout and diet regimen. It's easy to look back on past failures and dwell on the reasons why you or those programs failed to get you in shape.

Here's the deal: In order for any program to work, the negative must be banished from your mind. The only way to do this is to forget the past. Do not accept the past, forget the past! Accepting the past will make you think that it is just fine that you have failed in your physical fitness pursuits. It is not fine that you have failed because you are more important than to have failure run your thoughts.

At first it is hard to do this. A good way to practice this is to forget about recent problematic situations that you cannot control by dwelling on them and move on. If you are late for work one day, then set a goal and do not let it happen again. If you go out to dinner with friends and feel totally overwhelmed with temptation to resist those fried mozzarella sticks, remember that you are in control and that you and only you can sabotage your commitment. Do not sit and ponder on what has happened in the past. In doing this, you will

Sticking to a fitness regimen (a.k.a. commitment) has been proven to be the absolute most challenging thing for people who constantly seek to shape up. It's the reason why fitness is a multi-billion dollar industry and it's not about to decrease anytime soon.

So, why do so many people, possibly including you, fail with health and fitness goals? There are a few reasons why, but one of the biggest reasons is the "Buy In". In other words, unless you really have a powerful reason to get in shape and you're willing to put in the blood, sweat, and tears necessary to make it a reality, you are guaranteed to fail at it, case closed!

So, how do you create a "Buy In"? It may sound harsh, but one way is with scare tactics. You tie your reason for getting in shape to a fact such as, if you don't shape up, you'll likely end up getting sick and will die young. You do it by admitting to yourself that if you don't take care of yourself your family will likely lose you. You do it by being honest with yourself about the fact that the only way that anyone will be attracted to you is if you are attractive! You do it by not BS-ing yourself into thinking that people who are in good shape aren't treated better than those who are not! Listen, we hate these facts as much as many of you will (especially considering that we both were once obese) and we are sure we'll hear some of your rants about how wrong we are, but sadly enough, these are facts and it is what it is.

Another way to combat fitness failure is by having an accountability partner. Choosing a training partner who has similar goals as you is a great way to stay in the game and to make your goals a reality.

say to yourself, "maybe my diet and exercise program has failed, but this new program will not fail because my failure is in the past."

By not getting caught up in the past, one can see failure as a necessary step in achieving any goal. One cannot know success without also becoming acquainted with failure. Just be prepared for the next time and build up your willpower.

This technique can be used throughout your exercising career. If you fail to meet your ideal performance goals, then just forget about your failure that day and try it at the next workout session. If you fail at the next workout session, then forget about your failure and then try it at the third workout session. It's all about getting back in the saddle and not giving up!

Approach anything that you have failed at before as though you are trying it for the very first time. By exercising daily and following various nutrition guidelines, you will begin to notice that any type of setback has little or no effect on your motivation to succeed.

If you want your reality to be filled with success, then only think about the successes. If, however, you focus on failures, your physical fitness reality will be filled with failure and self-doubt.

Fail forward and you will realize your greatest fitness potential!

Here is a list of ways that you can avoid fitness failure and make your Body Sculpting goals a reality:

1. Create a scare tactic for yourself.

2. Find an accountability partner.

3. Make sure that your regimen includes the "Five Muscular Tiers," which are: Resistance Training, Cardiovascular Training, Nutrition, Supplementation, and Rest & Recuperation. By following the *Body Sculpting Bible* Program, you will fulfill this requirement.

4. Don't start your fitness regimen on New Years Day. It's a trend and trends end. Start it either before or after the holiday. Even a week apart is better than starting on this infamous day of destined fitness failures!

5. Be realistic with your goals. If you shoot too high, you could easily become frustrated and quit. Shoot for a doable goal, e.g. "I will lose three pounds by the end of this week" or "I will take my treadmill training to another level this week by increasing the speed by ½ MPH and adding a one-grade incline."

6. Make a pact with your family members. If you don't, self sabotage is imminent. If you all make fitness a part of your lives, all of your lives will surely be enriched.

Chapter 3
Training

For immediate Body Sculpting Bible support & coaching directly from James & Hugo, please visit www.BodySculptingBibles.com

3

Training is the first component inside the parenthesis of the formula for success. The way you train will ultimately determine the way you look. This is how you will be able to sculpt your body into a work of art.

There are two types of training: Anaerobic exercise (e.g. weight training), which uses glycogen as its main source of fuel, and Aerobic exercise (e.g. walking, bike riding, etc), which uses oxygen as its main source of fuel. We will discuss each separately and then go into detail about each type.

WEIGHT TRAINING

The anaerobic training that we will be using is weight training. Weight training is the number one way to re-sculpt your body. It is by far superior to any other form of exercise because *it is the only way that can shape your body and increase your metabolism permanently.* This is vital since a slow metabolism is at the root of obesity. We find it ridiculous how some so-called fitness authorities don't adhere to this simple yet very true concept. It is ludicrous how some "fitness experts" believe that aerobic exercise alone provides the key to the perfect physique. **These "authorities" are wrong** and should educate themselves by learning the facts.

Many women are concerned that weight training will make them muscle bound. This is not possible since women simply do not produce enough testosterone (the male hormone that is responsible for muscle growth) to achieve the Arnold Schwarzenegger look. What weight training will do is provide the firm, cellulite-free looking body that most women desire.

GOALS

Without goals we are dead in the water; we have nowhere to aim and nowhere to go. Therefore we need to set goals in order to achieve success.

Our ultimate body sculpting goals are as follows:

Gain: 5-10 pounds of muscle (or more depending on what you want) in order to tone up and increase your metabolism.

Lose: Enough fat to get down to between 12-16% body fat. Women **should never** go below 12% as going any lower would cause undesirable side effects such as the cessation of the monthly period (amenorrhea) and reduction of breast size.

Depending on where your physical fitness level is at this moment it may take you longer than six weeks to achieve these goals. However, don't feel bad about it: the important thing is that you will be moving forward. You will achieve these goals very quickly by being persistent and serious about your fitness program. Besides, remember that by doing nothing, in a year from now your body will look the same if not worse.

Now that you know where you're headed, let's see what the characteristics of a good weight-training program are.

CHARACTERISTICS OF A GOOD WEIGHT-TRAINING PROGRAM

In order for weight training to be effective, the following rules should be followed:

Sessions should be short: 60 minutes maximum. The maximum amount of time a weight training session should last is 60 minutes. After 60 minutes the levels of muscle building and fat burning hormones (like growth hormone and testosterone) begin to drop. In addition, the glycogen (stored carbohydrates) in your system, which is the fuel that your muscles use to contract, is depleted. If you weight train more than 60 minutes you will actually be wasting your time since you will no longer have the hormones or the fuel necessary to produce muscle growth. Continue to train past 60 minutes and you will get impaired recovery, which leads to overtraining, a condition where your body does not recover from its weight training sessions. This leads to loss of strength and muscle mass.

The rest between sets should be kept to a minimum; 90 seconds or less. Keeping your rest time in between sets and exercises to a minimum not only allows you to perform a prodigious amount of work within the 60-minute weight training window, but also helps to improve your cardiovascular system and most importantly maximizes the output of growth hormone, a powerful fat burning/muscle building hormone. Also, this rest interval promotes a muscle voluminizing effect in which water goes inside the muscle cells (not outside) and makes the muscles look more firm and toned. Do not confuse this with water retention outside of the muscle cells, which is what makes us look puffy and fat.

Sets of each exercise should consist of 8-15 repetitions. There are many reasons for this. First and foremost, it has been shown that it is within this range that growth hormone output is maximized. As we already know, this is a good thing since this hormone does exactly what we are looking for (increases muscle and decreases body fat). In addition, since you are performing so many repetitions, you get a great pump (blood rushing into the muscle) that provides nutrients to nourish muscle cells and helps them recover and rebuild faster. Finally, performing 8-15 repetitions reduces the possibility of injury dramatically since you will need to use a weight that you can control in order to perform the prescribed amount of reps. *(Note: This rule does not apply to the calves and abdominals as these muscles usually respond*

FAQ:
Can I ever go below or exceed the 8 to 15 repetition range?

ANSWER:
Absolutely! For all intents and purposes, the rep ranges that we recommend are for the workouts in the book. There may be times that you would benefit greatly by either doing more or fewer repetitions. It all depends on your goals and routine.

better to higher repetition ranges, in the order of 15-25 reps).

Training must be progressive. Progression means one more repetition than the last time the exercise was performed or a little bit more weight if you are able to do more than 15 repetitions for a particular exercise. It is important to understand that you will not be able to increase weight or the number of repetitions every session. However, progression comes in many forms, like performing more work within the 60-minute period. The overall goal of a training routine is to ensure progression over a period of time to bring about continuous improvements in muscle tone and definition.

Training must be varied. This principle is vital to ensure continuous gains in strength and muscle tone as well as to prevent boredom. Variation does not necessarily mean changing all of the exercises in your program. Variation can occur in the form of using different techniques to stimulate the muscle, changing repetition and set parameters, and even changing the rest between sets or simply changing the width of your grip placement on the bar to help isolate specific muscles. As you will soon see, the 14-Day Body Sculpting Workout makes full use of this principle since every two weeks your routine changes, providing you the variation that your body needs to keep achieving results.

Training must consist primarily of free weight basic exercises. Only free weight basic exercises provide the fast results you are looking for because they recruit the most muscle while you are performing them. Besides, the body is designed to be in a three dimensional universe. Whenever you use a machine you limit your body to a two-dimensional universe and consequently you limit the amount of muscle fibers that are going to do work. However, not all machines are bad. Some definitely have a place in our weight-training program because they allow you to isolate the muscle in a way that no free weights would allow you to do. However, our program should be mostly based on barbells, dumbbells and exercises where the body moves through space such as the dip, the pull-up and the squat. The best exercises for each body part are the following:

BACK

BASIC EXERCISES

Dumbbell one-arm row, pullover, pull-up, bent-over barbell row.

ISOLATION EXERCISES

Stiff-arm pull-down, low-pulley row.

CHEST

BASIC EXERCISES

Incline bench press (and its dumbbell version), flat bench press (and its dumbbell version), chest dip, and push-up.

ISOLATION EXERCISES

Chest fly (incline and flat versions), incline cable crossovers.

THIGHS AND BUTTOCKS

BASIC EXERCISES

Barbell squat (and its dumbbell version), ballet squat (and its dumbbell version), lunge, leg press.

ISOLATION EXERCISES

Leg extension.

HAMSTRINGS

BASIC EXERCISES

Stiff-legged deadlift (and its dumbbell version), leg press (feet high on the platform), lunge (how far you extend your leg when you do this exercise determines which leg muscle is activated the most. The farther away from the torso that you extend your leg, the more you hit the hamstrings).

ISOLATION EXERCISES

Lying leg curl, standing leg curl, seated leg curl.

FAQ:
I see all the regulars at the gym using machines. Are machines better than free weights?

ANSWER:
Free weights allow the muscles to be stimulated on many different levels. In order to prevent the free weights from wobbling around while you lift them, additional stabilizing and balancing muscles assist during the exercise, and you are fully working the entire muscle.

When you're exercising using a machine, you are restrained to a predefined range of motion. There are no stabilizing muscles involved, and you are strictly concerned with getting the weight from point A to point B. The bad side of this is you aren't getting the bonus of having additional muscles stimulated. The good side is that machines are great if you have an injury and need to isolate a muscle to avoid stressing it. You also may simply feel that you are being stimulated more with a machine than with free weights.

The best thing to do is use both free weights and machines. you can get the best of both worlds. As for the gym regulars: if you pay close attention, you'll find that they are lifting their fair share of free weights.

SHOULDERS

BASIC EXERCISES

Military press (and its dumbbell version), upright row (and its dumbbell version).

ISOLATION EXERCISES

Lateral raise, bent-over lateral raise, rear-delt machine.

BICEPS

BASIC EXERCISES

Dumbbell curl, barbell and dumbbell preacher curl, incline dumbbell curl, hammer curl, reverse curl, and E-Z bar curl.

ISOLATION EXERCISES

Concentration curl.

TRICEPS

BASIC EXERCISES

Barbell and dumbbell lying triceps extension, barbell and dumbbell overhead triceps extension, triceps dip, close-grip bench press (and its dumbbell version).

ISOLATION EXERCISES

Triceps pushdown, triceps kickback.

CALVES

(Note: For calves and abdominals there is really no distinction between basic and isolation exercises.)

Standing, seated, and donkey calf raise, calf raises on leg press machine, one legged or two legged calf raises with dumbbell.

ABDOMINALS

Crunches, leg raise, and knee-in, trunk curl and crunch, V-up.

AEROBIC TRAINING

Aerobic training such as walking or running on a treadmill is a good way to accelerate the fat burning process as long as it is not overdone and as long as it is used only in addition to a good weight training program. It should never be used as a substitute for weight training since it does not permanently increase your metabolism and does not have the ability to re-shape your body.

In order for aerobic exercise to be effective, it needs to be performed within the fat burning zone. The fat burning zone is the zone at which you are doing just the right amount of work to burn fat. Your pulse (how fast your heart is beating per minute) determines this zone. It is important to remain in this zone for a certain period of time. If you work harder or longer than what the formula recommends you will quickly become exhausted which will prevent you from continuing to perform the activity for a prolonged period of time, which is absolutely necessary in order to burn fat. On the other

FAQ:
Should I only weight train and leave the cardio to runners and endurance athletes?

ANSWER:
Absolutely not. Some fitness professionals will say that it is okay to only weight train, especially if your routine is made up of supersets. However, it's best that your fitness routine have a balanced approach and heart-healthy aerobics/cardio training is crucial.

hand, too low of an effort will not prompt your body to start its fat burning mechanisms.

To determine your fat-burning zone, use the following formula:

Fat burning zone = 220-(your age) x (.75)

For example, a 20-year-old woman would need to reach a pulse in the neighborhood of 150 beats per minute in order to be in the fat burning zone. It is important to remember that this is not an absolute figure, but an approximation. As long as you stay within 10 beats of the number that the formula dictates, you can rest assured that you will be burning fat.

In order for aerobic exercise to be an effective fat burner it needs to be performed at the appropriate times. There are two ideal times when aerobic exercise is most effective in burning fat. The ideal time is first thing in the morning on an empty stomach after drinking 16 to 24 ounces of water in order to prevent dehydration. When performed at this time you burn 300 percent more body fat than at any other time in the day because your body does not have any glycogen (stored carbohydrates) in the system to burn. Therefore, it has to go directly into the fat stores in order to get the energy necessary to complete the activity. The other time that aerobic exercise is effective would be immediately after a weight training session as your glycogen stores have already been depleted. Because of this, once you start doing your cardio, you will start burning fat as soon as you elevate your heart rate since it is the only fuel that will be available.

When aerobic exercise is not performed first thing in the morning or right after the weight training workout it takes your body approximately 20 to 30 minutes to start burning fat. This is how long it takes the body to deplete its glycogen stores and switch to a fat burning environment. Therefore, it is not as efficient to perform aerobic exercise alone at other times of the day because you would need to work out for 20-30 minutes just to get to the fat burning stage and then continue to work out for an additional 20 minutes to burn fat. This would mean a grand total of 50 minutes a day. In our opinion, aerobic exercise shouldn't be performed more than six times a week for 40 minutes maximum each session, in order to avoid losing muscle mass. Remember that more is not always better and this is especially true when it comes to aerobic exercise. As you will see, for this program (unless you are interested in fitness competition), the most you will be doing is three sessions lasting between 20 to 40 minutes each at the most.

Good forms of aerobic exercise include riding a stationary bike, fast walking (this can be done on a treadmill), climbing on a stair stepper, swimming, using a fitness rider or rowing machine, using any good cardio tapes like Tae-Bo, or any other form of cardiovascular activity that raises your heartbeat to the fat burning zone.

PUTTING IT ALL TOGETHER

Now we will learn how to put all this knowledge together in a workout program that will yield the results you are looking for. We present three different workouts. Which one you should choose will depend on your previous training experience and your fitness goals.

The first workout (the Break-In Routine) is to be used by women who have never done weight training before. This program is a break-in program that will not only allow you to get in shape quickly, but will also condition you to get in the shape necessary to be able to use the 14-Day Body Sculpting Workout.

The second workout (the 14-Day Body Sculpting Workout) is for women who have been weight training for at least 10 weeks and want to get into awesome shape (gain 5-10 pounds of muscle and reduce body fat to 12-16%).

The third workout (the Advanced 14-Day Body Sculpting Workout) is the most advanced workout to be used only by women who either have an interest in fitness competition or just want to look like a fitness competitor (gain 15-20 pounds of muscle and reduce body fat to 12%). This last workout requires at least 1 year of weight training experience in the gym and is the most rigorous and time-consuming workout. It will emphasize all angles of the muscle in order to produce the most stunning body sculpting effect. Therefore, this workout is reserved for the most serious fitness gals out there.

Before we present the 14-Day Body Sculpting Workout, let's discuss a few terms that you need to understand in order to execute the routine.

Repetitions or Reps: The amount of times that you perform an exercise. For instance, imagine you are performing a bench press. You pick up the bar, lower it, pause and lift it up. That action of executing the movement for one time counts as one repetition. If you perform that same movement a second time, then that is your second repetition and so on.

Sets: A set is a collection of repetitions that culminates in the muscle reaching muscular failure. Muscular failure is the point at which, due to a buildup of lactic acid in the muscle, it becomes impossible to perform another repetition with good form.

Rest Interval: The amount of time you rest between sets. For instance, a rest interval of 60 seconds means that after you finish your first set, you will remain idle for 60 seconds before going on to the next set.

Now that we have discussed these important terms, let's discuss the main techniques that make the 14-Day Body Sculpting Workout so effective.

Modified Compound Supersets: In a modified compound set, you pair exercises, usually for opposing muscle groups or for opposing muscle movements (e.g. push vs. pull). First you perform one exercise, rest the recommended amount of seconds and then perform the second exercise (i.e. first do biceps, then do triceps). Then rest the prescribed amount of time again and go back to the first exercise.

A modified superset for dumbbell rows and push-ups in which you perform 4 sets of each exercise will look like the following:

You will be resting 2 minutes plus the amount of time that it takes you to perform the other exercise, so you actually are resting a given muscle between 2.5 and 3 minutes. Using this technique of pairing exercises in a modified superset fashion not only saves time and keeps the body warm, it also allows for faster recovery of the nervous system between sets. This allows you to lift heavier weights than if you just stay idle for 2-3 minutes waiting to recover. An additional benefit of this technique is that it saves time and limits rest to a maximum of 90 seconds between sets.

Supersets: A superset is a combination of exercises performed right after each other with no rest in between. There are two ways to implement a superset. The first way is to do two exercises for the same muscle group at once (like dumbbell curls immediately followed by concentration curls). The drawback to this technique is that you will not be as strong as you usually are on the second exercise. The second and best way to superset is by pairing exercises of opposing muscle groups (antagonists) or different muscle movements such as back and chest, thighs and hamstrings, biceps and triceps, shoulders and calves, upper abs and lower abs. When pairing antagonistic exercises, there is no drop of strength whatsoever. As a matter of fact, sometimes your strength increases because the blood in the opposite muscle group helps you perform an exercise. For instance, if you superset dumbbell curls with triceps extensions, the blood in the biceps helps you do more weight during the triceps extensions. Because of this, we will only perform supersets where opposing muscle groups or opposing muscle movement exercises are paired. Supersetting not only allows you to do more work in a shorter period of time

SAMPLE MODIFIED COMPOUND SUPERSET				
EXERCISE	**PAGE NO.**	**REPS**	**SETS**	**REST**
MODIFIED COMPOUND SUPERSET # 1				
Back—Dumbbell One Arm Row	168	15-20	4	90 seconds
Chest—Push-Up (against the wall if unable to perform on the floor)	208	15-20	4	90 seconds

but it also increases endurance, creates an incredible pump (especially when you pair antagonistic exercises), and helps burn fat by elevating the heart rate to the fat burning zone (which also gives you cardiovascular effects). Also, because of the stress created by this technique, growth hormone levels go through the roof. Remember that this hormone is responsible for fat loss and enhanced muscle tone.

Giant Sets: Giant Sets are four exercises done one after the other with no rest between sets. Again, there are two ways to implement this. You can either use four exercises for the same muscle group or perform two pairs of opposing muscle group exercises. For the purposes of this book whenever we do Giant Sets, we will perform two pairs of opposing or different muscle group exercises with no rest (the exception is in abdominal work in which we will alternate between lower abs and upper abs).

A Giant Set for biceps and triceps in which you perform four sets of each exercise looks like this:

Giant Sets provide you with more of the same benefits that supersets offer. This is the most intense and powerful technique that we will use in our 14-Day Body Sculpting Workout. We need to be cautious when using Giant Sets since they are considered an

FAQ:
There is a lot to remember as far as reps, sets, rest times, as well as proper form. Can't I just stick to an easy routine?

ANSWER:
If you want to make radical and long-lasting changes to your body, you need to stick to the entire program and all of its details. No one said this was going to be easy. Once you get the hang of it, we promise that it will become second nature to you! All of the little details will help to make this program the most effective and powerful routine available.

extremely intense exercise protocol. Although the human body is capable of handling great intensity and stress, you should never push it to the edge. The Giant Sets protocol is a very powerful and results oriented training method, but should be used sparingly. With that said, the Giant Sets protocol will only be used for about two weeks. Have you ever heard the saying that "too much of a good medicine is bad?" This certainly applies to Giant Sets. This is really strong medicine in the fight against fat. Use it for more than two weeks and your body will no longer be able to recover; the nervous

SAMPLE GIANT SET				
EXERCISE	**PAGE NO.**	**REPS**	**SETS**	**REST**
GIANT SET # 1				
Thighs—Dumbbell Squat	168	8-10	4	No Rest
Hamstrings—Stiff-Legged Deadlift	208	8-10	4	No Rest
Back—Dumbbell One-Arm Row	170	8-10	4	No Rest
Chest—Push-up (against wall if unable to perform on floor)	198	8-10	4	60 seconds

SAMPLE SUPERSET				
EXERCISE	**PAGE NO.**	**REPS**	**SETS**	**REST**
SUPERSET				
Back—Dumbbell One Arm Row	168	15-20	2	No Rest
Chest—Push-Up (against the wall if unable to perform on the floor)	208	15-20	2	90 seconds

system will get burned out and will reach a state of overtraining (where your body can no longer recover from the workouts).

Now that we have discussed the three techniques that are the basis of the 14-Day Body Sculpting Workout, let's see what the routines look like.

HOW DOES THE 14-DAY BODY SCULPTING WORKOUT WORK?

The 14-Day Body Sculpting Workout is based on your body's physiology. From a physiological standpoint, it usually takes your body 14 days to get used to a new practice, whether that practice is a diet, a new exercise program or just getting up earlier in the morning. Getting used to a new practice, such as waking up early to exercise, is a great thing. However, getting used to an exercise program is not as great. Why? Once your body gets used to it, it will stop responding and your results (i.e. fat loss and increased muscle tone) will come to a screeching halt. That is the reason why most people who go to the gym experience great results initially, but later see and feel themselves going nowhere. The key to experiencing continued results is variation. However, it cannot be haphazard variation. You must have a planned scheme that will guarantee continual results; a scheme such as the one the 14-Day Body Sculpting Workout offers.

For the first two weeks you will use modified compound supersets. During this period, the body gets stronger as rest periods are abun-

dant and repetitions are at a higher range (12-15). Working out this way allows the nervous system to recover and the body to increase its strength. In addition, the high repetitions allow the body to start building more capillaries (necessary for the delivery of nutrients to the muscle cell) and prepare the joints for the heavier weights to come.

On weeks three and four you will start using supersets, a more intense technique that creates higher demands on the central nervous system, along with heavier weights and fewer reps (10-12) with a slightly higher number of sets. The increased volume and the shock to the body created by the increased stress of the weight training routine causes an increased output of growth hormone (which greatly enhances fat loss and muscle tone), and an increased metabolism.

When your body starts adapting to this rou-

FAQ:
Why 14 days?

ANSWER:
We found that our 14-day periodization program worked because its duration wasn't too long (so you wouldn't get bored) and it wasn't too short (so you wouldn't be constantly changing programs). It was "just right". The program has helped literally hundreds of thousands of people throughout the world make and keep amazing changes to their bodies.

tine, you further increase the intensity by increasing the number of sets again, using heavier weights (8-10 reps) and giant sets. Once again the body is shocked, growth hormone output goes through the roof and the metabolism is jolted. The routine is so intense that if you were to maintain it for more than 2 weeks you would enter a state of overtraining.

When your body has reached a level that gets fairly close to overtraining, you will give your body a chance to recover for the next couple of weeks by going back to week 1 where you use fewer sets, higher reps and have ample amounts of time to recover in between sets by using the modified compound superset technique. Are you going backwards? Not at all! With this program you are always moving forward. Even though you are going back to a less stressful type of training with less volume, you will notice that you will now be stronger on the same exercises. You will be able to use greater weight for the 12-15 repetition range for the following reason: In order for the body to prevent itself from going into overtraining during the two weeks of high volume and giant sets, it naturally built up its nervous system energies to the highest level possible as an emergency measure. Now that you have backed off on the stress, you'll have all of this extra energy the body will utilize to get even stronger. That is how your strength will increase. Then after two weeks of modified compound supersets, once again you'll begin to increase the stress on the body by continuing this results-producing cycle.

Why is it necessary to get strong and why should you lift heavier weights? Because building up your strength through progressive resistance training is the key to increased muscle tone and accelerated fat loss. Remember, if your strength stays the same, then your body will look the same and

you might as well consider yourself moving backwards.

Don't worry about looking like Arnold Schwarzenegger either; remember, a woman's body does not produce enough testosterone, the male hormone responsible for creating "mucho" amounts of muscle. Yes, you will still build beautifully lean and toned muscle tissue along with that cellulite-free look that you want, but the female hormone estrogen will make sure to maintain the femininity you desire.

BEST TIME TO WORK OUT

We recommend you work out in the morning as soon as you wake up. Drink 16 ounces of cold water before you start the workout and an additional 30 to 60 ounces during the activity. This is essential to prevent dehydration. We recommend working out first thing in the morning on an empty stomach because you will burn 300% more body fat this way. In the morning your body doesn't have any carbohydrates to burn. In the absence of carbohydrates, your body goes straight to the fat stores (triglycerides) in order to get the energy necessary to do the work. Another good reason to work out in the morning is the fact that at this time growth hormone levels are at their highest levels. Working out in the morning will allow you to expedite the fat loss process for dramatic results. However, we do understand that certain obstacles such as work constraints and other situations might not permit everybody to train in the morning. In this case, do your cardio or weight training three hours after any meal (If your last meal was at 3:00 pm, then your exercise session should be at 6:00 pm).

If you follow the Advanced 14-Day Body Sculpting Workout you will be doing cardio and abs first thing in the morning and weight training at some other time during the day.

However, if this is impossible due to your schedule, then perform abs before the weight training workout and cardio right after the weight-training workout is completed. *(Note: If you do decide to work out in the morning, please make sure that you properly warm-up and stretch. This will not only ensure that you are wide awake but will also prevent injuries and potential accidents.)*

WORKOUT CLOTHING

When you go to the gym, you should be wearing comfortable clothes that allow your body to move freely without constraints. Therefore, rigid clothes like jeans are definitely out of the question. You also need to choose clothes based on the climate you live in and environmental conditions. You should wear extra layers of clothing if your environment is cold helping to keep your body temperature on the warm side and prevent possible injuries. Also wear nice comfortable cross training shoes along with a thick absorbent pair of socks. Never train in your bare feet or with sandals as you could seriously injure your feet if you ever dropped a weight on them.

HOW FAST SHOULD YOU LIFT THE WEIGHT?

This next section covers a fascinating topic that has caused debate among many people in the fitness industry: "Should I lift the weight fast? Should I lift the weight slow? Should I move the weight fast or slow on the positive (concentric) portion of the rep? Should I move fast or slow on the negative (eccentric) portion of the rep?" All of these are very good questions and should be researched. We have done the research and will now explain each one in detail.

We have found that slow lifting is usually only good for beginners who have never lifted a weight before. It helps them to learn and master the movement and prevents them from using bad exercise form. However, as you become more advanced, science and our own experience indicate that you should lift the weight as quickly as possible without sacrificing form and without involving momentum (jerking and bouncing of the weights). You create more force by lifting fast and therefore more muscle fibers need to be activated. By ensuring that you are not using momentum to help you move the weight, you can be sure that the force generated during the movement will be created solely by your muscles. This is what helps stimulate your muscles to grow creating the tone and shape that you desire. While some might believe that super slow lifting is beneficial because it is difficult to perform and painful, it is not the best way to stimulate muscle growth. Super-slow lifting accumulates too much lactic acid within your muscles and fatigues them before they reach real momentary muscular failure.

Science tells us that Force = Mass (in this case the weight you are lifting) times Acceleration (the increasing speed at which you lift the weight). Therefore, the best way to lift weights is to lift them fast, with total control of the weight and void of momentum. Since you won't be jerking the weights or using ballistic movements during exercise, the risk of getting injured is not any greater than the risk of getting injured lifting super slowly.

One last point about lifting speed. If you are lifting a weight that only allows you to do eight repetitions, if you're looking in the mirror, it will look like you are lifting the weight slowly even though you are lifting it as fast as possible. This is due to the fact that the heavier the weight, the slower you will be able to move it, even though you are trying to accelerate it as fast as you can. This is amazing! I'm sure you've heard people's concerns about how lifting heavier weights is dangerous, right? It is actually the opposite. When you lift lighter

> **FAQ:**
> *I've read that varying your lifting speed can actually be beneficial.*
>
> **ANSWER:**
> It definitely is. Just like the 14-Day Body Sculpting Program changes every 14 days, which makes sure your muscles are never expecting what's coming, you can change your lifting speed to increase results. The speed at which you lift the weight from point A to point B can have huge effects on your muscles, as it can increase the amount of concurrent time your muscles are under tension during each set. The key here is to switch things up from time to time.

weights, you have the ability to move the weights, very quickly and sloppily because little stress is put upon the muscles, tissues and joints. This creates a greater risk for injuries to occur. When you lift heavier weights, you are forced to go slower with the weights and to use controlled form during movement. Lifting heavier weights will stimulate more muscle fibers while limiting the chance for injuries (assuming that the maximum amount of weight lifted is one that allows for a minimum of eight repetitions; heavier weights may indeed cause connective tissue injury).

MUSCLE SORENESS

Muscle soreness is caused by micro trauma to the muscles and is a good indicator that the workout you performed was effective. If you have never exercised before, you will experience higher levels of soreness than usual at the beginning of your program. That is okay. As your body gets used to the exercise pro-

gram the muscle soreness will subside to tolerable levels. You just need to persevere through those first few weeks. Do not confuse this type of soreness with overtraining.

There are several degrees of soreness.

- Delayed onset muscle soreness
- Typical mild muscle soreness
- Injury-type muscle soreness

The first type of soreness is Delayed Onset Muscle Soreness (DOMS). The term DOMS refers to the deep muscular soreness usually experienced two days after (not the day after) the exercise has been done. DOMS prevents the total muscular contraction from occurring within a muscle. This type of severe soreness is caused when you either embark on an exercise program for the first time or when you train a body part harder than usual. It can last for a couple of days for an advanced well-conditioned athlete or for as long as a week for a beginner. If this type of soreness is affecting you and it is time to work out again, the best thing to do is not to rest but to exercise the affected body part in an active recovery routine. In active recovery routines all of the loads are reduced by 50 percent, and the sets are not taken to muscular failure. For example, if you are to perform an exercise for 10 repetitions, divide the weight that you usually use for that exercise by two and that is the weight you will use for your active recovery routine. Also, stop performing the exercise even though you may not reach muscular failure at the tenth rep. The reason for this type of workout is to restore full movement in the muscle, helping to remove the lactic acid and other waste products building up within the muscles. It also forces high concentrations of blood into the damaged area of the muscles and nourishes the muscles for repair and growth. We find that doing this is always beneficial; by the next day you will not be as sore or stiff as you ordinarily would have been if you had skipped a workout in order to wait for the pain to subside.

The second type of soreness is the typical mild muscle soreness experienced the day after a good workout. While scientists are still unable to pinpoint the true cause of such soreness, the explanation generally accepted is that it is caused by micro trauma at the muscle fiber level and by an excess of lactic acid. At any rate, what's important is that this is good soreness considering it is of a mild nature and muscle function is not impaired as it is with DOMS. The pain generally lasts a day for advanced athletes and up to three days for a beginner. This soreness, on average, indicates that you had a good workout the day before because you created the trauma necessary to trigger adaptation (e.g. muscle growth). When you are no longer experiencing this type of soreness, it is a good indication that your body has successfully adapted to the training program. This is not one of the goals you will be striving for, as it leads to no gains. This is the reason why our program changes on a consistent basis.

The third type of soreness is the one caused by injury. This soreness is entirely different in nature from the ones described above, as it is usually immobilizing and triggers very sharp pain within the muscles and/or joints. Depending on the nature of the injury, the pain might either be experienced constantly or only when the joints are moved or the muscles contract. These injuries often become apparent as soon as they happen. Other times they appear either the day after and even sometimes days after the activity. If you suddenly become injured, the first thing that you should do is apply the RICE principle (Rest, Ice, Compression and Elevation). After consulting a doctor, he/she might allow you to continue training, carefully working around the injury (in other words, utilizing exercises that work around the injured muscle(s), without over stepping the range of motion that triggers the pain). More serious injuries, such as a muscle tear, may involve complete rest of the injured and surrounding areas and, depending on the severity, possibly surgery. The best way to prevent this type of injury, pain and soreness, is by cycling your exercise parameters and by constantly practicing good form.

BREATHING WHILE PERFORMING AN EXERCISE

The correct way to breathe while performing an exercise is to exhale (breathe out) while you are forcing the weight up (the concentric phase or muscle contraction) and to inhale (breathe in) while you are lowering or releasing the weight (the eccentric phase or the negative portion of the exercise). For example, if you are doing a bench press, you exhale while you push the weight up away from your body and inhale while you lower the weight down towards your chest.

WARMING UP BEFORE TRAINING AND STRETCHING

People always ask us, "What is the best time for stretching?" Our answer is, the best time

---

FAQ:
I am concerned that I am not breathing correctly during exercise.

ANSWER:
The most important thing to do is just make sure you're breathing! Don't hold your breath. Lots of people (especially beginners) can quickly become overwhelmed with all of this new information to retain. Stop worrying so much about what

---

you're not doing right and just do the best you can. When it comes to breathing, your body has a wonderful ability to make sure you're breathing so you don't pass out.

When you are weight training, the rule is to exhale during the exertion and inhale during the descent. If you mess up here and there, just practice!

for stretching would be after your body temperature has increased and the blood has begun circulating within the muscles. This is achieved by performing exercise that raises your heart rate and circulates the blood at an increased rate. If you fail to adequately do this, you run the risk of tearing a muscle or causing bodily injury. Are you up for an experiment? Wet a rubber band with water and put it in the freezer. After two hours, take it out and try to stretch it to its limit. Pay attention and you will discover that the rubber band easily breaks. The same process can easily happen to your muscles if you stretch them without sufficiently warming them up. Having said that, before you begin the weight training workout, spend 15 minutes in warming up followed by light stretching.

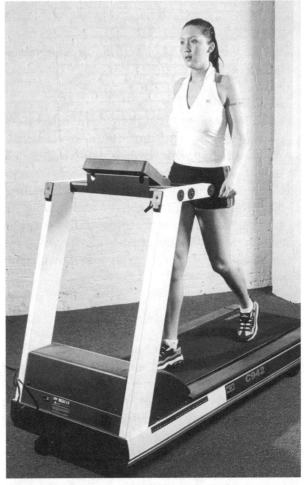

Before stretching, perform approximately six minutes worth of aerobic activity to get the blood flowing and to increase your body temperature.

FAQ:
I am getting a lot of mixed messages about stretching: do it, don't do it. What's the definitive answer?

ANSWER:
Stretching is great! There is just a time and place to do it. Stretching is essential to make sure your body is flexible and mobile. If you sit for long periods of time, you know how quickly you can become stiff and achy. Stretching allows the muscles, joints, and connective tissues to remain limber and mobile. Don't forget that weight training is itself a form of stretching. It's false that bodybuilders aren't flexible. We have seen lots of huge guys and girls do full Chinese splits!

It takes work to increase and maintain your flexibility. Just make sure that you are fully warmed up before stretching. You can stretch between sets or at the end of your workout.

SELECTING THE WEIGHT FOR EACH EXERCISE

The weight you select for each exercise depends on the amount of repetitions you need to do for a particular set. If you need to do between 10-12 repetitions for one set, pick a weight where you fail (the point at which completing another repetition becomes impossible) between 10-12 reps. This takes a bit of practice but after a while you will become extremely accurate when it comes to choosing the correct weight for a particular repetition range. If you pick a weight that allows you to do more than 12 repetitions, you'll need to increase the amount of weight being lifted. If you reach failure before hitting the tenth rep, you'll need to decrease the amount of weight being lifted. For example, if you were doing four sets of an exercise, as you continue to work through the sets, fatigue will set in and you may not be able to continue using the weight that you chose to lift during the first set. When you get to the point where you can no longer lift a particular weight for a pre-determined repetition range, simply decrease the weight and prepare yourself for the next set.

OVERTRAINING

Overtraining is a condition caused when the body is taxed beyond its ability to recover. The main causes may include long workouts, an overload of training volume (too many sets and reps), a bad diet lacking nutrients, lack of sleep, etc. People experiencing this condition might notice such symptoms as a loss of muscle mass, weakness, trouble sleeping, loss of appetite, a lethargic and constant tired feeling and feelings of depression.

It is impossible to overtrain with our weight training program (assuming you follow the nutrition and rest practices prescribed) because after you stress the body's recuperative capabilities to the maximum (by doing supersets for two weeks and then moving on to giant sets for two more), you back off into the less stressful modified compound supersets. In addition, you get a rest day after every day of lifting (unless you are using the advanced version) and you also get the weekends off. During rest days, you concentrate on fat burning aerobic exercise (which aids in the recuperation process by removing the lactic acid created by weight training) instead. We use Sunday as our total inactivity day; you can choose any day of the week as your rest day. This day serves to rest the body and the mind.

Finally, the ample nutrients provided by the diet, along with the recommended supplements, eliminate the possibility of getting overtrained.

Provided that you follow the training program as laid out, in conjunction with the nutrition and rest components, for the purposes of this book, overtraining is a state of mind and does not exist.

SKIPPING WORKOUTS

Skipping workouts is unacceptable. You hear it all the time, people constantly making excuses about how they have not time to exercise. Baloney! Unless you are in a situation where you are on call 24 hours a day and are being utilized at least 23 hours out of the 24, then we are more than sure that you can find the time to train. The fact of the matter is that some people don't want to spend the time exercising, so instead, they make excuses about how busy they are. We don't care if you only have 15 minutes to allocate towards exercise, it's still 15 minutes of exercise!

FAQ:
What is the best type of warm up? Would running on a treadmill suffice?

ANSWER:
Running on a treadmill would be enough for leg training, but it wouldn't warm up the upper body at all. The absolute best way to warm your muscles, joints, and connective tissue prior to weight training is to actively practice the exercise movement you will execute. In other words, if you are going to do heavy squats, your warm up should be doing a squat with your body weight only at high repetitions, or even a 45 pound Olympic bar for the same amount of reps. The key here is to warm up the muscles you are about to train, not to exhaust them. You don't want too much time doing reps with lots of weight. Listen to and feel your body as you warm up.

For example, if you were planning on doing three working sets of 10 repetitions using 225 pounds, your warm up sets might look something like this:

1st set: 45 pound bar, 5 reps

2nd set: 95 pounds (25 pound plates on each side of bar), 4 reps

3rd set: 135 pounds (45 pound plates on each side), 3 reps

4th set: 185 pounds (45 & 25 pound plates on each set), 2 reps

If you still feel a bit stiff, you could do one more set with the same weight and reps you used in the last warm-up set.

If you are interested in completely changing the way you look and feel, all the excuses in the world can not hold you back from doing what it takes to fit a workout into your schedule. All you need is the vision, the motivation and the determination to do so.

Skipping workouts will severely jeopardize your toning and fat burning efforts, in addition to destroying your body sculptor's mindset. However, if for some reason you are not able to train (let's say because all the gyms in the world are closed on that day, and you have no gym at home and don't know anyone with one),

then remember back to what your grandparents use to say, about how they had to walk over five miles just to get to work, in the snow, with no shoes or socks! In all seriousness, if you miss a workout one day, simply make up the skipped session the next day. This might mean training twice in one day (doing your cardio session in the morning and weights in the afternoon) or sacrificing your Sunday rest day.

If you miss a workout for whatever reason, don't beat yourself up about it. Just realize that tomorrow is a new day and you will be able to make up the skipped session. However, don't

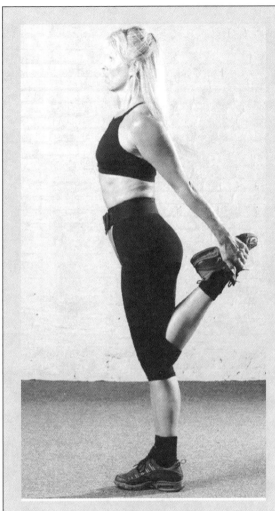

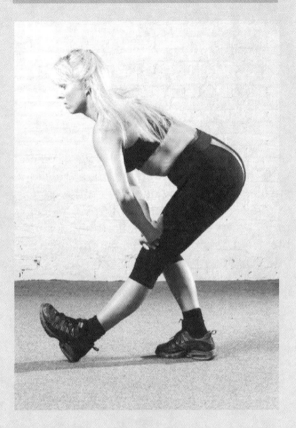

Stretch your **thighs** by grasping a pole with one arm and bending the opposite leg, bringing your foot towards your buttocks (if you grasp the pole with the left hand, then bend the right leg). Grasp your ankle with the free hand and slowly lift your foot as comfortably as possible. Hold this position for a count of five and repeat with the other leg.

Stretch your **hamstrings** by stepping forward with your left heel while bending your right knee. Keep your left leg straight and toe pointed up. Placing your hands on your left thigh, bend forward at the waist and feel the stretch in your hamstring. Hold this position for a count of five and repeat with the opposite leg.

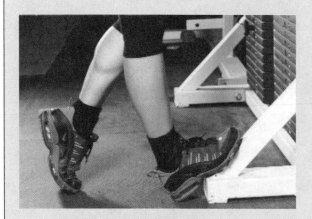

Stretch your **calves** by grasping a pole with both arms, standing on a raised surface, and placing one foot on the edge of the surface in order to allow your heel to go down as far as comfortably possible. Hold this position for a count of five and repeat with the other leg.

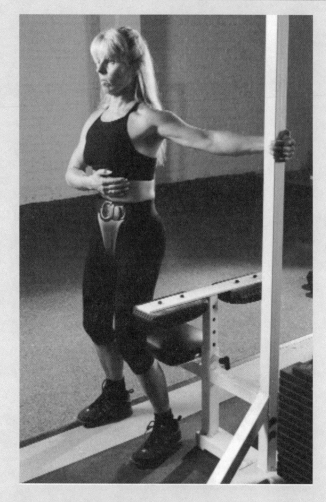

Stretch your **chest** by grasping a pole with one of your arms, ensuring that this arm is parallel to the ground. Slowly turn away from the pole and allow your arm to be as far behind the body as possible. Ensure that you do not overextend your chest by going as far away as is comfortably possible. Hold this position for a count of five and repeat with the other arm.

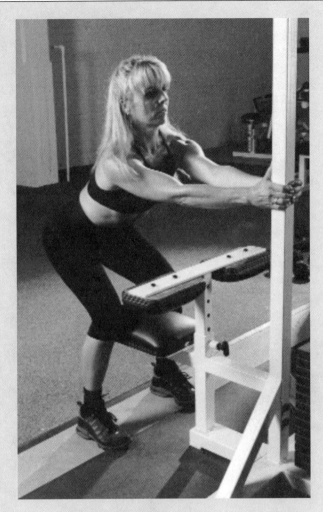

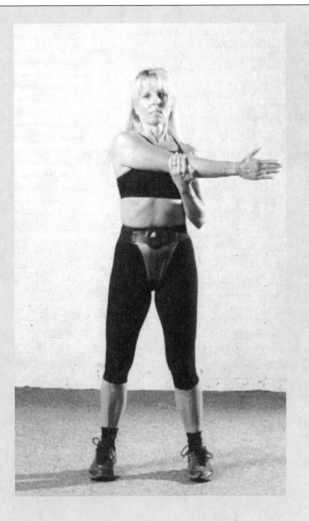

Stretch your **back** by grasping a pole with both arms, bending your knees, and sitting back in order to fully extend your arms and achieve a stretch in your lats and lower back. Hold this position for a count of five.

Stretch your **shoulders** by grasping one of your wrists with the opposite hand. Without moving your torso, begin to pull your arm as far as possible. Hold this position for a count of five and repeat with the other arm.

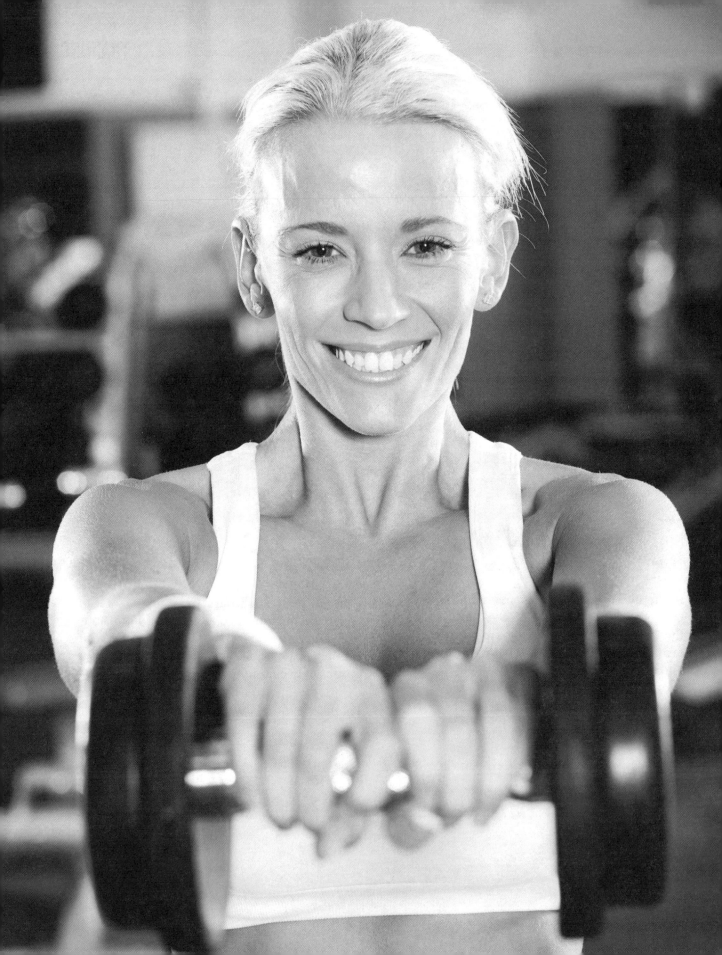

Chapter 4
Nutrition

For immediate Body Sculpting Bible support & coaching directly from James & Hugo, please visit www.BodySculptingBibles.com

4

THE **BODY** **SCULPTING** **BIBLE** FOR **WOMEN**

The second component of the formula for success is nutrition. Nutrition is what gives us the raw materials for recuperation, energy, and growth. Without a good diet, your dreams of achieving your ideal body will never be reached. Please pay close attention to the following sections.

If you truly wish to succeed and reach all of your body-sculpting goals quickly with no delays, then you must make sure to follow the nutritional guidelines. Too many people neglect to follow these guidelines and, because of that, never reach their goals of creating a beautiful physique. You could train like a maniac but if you fail to pay attention to your nutrition, you will fail.

Let's discuss the characteristics of a good nutritional program, beginning with the nutritional basics.

NUTRITION BASICS

There are three macronutrients that the human body needs in order to function properly:

CARBOHYDRATES

Carbohydrates are your body's main source of energy. When you ingest carbohydrates, your pancreas releases a hormone called insulin. In addition to regulating our blood sugar, insulin is very important because:

- It grabs on to the carbohydrates and either stores them in the muscle and liver for future use (this is called glycogen which is stored carbohydrates) or stores them as fat.

- It grabs on to the amino acids (protein) and shelters them inside the muscle cell for recovery and repair. This is called increasing protein synthesis.

- While the above is an oversimplification of the many actions of Insulin, for our purposes of discussion those are its main functions.

Most people who are overweight and are on low fat/high carbohydrate diets are in that condition because they eat an overabundance of carbohydrates. Too many carbohydrates cause your body to release huge amounts of insulin. When there is too much insulin in the body, your body naturally turns these excess carbohydrate calories into fat, thus creating a human fat storing machine. Therefore, it is important that we eat the right amount and types of carbs.

COMPLEX AND SIMPLE CARBOHYDRATES

Carbohydrates are divided into two categories: complex carbs and simple carbs.

The **complex carbohydrates** are hundreds of sugar units linked together in single molecules (reason they are called complex) and typically give you more sustained energy (provided they have a medium to low Glycemic Index (GI)) as they take more time to be broken down by the body. Note: Complex carbohydrates with a high GI behave more like a simple sugar, which is digested quickly.

There are two types of complex carbs, which you will be eating in small portions frequently throughout the day:

- **Starchy carbs** provide you with raw energy that your body can use. Good sources are oatmeal, grits, brown rice, lentils, sweet potatoes, and cream of wheat.

GLYCEMIC INDEX

In order to understand the proper carbs to consume, you must understand the details of the Glycemic Index. The Glycemic Index (or GI for short) is a measure of how quickly your blood sugar rises after ingesting a carbohydrate. Basically, once you consume a carbohydrate and it gets digested it gets turned to glucose (blood sugar). Blood sugar is used by the body to manufacture ATP (Adenosine Tri-Phosphate), which is the molecule that the body uses to power up all of its functions. You can think of ATP as your body's fuel, as without ATP, your organism would not be able to function.

The way that GI works is that each food is assigned a value, typically from 0-100, based on how fast blood sugar increases in the next two hours after consuming a carbohydrate. A value of 100 would represent a food that increases blood sugar very rapidly, such as a straight glucose drink. A value of 59, like the one from brown rice, means that the blood sugar response is moderate. Therefore, for the purposes of blood sugar control and fat loss, brown rice is a much better choice than a glucose drink.

That is because how quickly a carbohydrate is turned into glucose and released in the bloodstream affects the amount of insulin that the pancreas will release to control blood sugar levels. Too quick of a conversion and your insulin levels skyrocket, a bad situation if you are trying to lose body fat since fat loss cannot occur in the presence of high insulin levels. Such a hormonal environment triggers fat storage. Therefore, it stands to reason that if a carbohydrate is released slowly into the blood stream, then less insulin is released and fat loss is maximized.

So is controlling GI the main key to losing body fat? Yes and no. Understanding the effect of foods on your blood sugar is important as several studies have shown that eating low GI carbohydrates throughout the day suppresses appetite and provides more stable energy levels as blood sugar is better controlled (Note: sudden drops in blood sugar make you feel hungry and lethargic). In addition, eating low GI foods allows for more consumption of food without body fat storage and for a leaner you due to body fat loss.

What's a Low GI Food?

While there are many opinions out there on what a low GI food is, typically a food under 55 is considered low, a food under 70 is medium and anything over 70 is high. However, we must understand that what you eat in conjunction with your carbohydrates will affect your GI. Every time you eat a protein with a carbohydrate the total GI of the meal will go down since protein is a very complex molecule and thus slows down the digestion of the carb. Fats also have this effect. Since you will not be eating just a carbohydrate in the Body Sculpting Bible nutrition plan, then the raw GI number should only be used as a guideline. Besides, GI does not provide us with the whole answer as to which carbohydrate is best for us in order to lose fat.

What GI Does Not Take Into Account

An important reason why we cannot take GI as the only measure of whether a carbohydrate that we choose will help us lose fat or not is because GI does not take into account the different ways in which the body handles complex carbohydrates from starches like brown rice (or grains like oatmeal) vs. a simple carbohydrate like an apple.

- **Fibrous carbs** cannot be absorbed, but are rich in vitamins and minerals. In addition, fiber cleans up your intestines, which allows for better absorption of the nutrients that you get from digestible foods. Mixing fibrous sources with starchy sources lowers the rate of digestion of the starchy carbs, thus lowering their GI. Good sources are: asparagus, squash, broccoli, green beans, cabbage, cauliflower, celery, cucumber, mushrooms, lettuce, red or green peppers,tomato, spinach, and zucchini.

Simple carbohydrates are made up of one, two, or three units of sugar)at the most) linked together in single molecules, and thus, give you immediate energy as they are released more readily in the body. Good sources are: apples, pears, cantaloupes, oranges, cherries, strawberries, grapefruit, lemon, nectarines, peaches. Higher sugar fruits like grapes or bananas are best for after a workout if desired.

Though the glycemic index categorizes most fruits as low GI, as you will see, the simple sugar found in fruits called fructose is metabolized differently than the sugars from starches. To understand how the process differs, first let's see how the body uses glucose.

If blood glucose levels are low, the body uses the glucose it gets from foods and bums it immediately for energy. This is one of the reasons why after a workout, the body utilizes carbohydrates so efficiently. Now, assuming that there is no immediate need for energy, glucose is then converted into glycogen and stored in the liver or the muscles. The liver can hold roughly100 grams of glycogen but the muscles, depending on how muscular you are, may store between 200-400 grams. The key point to remember: The glycogen from muscles can only supply energy to the muscles when they are contracting (so muscle glycogen gets depleted badly during a weight training workout). Liver glycogen however, can supply energy to the entire body. It is key to remember this in order to understand how fructose does not help with fat loss.

The way that the body gets fat when there is an excess of carbohydrates is that if all of the glycogen stores in the body are full, then the extra glucose is converted to fat by the liver and stored as adipose tissue (bodyfat), probably around your waist.

Now that you understand how glucose is used and how fat can be stored in situations where all glycogen levels are full, lets go back to the fruits. What happens with fructose is that the muscles do not have the enzyme required to turn fructose into glycogen. The liver does, so fructose replenishes the liver. It does not take much to replenish a liver of glycogen as it can hold around 100 grams only. Therefore, if you overdo the fruits, you will fill up your liver glycogen and this causes the body to release an enzyme signaling the body that glycogen stores are full. Since the liver has to supply energy for the whole body, the body uses its glycogen stores as the fuel gauge. When the tank is full, so to speak, that is when any extra fuel gets stored away. Because of this, we suggest that fruits are limited and even eliminated If on an aggressive fat loss diet. By the way, if you are wondering why most fruits can be so low GI and still cause so much damage is because fructose leaves the liver as fat and fat does not raise insulin levels.

CARBOLHYDRATE CONSUMPTION RECOMMENDATIONS

It is recommended that you eat mainly medium (less than 65 GI) to low (less than 55 GI) glycemic complex carbs throughout the day, as they are responsible for creating consistent energy levels for peak performance and daily functions.

If you must eat fruits, minimize your consumption to two servings per day at times where some of your liver glycogen has been depleted. The best times are the morning with breakfast and right after a workout. This will help to speed up the recuperation time and aid in the production of lean muscle tissue. Ingesting simple carbs throughout the day is not recommended as if your liver glycogen is full, then you will risk storing body fat.

Now that we have covered all that there is to know regarding carbohydrates, let's talk about the major building blocks in the body, which are proteins.

PROTEIN

Every tissue in your body is made up of protein (i.e. muscle, hair, skin, and nails etc.). Proteins are the building blocks of lean muscle tissue. Without it, building muscle and burning fat efficiently would be impossible. Protein helps to increase your metabolism every time you eat it by 20% and it time-releases carbohydrates (glucose) by lowering their glycemic index, so you get sustained energy throughout the day.

During the 14-Day Body Sculpting Program, you should consume between 1-1.5 grams of protein per pound of lean body mass. (In other words, if you are 200 lbs and have 10% body fat, you should consume at least 180 grams of protein, since your lean body mass = 180 lbs.) Most people should not consume more than 1.5 grams per pound of lean body mass as this is unnecessary and the extra protein will be turned into glucose and used for energy, excreted out of the body, or provide excess calories that may get turned into fat. (Note: While protein itself is very unlikely to be stored as fat, a consistent caloric intake higher than

that required for your body to function will lead to an increase in body fat over time).

Good examples of protein include: salmon, lean ground turkey, founder, grouper, halibut, cod, round steak, chicken breast, tuna fish (spring water), turkey breast, whey protein, and egg substitutes.

All proteins are low in glycemic index and by combining a carbohydrate with a protein the combined glycemic index of the whole meal goes down as a result. The proteins included here were selected due to their low fat content and their digestibility.

Note: Avoid deli meats as they are high in sodium. If you are eating salmon, eliminate two servings of good fats.

FATS

All the cells in the body have some fat. Fats are responsible for lubricating your joints. In addition, hormones are manufactured from fats. If you eliminate the fats from your diet, your hormonal production will drop, and a whole array of chemical reactions will be interrupted. Your body will start accumulating more body fat than usual to keep functioning. Because your testosterone production is halted, so will the production of lean muscle mass. Therefore, in order to have an efficient metabolism, we need to consume a small amount of certain fats.

There are three types of fats: Saturated, polyunsaturated, and monounsaturated.

Saturated Fats are associated with heart disease and high cholesterol levels. They are found to a large extent in products of animal origin. However, some vegetable fats are altered in a way that increases the amount of saturated fats in them by a chemical process known as hydrogenation. Hydrogenated vegetable oils are generally found in packaged foods as they extend the shelf life of the food item. However, in return, these fats, when consumed, cause your body to be resistant to insulin (which in turn causes issues in controlling your blood sugar) and also increase your cholesterol dramatically.

Palm oil and palm kernel oil, which are also frequently used in packaged foods, and non-dairy creamers are highly saturated. These oils are also many times hydrogenated. If you read the ingredient label of an item and see that it says "partially hydrogenated (name of oil)", then immediately put that item back on the shelf. Consider partially hydrogenated oils poison to your body.

Polyunsaturated Fats make up most of the fats in vegetable oils, such as corn, cottonseed, safflower, soybean, and sunflower oil. Also, flaxseed oil and fish oils are polyunsaturated. These last two fats are usually high in the Omega 3 Essential Fatty Acids (EFAs). What are Omega 3 EFA's? Omega 3 EFAs are one of the two essential fats that the body needs. "Essential" means that the body cannot produce it on its own and therefore must be obtained from diet. The other kind of EFAs the body needs are the Omega-6 oils. Flax and fish oils are high on the Omega 3, which help improve immune system, energy production, insulin, sensitivity, and hormonal production. In addition, they have been shown to have antilipogenic properties (help prevent fat storage) as well as help to burn body fat, and assist in improving recovery by having anti-inflammatory properties and by protecting muscle from being broken down. Omega-6 oils are also beneficial to the body by reducing post training inflammation. These oils, however, are more easily found in most vegetable oils, butter, poultry and eggs so we don't see a need to supplement them further.

Monounsaturated Fats make a positive Sources of these fats are virgin olive oil and peanut oil. 20% of your calories should come from good fats. Any less than 20% and your hormonal production goes down. Any more than 20% and you start accumulating plenty of fat.

Good sources of fat are the natural fat from the egg yolk of organic eggs (good saturated fat), extra virgin coconut oil (good saturated fat), extra virgin olive oil (good monounsaturated fat), organic peanut butter (good monounsaturated fat), fish oils (good polyunsaturated fat) and flaxseed oil (good polyunsaturated fat).

WATER

Water is by far the most abundant substance in our body. Without water, an organism would not survive very long. Most people who come to us for advice on how to get in shape, almost always underestimate the great value of water.

Water is good for the following reasons:

- Over 65% of your body is composed of water (most of your muscle cells are composed of water).

- Water cleanses your body of toxins and pollutants that can make you sick.

- Water is needed for all of the complex chemical reactions that your body performs on a daily basis. Processes such as energy production, muscle building, and fat burning all require water. A lack of water would interrupt all of these processes.

- Water helps lubricate the joints for increased mobility and decreased joint pain.

- When the outside temperature increases, water serves as a coolant to lower body temperature to where it is supposed to be.

- Water helps control your appetite.

Have you ever felt like you were still hungry after eating a huge meal? This might very well be an indication that your body is beginning to dehydrate. You will notice that by drinking water at that time, your cravings will miraculously stop.

- Cold water increases your metabolism and aids in the breakdown of body fat.

In order to determine how much water your body needs each day, multiply your lean body weight by 0.66. This indicates how many ounces of water your body needs in a day for optimum function.

CHARACTERISTICS OF A GOOD NUTRITION PROGRAM

Now that we have discussed the main nutrients that your body needs day in and day out to function, let's discuss what makes up a good nutrition program.

Nutrition Chart and Glycemic Index

STARCHY CARBOHYDRATES			
Eat with all 5-6 meals throughout the day. Around 25-27 grams of carbohydrates per serving. 1 serving per meal.			
FOOD ITEM	**SERVING SIZE (MEASURE DRY)**	**GLYCEMIC INDEX**	**DESIRABLE**
Old Fashioned Oats	1/2 cup dry	Low	Highly
Cream of Rice	1/4 cup dry	High	Good After Workout Only
Cream of Wheat	4 tablespoons dry	Medium	Good
Baked Potatoes	4 ounces cooked	Medium	Good
Sweet Potatoes	4 ounces cooked	Medium	Good
Rice (Brown Whole Grain)	1/2 cup cooked	Medium	Good
White Rice	1/2 cup cooked	High	Good After Workout Only
Spaghetti	4 oz cooked	Low	Good in GI but too many carbs for a small serving.
Whole wheat flour bread	2 slices	High	Not a great choice but okay in moderation.
Corn	3/4 cup	Medium	Good
Peas	1 cup	Medium	Good
Low GI=1-55 Medium GI=56-69 High GI=70-100			

SIMPLE CARBOHYDRATES

If you must, eat 1 serving with Breakfast and 1 after workout as even though they are low to medium in GI, too many simple sugars from fruits in the diet throughout the day can prevent fat loss. If your post workout meal is breakfast, then just consume 1 serving per day of fruits.

Around 10 grams of carbohydrates per serving. If breakfast is the post workout meal: 1 serving per day with post workout meal. If post workout meal is not breakfast: 1 serving with breakfast and 1 serving with post workout meal.

FOOD ITEM	SERVING SIZE	GLYCEMIC INDEX	DESIRABLE
Apples	1/2	Low	Good
Oranges	1/2	Low	Good
Grapefruit	1/2	Low	Good
Cherries	7	Low	Good
Pears	1/3	Low	Good
Bananas	1/3	Medium	After Workout Only
Lemons	1	Low	Good
Cantaloupe	1/4 melon	High	After Workout Only
Strawberries	1 cup	1 cup	Good
Apricots	3	Medium	After Workout Only
Grapes	1/2 cup	Low	Good
Mango	1/3 cup	Medium	After Workout Only
Papaya	1/2 cup	Medium	After Workout Only

Low GI=1-55 Medium GI=56-69 High GI=70-100

FIBROUS CARBOHYDRATES

Eat at least 1 serving with lunch and 1 serving with dinner though more can be consumed if desired; consider these free foods as they do not get absorbed.

Around 10 grams of carbohydrates per serving. At least 1 serving at lunch and 1 serving at dinner.

FOOD ITEM	SERVING SIZE (MEASURE COOKED)	GLYCEMIC INDEX	DESIRABLE
Broccoli	1 cup	Low	Good
Green Beans	1 cup	Low	Good
Asparagus	12 spears or 1 cup	Low	Good
Lettuce	1 head raw	Low	Good
Tomatoes	2 cups chopped	Low	Good
Green Peppers (chopped)	1-1/2 cups raw	Low	Good
Onions	1/2 cup	Low	Good
Mushrooms	1 cup	Low	Good
Cucumber sliced	3 cups	Low	Good
Cauliflower	2 cups	Low	Good
Spinach	4 cups	Low	Good
Cabbage	2 cups	Low	Good
Carrots	1/2 cup sliced	High	After Workout
Low GI=1-55 Medium GI=56-69 High GI=70-100			

PROTEINS

FOOD ITEM	SERVING SIZE (MEASURE COOKED)	GLYCEMIC INDEX	DESIRABLE
Chicken breast (skinless)	3 ounces	Low	Good
Turkey	3 ounces	Low	Good
Veal	3 ounces	Low	Good
Top Sirloin	3 ounces	Low	Good
Tuna	3 ounces	Low	Good
Wild Alaskan Salmon	3 ounces	Low	Good
Egg Whites (in carton)	1 cup	Low	Good
Whey Protein	1 scoop	Low	Good
Orange Roughy	3 ounces	Low	Good

GOOD FATS

Around 5 grams of fats per serving. 1 serving at lunch, dinner, and any other meal except post workout meal.

FOOD ITEM	SERVING SIZE	GLYCEMIC INDEX	DESIRABLE
Fish Oils	1 teaspoon	Low	Good
Flax Oils	1 teaspoon	Low	Good
Extra Virgin Olive Oil	1 teaspoon	Low	Good
Natural Peanut Butter	2 teaspoons	Low	Good

All fats are low in glycemic index and by combining a carbohydrate with a protein the combined glycemic index of the whole meal goes down. The fats included here were selected due to their high essential fatty acids content and their health properties.

NOTES: Avoid cooking with flax oil as the heat degrades the oil. Bake and broil instead of frying. Also, if eating salmon, eliminate 2 servings of good fats as salmon is high on EFAs.

The complete list of the glycemic index and glycemic load for 750 foods can be found in the article "International tables of glycemic index and glycemic load values: 2002," by Kaye Foster-Powell, Susanna H.A. Holt, and Janette C. Brand-Miller in the July 2002 American Journal of Clinical Nutrition, Vol. 62, pages 5–56. <http://www.ajcn.org/cgi/content/full/76/1/5>

Your nutrition plan should be based on eating small and frequent meals throughout the day. Why? Because when you feed your body several times a day, your metabolism greatly increases. In addition, whenever three hours go by without any food consumption, your body switches to a catabolic state (a state in which your body starts burning muscle for energy!). The body actually believes that it is starving and in an attempt to protect itself from starvation, begins to feed itself by cannibalizing on your lean muscle tissue! It also lowers its metabolic rate (rate at which the body burns calories) and begins to store ingested calories as fat for future use. Bad scenario to be catabolic! The diet industry has made us think that the key to losing fat requires an extreme restriction of calories. You can see how much this theory has worked as America continues to gain weight!

Another reason to eat frequent meals is to manage blood sugar, insulin management, and energy levels. Larger infrequent feedings result in larger releases of insulin, with blood sugar crashes resulting in low energy levels 30 minutes to an hour after the meal is eaten. In addition, whatever calories the body cannot use at that time are stored for future use as body fat. Also, when you fall into the state of low blood sugar, you get lethargic and may start to crave sweets. Smaller, more frequent feedings spike the metabolism and maintain a more stable blood sugar pattern that results in better utilization of nutrients, more stable energy, and reduced cravings (or even no cravings) throughout the day.

During the 14-Day Body Sculpting Program, you will be eating four to five meals a day or five to six if you are following The Advanced 14- Day Body Sculpting Program) at two and a half to three-hour intervals.

Your meals should contain carbohydrates, protein and fats in the correct ratios. When you eat a meal that does not make up the proper balance of nutrients (for example an all carbohydrate meal; such as a pasta meal), you will not yield the desired results. Every macronutrient has to be present for the body to absorb them and use them properly and efficiently. Without boring you with the effect of food on the body's biochemistry, let's just say that if you solely eat carbohydrates as a meal, your energy levels will crash in about 30 minutes, and your body will store any carbs that were not used as body fat. Conversely, if you only eat protein all the time, you will lack the energy. Therefore, by eating a meal with one serving of starchy carbohydrates, a serving of fibrous carbohydrates and a serving of protein, you will have most of the macronutrients that your body needs. Once you add a tablespoon of either extra virgin olive oil or flaxseed oil to one of your vegetable servings of the day, then you have covered all of your macronutrient requirements.

No smoking and limited alcohol consumption. Both offer health problems which are not in line with what you are trying to accomplish. Alcohol in particular adds seven empty calories per gram to your diet, which is not a good situation when you are trying to control your caloric intake.

Increase your intake of protein. Proteins are the building blocks of all living organisms. If you are trying to build a structure such as the Empire State Building any construction contractor will tell you that they will need way more raw material to build such a large structure than to build a regular house. The same thing happens with body sculpting. Several researchers have discovered that the protein needs of people engaged in weight training activities exceed those of sedentary people. While most researchers are still debating on the amount, most of us in the field agree that 1-1.5 grams of protein per pound of lean body mass is just about right for any hard training. "Now what about kidney damage?" some may ask. Well, according to research conducted in the year 2000 called, "Do Regular High Protein Diets Have Potential Health Risks on Kidney Function in Athletes?" published in the International Journal of Sports Nutrition (Jacques R. Poortmans and Oliver Dellalieux. *International Journal of Sports Nutrition*, 2000, 10), higher protein intakes do not pose a threat to healthy kidney function. Having said that, the same is not true if you already suffer from a kidney condition.

Reduce your intake of bad fats and bring on the good fats. Bad fats are things like butter, cooking oils, and saturated fats such as the ones found in meats. However, ensure adequate intake of good fats such as flaxseed oil, extra virgin olive oil and natural peanut butter. One tablespoon of flaxseed oil a day covers all of the essential fatty acid requirements of most people.

Reduce your intake of sugars. Foods laden with sugar cause a sharp rise in insulin levels. Insulin is a good hormone when it is not present in excess as it carries the amino acids from the protein into the muscle cells so that they can be used for growth and repair. It also carries carbohydrates into the liver and muscle cells for storage as glycogen (stored carbohydrates) that can be used for future occasions. However, in excess, once the body's reserves of carbohydrate storage are full, insulin turns these carbs into fat!

In addition, the excess insulin production will also take the carbs away from the blood stream too quickly creating a situation of low blood sugar. In this case you feel tired, groggy, and usually crave sweets. It is a vicious cycle that guarantees fat gain and possibly insulin resistance and diabetes later on. So this means that you need to eliminate all sorts of junk food from your diet. That alone will cause you to eliminate empty calories that are not used by the body and are turned into fat. Also, foods that are high in sugars and fats are the worst as when both these macronutrients are present it is extremely easy for insulin to carry triglycerides (fats) into the adipose tissue stores (fat cells). Also, regular sodas are out as well as fruit juices. Fruit juices you say? Yes. Most fruit juices are really high in sugars typically in the order of 30-40 grams per eight - ounce servings! In addition, do you know that three eight-ounce glasses of orange juice are enough to fill up your glycogen stores? Remember that once liver glycogen is full, any extra blood sugar gets stored in places that won't make you look great in a bathing suit.

If you are interested in gaining muscle, have the correct post workout nutrition meal. The most important meal is the post workout meal. This meal should consist of a high glycemic complex carb and preferably some sort of fast released liquid protein such as Whey Isolate. Surprised? Well, only after a workout it is beneficial to have a large release of insulin as in this manner glycogen levels get replenished quicker, and repair and growth occur. If you cannot do away with fruits, this is the time to have a serving of simple carbs as well. There are many post workout preparations that are effective as long as there is minimum fat and fiber in the meal as both fats and fiber reduce the speed at which the food is released. A good example of a post workout meal is cream of rice with whey protein isolate. cream of rice has a high glycemic index that it makes it perfect to create the high insulin environment needed for glycogen replenishment after a workout. A trick that we learned from Mr. Central Florida Todd Mendelsohn (from www.musclebuildingdiet.com) is that you can have a serving and a half of cream of rice

(1/4 cup uncooked) mixed with whey protein isolate (a very fast released protein) as the ideal meal after a workout. It will replenish all glycogen stores immediately as well as provide the body with amino acids that it needs. By replenishing glycogen store and providing the body with the amino acids that it needs at this crucial time you accelerate your body sculpting results tenfold!

DESIGINING YOUR BODY SCULPTING DIET

Now that we have discussed what foods to eat and in which amount, we can move on and design our diet. However, we realize that not everyone is at the same level. Some of you may already be following a program that is close enough to what we recommend here while others find this information to be completely new to them. Because of that, we have created three levels from which to start.

If you are completely new to this please choose the Break-In Body Sculpting Diet Plan. By slowly changing your diet in this manner, you will not find the changes so overwhelming. If you already follow a set diet and you just need to fine tune it, then just go straight to the Body Sculpting Diet Plan. If you have been following a great diet for a while, already look great and want to take it to another level, such as the look of a fitness or figure competitor, then follow the Advanced Body Sculpting Diet Plan. Please keep in mind that the Advanced Body Sculpting Diet Plan is more restrictive as it is designed with the goal of achieving an incredible level of fitness and leanness.

BREAK-IN BODY SCULPTING DIET PLAN

Usually people associate diets with starvation plans or days of agony and pain. However that is not the correct definition of a diet. The word diet refers to the food choices that we make on a daily basis. In this book, we are going to teach you a program that you will be able to use for the rest of your life to help keep you in tip-top shape. The reason our diet works is because of our food choices, the timing of meals and the back and forth switching in caloric intake. We don't expect you to change overnight. As a matter of fact, this is the reason why we feel that 99 percent of dieters fail. Our goal is to have you succeed just as we did. While it is possible for some people to make drastic changes in a small amount of time, we realize that most people do better by making incremental and progressive changes that will eventually get them to reach their desired goals. That is the way that we are going to teach you to change your "diet." Small incremental steps with huge rewards!

BABY STEPS, GIANT RESULTS: THE NO-PAIN, ALL-GAIN PLAN TO A PERFECT DIET

In keeping with our 14-day philosophy, we will make incremental changes to your diet every two weeks. Remember that this is how long it takes to create a new pattern as well as how long it takes the body to get used to something new. Every 14 days we are going to set a goal. Each goal will build upon the success of the previous one. It is imperative that you use your determination and all of the Chapter three techniques in order to ensure the success of the program. By achieving a new goal every two weeks, you will end up with the diet that will yield the consistent fat loss/muscle toning results that you are looking for. In other words, you will end up with the exact same diet that we discussed in the sections above!

(Weeks 1-2) Cut the fat.
For the first two weeks we just want you to start looking at the labels of food that you consume and try to start cutting out as many fats

as possible. Make some instant changes in your current routine, for example:

If you fry things, start steaming or broiling as a healthy alternative.

If you use salad dressing with a high-fat content, substitute them for low-fat or non-fat choices.

Select lower fat choices for meats. For instance, if you consume corned beef, substitute skinless chicken or turkey instead. If you consume chicken with the skin, start removing the skin (this has the most fat). If you like red meats, then buy the lean cuts.

Your taste buds will get used to your new low fat eating habits in the two-week period..

(Weeks 3-4) Eliminate refined sugars.

Now it's time to eliminate the refined sugars from your diet. Where are the refined sugars? They are everywhere! Therefore, in order to accomplish this goal, do the following:

- Eliminate regular sodas because they contain large amounts of sugars. Instead drink diet sodas (however, they contain Aspartame, and some research indicates that high consumption of Aspartame may cause cancer and many, many other potentially serious side effects in the long term. It may be a good idea to switch to a non-carbonated beverage).

- Eliminate the use of table sugars.

- Eliminate the consumption of sweets (except on the day that you have your cheat meal).

(Weeks 5-6) Incorporate an abundant amount of water.

Start drinking much more water than you have previously consumed. We have already explained the reasons for consuming water. In order to accomplish this goal do the following:

Substitute water for all types of drinks (including diet sodas and fruit juices, even if they claim to be natural). natural). Every time you get thirsty, drink water.

Drink at least an eight ounce glass of water with every meal.

Drink approximately 16 ounces or more of water during your workout.

(Weeks 7-8) Caloric intake control and macronutrient management.

During these next two weeks, we will get closer than ever to the ideal diet. The good news is that after these two weeks, dieting will cease to get more complicated and you will continue to see some truly unbelievable results.

In order to jump on the fast track for results, without hesitating, do the following:

Start following the Low Calorie Diet prescribed in the Body Sculpting Diet Plan section.

Write down everything that you eat, along with the serving size.

Use the tables found in the Choosing What to Eat section (or Appendix B) in order to select your foods and know what your serving sizes look like.

For instructions on how to proceed after week eight, read the Caloric Cycling section presented in the Body Sculpting Diet Plan section.

WEEKS 1-2: CALORIES:LOW (Approximately 1200 calories)

Around 120 grams of carbohydrates (mostly complex with simple carbs being saved for after the workout)

Around 120 grams of protein

Around 26 grams of fats

MEAL #1 (7:30 AM) BREAKFAST (POST-WORKOUT)

Choose 1 serving of Proteins
Choose 1 serving of Starchy Carbs
Optionally, you may choose to add 1 serving of Simple Carbs in the form of Fruit, if you can't live without them.

MEAL #2 (10:30 AM) MORNING BREAK SNACK

Choose 1 serving of Proteins
Choose 1 serving of Starchy Carbs
Choose 1 serving of Good Fats

MEAL #3 (1:30 PM) LUNCH TIME

Choose 1 serving of Proteins
Choose 1 serving of Starchy Carbs
Choose 1 serving of Fibrous Carbs
Choose 1 serving of Good Fats

MEAL #4 (3:30 PM) AFTERNOON BREAK SNACK

Choose 1 serving of Proteins
Choose 1 serving of Starchy Carbs

MEAL #5 (6:30 PM) DINNER

Choose 1 serving of Proteins
Choose 1/2 serving of Starchy Carbs
Choose 1 serving of Fibrous Carbs
Choose 1 serving of Good Fats

WEEKS 3-4 CALORIES: HIGH (Approximately 1500 calories)

150 grams of carbohydrates (mostly complex with simple carbs being saved for after the workout)

150 grams of protein

33 grams of fats

MEAL #1 (7:30 AM) BREAKFAST (POST-WORKOUT)

Choose 1 serving of Proteins
Choose 1 serving of Starchy Carbs
Optionally, you may choose to add 1 serving of Simple Carbs in the form of Fruit, if you can't live without them.

MEAL #2 (10:30 AM) MORNING BREAK SNACK

Choose 1 serving of Proteins
Choose 1 serving of Starchy Carbs

MEAL #3 (1:30 PM) LUNCH TIME

Choose 1 serving of Proteins
Choose 1 serving of Starchy Carbs
Choose 1 serving of Fibrous Carbs
Choose 1 serving of Good Fats

MEAL #4 (3:30 PM) AFTERNOON BREAK SNACK

Choose 1 serving of Proteins
Choose 1 serving of Starchy Carbs

MEAL #5 (6:30 PM) DINNER

Choose 1 serving of Proteins
Choose 1/2 serving of Starchy Carbs
Choose 1 serving of Fibrous Carbs
Choose 1 serving of Good Fats

MEAL #6 (8:30 PM) LATE SNACK

Choose 1 serving of Proteins
Choose 1/2 serving of Starchy Carbs
Choose 1 serving of Fibrous Carbs
Choose 1 serving of Good Fats

THE 14-DAY BODY SCULPTING DIET PLAN

CALORIC CYCLING

Congratulations for making it this far, ladies!. By now, between the training and the diet you have seen some extremely favorable changes in the way that you look and feel. Great! Now we will give you the secret for creating even more powerful and consistent results. The secret is caloric cycling. By incorporating the following cycling principles in your diet, you ensure that you'll never reach the nasty fat loss plateaus that most dieters encounter.

In the training section we discussed how the body will quickly adapt to an exercise program and stop responding to the routine. When this happens, your results cease and your efforts are simply wasted. The same principle applies to your diet.

In order to keep your metabolism efficiently burning body fat and building your body, caloric cycling will play an essential role in the program. As a matter of fact, recent research points to the fact that you can lose faster (up to twice as fast) by cycling your calories than by not cycling them.

Here's how to cycle calories:

If you have been on the Break-In Plan, follow the High Calorie Diet found on page 78 for the next two weeks.

Go back to the Low Calorie Diet found on page 78 for the following two weeks.

Alternate every two weeks in this manner for fantastic results.

Continue writing down everything that you eat as well as the serving sizes in order to ensure that you don't go over the allotted macronutrient intake per meal.

Presented below is the 14-Day Body Sculpting Diet Plan. For the first two weeks you will follow the Low Calorie Diet and for the next two weeks you will follow the High Calorie Diet.

STRIVE FOR CONSISTENCY, NOT PERFECTION

Many times we see dieters start out doing great. However, there comes a day that for some reason or another they lose a workout or they blow their diets. After that day, they become so discouraged that they continue missing workouts or destroying their diets with self-sabotage. Many weeks go by before they get back on track (if ever). In the meantime, muscle size fades, and the fat pounds pile up. Please remember the following: We are all human, and we are entitled to make mistakes. Always strive for perfection, but if for some reason things don't go as well as they should on a given day pick up and then move on. Forget about it and jump right back into your program. If you blow a meal one day, don't make it any worse by eating incorrectly all day long. If you miss a workout, don't wait until next Monday to start over. Just continue with your program the way it is laid out. Pick up from where you left off! In the end your determination and consistency will enable you to win the battle of the bulge.

TROUBLESHOOTING YOUR CALORIC INTAKE

The optimum fat loss per week is two pounds. Any more than two pounds per week and you will lose muscle, which will result in the loss of muscle tone, which in turn yields a saggy look and a significantly lower metabolism. Having said that, we need to point out the fact that while most women burn from 1200 to 1500 calories some have a higher than usual metabolism. Therefore, some women may find themselves losing more than two pounds a week at the prescribed number of calories and others may find themselves gaining weight. If this is the case, don't panic! If you find you are losing too much, simply add one serving of carbs, one serving of proteins, and one serving of good fats to your diet (both on low and high calorie weeks). In this manner, your diet will fluctuate between 1450 and 1750 calories. After two weeks you should assess how this is working by measuring your lean body mass. If you are still losing too much weight after two weeks, again increase your food intake by an additional serving of carbs, proteins and fats. Repeat the process until you reach the caloric intake that allows for two-pound fat loss while at the same time adds muscle tone/size.

The reverse applies if you are suddenly gaining weight. If you are gaining, cut your calories by 1/2 serving of just carbs and proteins for both the lower calorie diet and the higher calorie diet. You'll notice that we did not cut the calories by quite as much (since we cut no good fats), as your metabolism might only need a 200 calorie deficit. If you find that you are still gaining, even after the 200 calorie cut, you may than decrease your calories by the additional 200 calories. Don't jump the gun, though. Give your body the two-week opportunity to adjust before decreasing your calories.

CAUTION

The diet plans in this book are designed for women with sedentary lifestyles. If you are into marathon running or any sort of high endurance sport, then you may need to double or even triple the amount of carbohydrates that are prescribed in this program.

STARCHY CARBOHYDRATES APPROVED LIST

Around 25-27 grams of carbohydrates per serving. Amount of servings depends on whether it is a low, medium or high carbohydrate day.

FOOD ITEM	SERVING SIZE (MEASURE DRY)	GLYCEMIC INDEX	DESIRABLE
Old Fashioned Oats	1/2 cup dry	Low	Highly
Cream of Rice	1/4 cup dry	High	Good After Workout Only
Cream of Wheat	4 tablespoons dry	Medium	Good
Baked Potatoes	8 ounces cooked	Medium	Good
Sweet Potatoes	8 ounces cooked	Medium	Good
Rice (Brown Whole Grain)	1/2 cup cooked	Medium	Good

PROTEINS

Eat with all 6-8 meals throughout the day. Around 28-30 grams of protein per serving. 1 serving per meal.

FOOD ITEM	SERVING SIZE (MEASURE COOKED)	GLYCEMIC INDEX	DESIRABLE
Chicken breast (skinless)	4 ounces	Low	Good
Turkey	4 ounces	Low	Good
Veal	4 ounces	Low	Good
Top Sirloin	4 ounces	Low	Good
Tuna	4 ounces	Low	Good
Wild Alaskan Salmon	4 ounces	Low	Good
Egg Whites (in carton)	1-1/4 cup	Low	Good
Whey Protein	1-1/4 scoop	Low	Good
Orange Roughy	4 ounces	Low	Good

WEEKS 1-2: CALORIES: MEDIUM (Approximately 2200 calories)

MEAL #1 (8:30 AM)
Carbs 54 grams; Protein 45 grams; Fats 17 grams

1 cup egg substitute	160 calories
1 cup of dry oats	300 calories
1 tablespoon Flaxseed Oil	130 calories

MEAL #2 (10:30 AM)
Carbs 20 grams; Protein 20 grams; Fats 4 grams

Protein Drink	195 calories

MEAL #3 (12:30 PM)
Carbs 50 grams; Protein 48 grams; Fats 8 grams

8 ounces chicken (weighed prior to cooking)	120 calories
1 cup salad	80 calories
(lettuce, tomato, carrot, cucumber, green peppers, etc.)	
10 oz baked potato	200 calories

MEAL #4 (2:30 PM)
Carbs 20 grams; Protein 20 grams; Fats 4 grams

Protein Drink	195 calories

MEAL #5 (4:30 PM)
Carbs 45 grams; Protein 48 grams; Fats 5 grams

(Pre-Workout Meal; to be eaten at least two hours before the workout)

8 oz Chicken, turkey breast or tuna	240 calories
(weighed prior to cooking)	
1 cup brown rice	180 calories

6:30-7:30 PM WEIGHT TRAINING WORKOUT

MEAL #6 (7:30 PM)
Carbs 42 grams; Protein 50 grams; Fats 0 grams
(Bring this meal to gym)

50 grams of protein from whey isolate product	200 calories
7 tablespoons of cream of rice	175 calories

DAILY TOTALS
Calories: 2175; **Carbohydrates:** 231 grams;
Protein: 231 grams; **Fats:** 38 grams

WEEKS 3-4 CALORIES: HIGH (Approximately 2700 calories)

MEAL #1 (8:30 AM)
Carbs 81 grams; Protein 50 grams; Fats 20 grams

1 cup egg substitute	160 calories
1.5 cup of dry oats	450 calories
1 tablespoon Flaxseed Oil	130 calories

MEAL #2 (10:30 AM)
Carbs 20 grams; Protein 20 grams; Fats 4 grams

Protein Drink	195 calories

MEAL #3 (12:30 PM)
Carbs 50 grams; Protein 48 grams; Fats 8 grams

8 ounces chicken (weighed prior to cooking)	120 calories
1 cup salad	80 calories
(lettuce, tomato, carrot, cucumber, green peppers, etc.)	
10 oz baked potato	200 calories

MEAL #4 (2:30 PM)
Carbs 20 grams; Protein 20 grams; Fats 4 grams

Protein Drink: 1 serving Lean Mass Matrix	195 calories

MEAL #5 (4:30 PM)
Carbs 48 grams; Protein 48 grams; Fats 5 grams

(Pre-Workout Meal; to be eaten at least two hours before the workout)

8 oz chicken, turkey breast or tuna	240 calories
(weighed prior to cooking)	
8 oz sweet potatoes	200 calories

6:30-7:30 PM WEIGHT TRAINING WORKOUT

MEAL #6 (7:30 PM)
Carbs 42 grams; Protein 50 grams; Fats 0 grams
(Bring this meal to gym)

50 grams of protein from whey isolate product	200 calories
7 Tablespoons of cream of rice -	175 calories

MEAL #7 (9:30 PM)
Carbs 18 grams; Protein 40 grams; Fats 5 grams

Protein Drink	390 calories

DAILY TOTALS
Calories: 2735; **Carbohydrates:** 301 grams;
Protein: 276 grams; **Fats:** 49 grams

GOOD FATS
Around 5 grams of fats per serving. 1 serving in breakfast, lunch and dinner.

FOOD ITEM	SERVING SIZE	GLYCEMIC INDEX	DESIRABLE
Fish Oils	1 teaspoons	Low	Good
Flax Oils	1 teaspoons	Low	Good
Extra Virgin Olive Oil	1 teaspoons	Low	Good
Natural Peanut Butter	2 teaspoons	Low	Good

BODYWEIGHT CHARTS
If all of the math above is making you dizzy, no need to worry as the table below provides you with all of the macronutrient requirements that you need depending on your LBM and also on whether you are doing a Low, Medium or High Carbohydrate Day.

	Carbs (g)			Protein (g)	Fats (g)
LBM	LOW DAY	MEDIUM DAY	HIGH DAY		
70	35	62	105	105	21
75	38	66	113	113	23
80	40	70	120	120	24
85	43	75	128	128	26
90	45	79	135	135	27
95	48	84	143	143	29
100	50	88	150	150	30
105	53	92	158	158	32
110	55	97	165	165	33
115	58	101	173	173	35
120	60	106	180	180	36
125	63	110	188	188	38
130	65	114	195	195	39
135	68	119	203	203	41
140	70	123	210	210	42
145	73	128	218	218	44
150	75	132	225	225	45
155	78	136	233	233	47
160	80	141	240	240	48
165	83	145	248	248	50
170	85	150	255	255	51

ADVANCED BODY SCULPTING DIET PLAN

Some of you girls want to attain an extreme level of fitness; a level achieved by only a handful of women that choose to take the Body Sculpting Lifestyle to the next level.

If you fall in this category and want to look like a competitive figure or fitness athlete, then this section is for you. Be warned however that in order to achieve such look, an extreme amount of discipline is required. You have to keep In mind that the more extreme you want to look, the more disciplined and restrictive you need to be about your nutrition. You will also have to spend more time in the gym as well, following a routine like the Advanced Body Sculpting Workout where you do weights and cardio for 6 days a week.

If this still appeals to you, then the diet strategy provided in tills section is just right for you and will provide you with the desired results.

CARBOHYDRATE CYCLING FOR EXTREME BODY SCULPTING

The key to convincing the body to go extremely low in body fat is to deprive it of carbohydrates temporarily. In this manner, your body has to use more fat than usual in order to meet its energy needs. Now, we are not talking about a zero carbohydrate diet or anything along those lines. We are talking instead of creating a state of moderate carbohydrate depravation followed by a state of moderate carbohydrate loading in order to prevent the metabolism from adjusting downwards (as if you did low carbs all of the time the body would adapt by lowering its metabolism to prevent further fat burning). So if you compared your glycogen stores (stored carbohydrates in the liver and muscles) against the gas tank of a car, you would want to run with the tank in medium at all times.

How is this accomplished? By having a low carbohydrate day followed by a medium carbohydrate day and then followed by a high carbohydrate day.

> **Day 1: Low Day**
> **Day 2: Medium Day**
> **Day 3: High Day**
> **Day 4: Start Over At Day 1**

How to Determine Your Low, Medium, High Carbohydrate Days

In order to determine how many carbohydrates you will need on any given day, you'll need to know what your lean body mass is.

Lean Body Mass (LBM) = (Total Weight - Fat Weight)

You can calculate your fat weight by using a pair of skin fold calipers on yourself (such as the Accu-Measure) or by having a trainer at your health club (if you are a member at one) check it for you. As an alternative, go to Appendix F: Tracking your Progress, where we present some formulas that you can use.

Once you have your LBM, you can use the formulas below to figure out the carbohydrate-grams you need per day.

> **Low Carbohydrate Day = LBM x 0.5**
> **Medium Carbohydrate Day = LBM x 0.88**
> **High Carbohydrate Day = LBM x 1.5**

The carbohydrate sources you will be choosing from will be mostly low to medium glycemic starchy ones (except for the cream of rice after a workout which is high glycemic) as these sources work best for insulin release control, loading muscle glycogen, and energy purposes. For best results, stick to the carbohydrate choices presented in the Approved List.

EATING ON THE RUN: FAST FOODS

In today's times, the fast paced living of our society can really tax our abilities to plan and prepare. This preparation certainly includes the scheduling of food consumption. If for one reason or another, our time constraints don't allow us to take the time to prepare all of the food we need for the day, or if we simply run out of food, there is a solution. You can go to fast food restaurants. Now, aren't fast foods bad if you are trying to get in shape? Well, the answer is "no" as long as you choose wisely.

The rules for eating in fast food restaurants (or any other type of restaurant) are:

- If it is not your cheat day (see The Sunday Reward section), refrain from fatty choices such as French fries.

- Drink between 8-16 ounces of water before you get to the restaurant and then drink an additional 8-16 ounces while you eat. This will prevent you from feeling hungry and falling to temptation. If you find that temptation is strong remember two things:

    a) There is nothing better than being in shape.

    b) You control everything that goes into your mouth. Food does not and should not control you!

- Always combine a serving of low fat protein (in the case of fast food restaurants, this is either skinless chicken or turkey) with a small serving of carbs. Remember that if you are eating a chicken or turkey sandwich, the bread will count as the carbs.

- Salads in addition to a serving of protein and a serving of starchy carbs are always good since they provide fiber and fill you up. However, avoid using high fat/high sugar dressings.

- Refrain from using high carbohydrate sauces or mayonnaise.

Basically, if you stick to the five rules discussed above, no matter where you find yourself, you won't have a problem finding something to eat. Bon Appetite!

How to Determine Your Protein Levels

Because you will be training hard, you will need 1.5 grams of protein per pound of LBM split over 6 meals per day in order to preserve and enhance muscle tone.

Protein Grams = LBM x 1.5

As far as protein choices, all of the ones discussed in the nutrition section are fair. However, due to the fact that you will need more protein, the serving sizes are bigger.

How to Determine Your Fat Grams

In the absence of carbohydrates, one's needs for good fats increases. In addition, remember that good fats help to preserve muscle tissue, produce energy and also aid in the burning of body fat.

To determine how many grams of good fats your body needs, here is the formula:

Good Fats = LBM x 0.3

As far as good fats choices, all of the one discussed in the nutrition section are fair.

DESIGNING YOUR DIET

Designing your Advanced Body Sculpting Diet plan is easy.

1. First, divide your protein requirements by 28. That will give you the number of meals that you will need per day. If the resulting number is a decimal, just round to the nearest tenth. So for instance in the case of a woman with 140-lbs of LBM, 210 divided by 28 equals 7.5, so in this case, just have eight servings of protein per day (eight meals). In the case

of a 135-lb woman, 203 divided by 28 yields 7.25 so therefore seven servings of protein are required in this case, which yields seven meals.

2. Now that you know the number of meals that you will have, divide the amount of carbohydrates by 25. This will give you the approximate amount of carbohydrate servings that you need per day. Follow the same rounding protocol as described above for proteins. If you only are allowed two servings, then add them to Meal 1 and your Post Workout Meal (PWM). If Meal is your Post Workout Meal then you just need to add the second serving to Meal 3. If you have three servings of carbs, then add them to meals 1, 2, and your post workout meal. Again, if Meal 1 is your PWM, then you would have carbs at meals 1, 2, and 3. Continue this same pattern for the amount of servings that you have.

3. For fats, divide the grams of fats by five and that gives you the number of teaspoons of EFAs that you need in your diet, keeping in mind that if salmon is consumed, two of those teaspoons can be eliminated. As long as you do not add these to your PWM, then you can add them to any of the other meals.

4. For vegetables, there is no need to count, so just add them at will to at least two meals. On low carb days, feel free to add them to all of your carb free meals.

DIETING TO ADD MUSCLE MASS

The Body Sculpting Diets in this book are designed to help women add some muscle

BEVERAGE TIPS

Many dieters, due to their lack of nutrition knowledge, can literally just blow their diets without realizing that they're doing it. The culprit? Drinking the wrong types of beverages.

- Drink plenty of water daily. Your recommended fluid intake should be 0.66 x body weight in ounces per day.

- Absolutely no regular sodas or fruit juices, even the ones that claim to be all natural, as there are way too many simple carbs in these beverages. For example, the average soda contains 40 grams of sugar while an 8-ounce serving of the average fruit juice contains between 25-35 grams of simple carbs! Therefore three 8 ounce glasses of orange juice would fill up your liver glycogen immediately!

- Crystal Light beverages, and decaffeinated tea/coffee are OK as long as they are used in moderation; your main beverage should be water.

- Try to avoid all alcohol. An occasional glass of red wine is OK provided that you are of legal drinking age.

COOKING TIPS

If you want to achieve your Body Sculpting goals, proper food preparation is essential! Follow the guidelines below to ensure proper food preparation:

- Eat vegetables raw or slightly steamed. If boiling, be careful not to overcook or you will lose the nutritional value of the vegetables.

- Do not fry. Always broil, grill, steam or bake (broiling, grilling and steaming are better as they allow fat to drain while cooking).

- Trim all fat from meat and remove skin from poultry prior to cooking.

- Do not use salts, butter, oils, or sugar while cooking. Experiment with herbs, non-salt seasonings, lemon Juice, vinegar, garlic and pepper, even a touch (1 Tbsp; not a bottle) of some white or red wine. Occasional use of salsa, low sodium soy sauce, catsup, and mustard to enhance meats and vegetables is OK if used sparingly (1 Tbsp). Minced white or green onions are also excellent for seasoning.

TIPS FOR CHOOSING FOODS

1. Always try to use natural foods. Avoid using canned or pre-prepared types of foods as they usually contain too much fats, sodium and carbs.

2. Always choose low fat protein sources. If you eat really low fat meals, don't worry about incurring a fat deficiency since the supplements program takes care of the need for essential fatty acids. Besides, there are trace amounts of fats even in the low fat protein sources that we choose.

3. If you choose to include skim milk in your diet, remember that it not only has protein (8 to 9 grams for every 8 ounces of milk) but also simple carbs (12 to 13 grams for every 8 ounces of milk). Therefore, count milk as both. Note that since the carbs in milk are simple carbs, this food item should only be used in the post workout meal. Guys interested in competing or following the Advanced Body Sculpting Diet, should however eliminate any dairy products from the diet as these products tend to make you retain water and the lactose in them make it harder to get to the desired low body fat percentage required for contest condition. In addition, whole wheat products should also be minimized during this phase as they may contain pytho-estrogens that make it harder to lose fat.

4. Try to include fibrous carbs in at least two meals.

5. Post Workout Meal should contain high glycemic complex carbs combined with fast released proteins such as whey protein isolate. Fats and fibers should be eliminated from this meal ideally to facilitate maximum insulin release and thus improve recovery and muscle growth.

while stripping body fat at the same time. For those women who have a faster metabolism and are just interested in gaining muscle as their body fat is already low then all of the advice in this applies to them with the following modifications to the training and nutrition programs.

EATING TO GAIN MUSCLE WEIGHT

Eating to just gain muscle (as opposed to gaining muscle and losing body fat) follows the same prescriptions above except that the total caloric intake will be higher, for most people in the other of 2200 calories for two weeks and 2700 for the next two.

Two sample meal plans guaranteed to pack on the muscle are presented on page 82.

DO I NEED TO MEASURE MY FOOD INTAKE AND LOG IT IN A DIARY FOREVER?

Not at all. Typically you will notice that after the first six-week cycle, you pretty much know how much food you need to take in everyday. The reason for measuring and keeping track of the foods that you eat during the first six weeks is to give you an idea of how much food you need in order to get in shape. Without tracking at the beginning of the program, it would be impossible to determine the correct quantity of nutrients your body needs in order to lose weight and tone up. However, since after six weeks you already know how much food you need, you can start building your meals based on a visual inspection alone. However, just be cautious not to progressively put more food on the plate. If you start to see that your weight is beginning to climb, track your food intake for the next three days and see how much you are deviating from what you should be having.

ADD A CHEAT MEAL TO THE MIX

If you are not following the Advanced Body Sculpting Diet, you may cheat on your diet for one meal on Sunday (e.g. FORGET CALORIE COUNTING and eat whatever you want—within reason, of course—for that one meal). You can only reward yourself in this way if you have stayed on track the rest of the week. One cheat meal a week may actually be beneficial since it confuses your body and increases your metabolism. By cheating, you prevent your body from adjusting to the diet, which would lower metabolism. It also removes the psychological fear that you will never again be able to eat bad foods. However, having said that, we must caution that some people (us included) find it hard to go back to good dieting if they incorporate cheat foods in their diets once a week. They fall into a non-stop bingeing rage with these foods that may last for weeks. Do not feel bad if you fall into this category. It is natural to crave foods that are bad, considering that they taste so darn good. If you fall into this category and feel tempted or need to still build your will power of resistance, then stick to a healthy diet and stay away from cheat meals until you have reached a confident level of empowerment. We have actually learned to do just fine without cheat foods at all.

However, we are human beings and bringing balance in our lives includes allowing us to look forward to tiny breaks. This cheat meal has proven to have an extraordinary affect with helping people avoid retreating from their healthy eating regimen. Call it moderation without complete deprivation. Look forward to the weekend cheat meal and allow the cheat meal to will away the desire to slip up during the week. Allow that cheat meal to break the monotony and then get right back on track for healthy eating during the week!

The Importance of Preparing Food Beforehand

Preparation is crucial to the success of your dietary program. If you are not prepared, you will fail. Life is too hectic nowadays to be eating five or six times a day without a little bit of preparation.

One thing you can do is prepare your food the night before and store it in individual containers that have a section for complex or simple carbs, a place for fibrous carbs, and a place for protein. You also can prepare protein shakes the night before and store them individually in containers that you can purchase at the grocery store. When the following day comes, all you have to do is take out the container that has breakfast, heat it up, and eat. Then grab the container for lunch and two protein shakes, put them in the cooler, and go to work. Take a water bottle everywhere you go. No need to dehydrate while at work. When you come home, take out the container holding dinner, re-heat it, eat it and prepare the food for the following day.

If you think you will be able to stick to the plan without being prepared, you place yourself at risk. You will either end up eating the wrong kinds of food, or missing meals. You will definitely spend more money, because eating out is not cheap. Therefore, remember to be prepared!

Meal Frequency and Work

Choose from among these alternatives to make sure you have five or six meals a day:

- Have lunch and dinner as real meals and keep the rest of the meals as either meal replacement protein shakes or protein bars; preferably meal replacement shakes as most protein bars have too much fats and sugars.

- Have real food for your breakfast, lunch and dinner and and meal-replacement protein shakes for the other two meals.

- Have all of your meals as real meals by convincing your boss to allow you to have three 20-minute breaks instead of a full hour lunch break so you can eat all of your meals.

Emotional Eating

In our fast-paced, high-stress society many people resort to emotional eating for comfort. This is a dangerous activity; if this happens very often the weight will begin to pile on. Also dangerous is the fact that emotional eating usually occurs at night after work.

If you feel like you engage in emotional eating, remember that you need to write down everything you eat during the first eight weeks of this program. During the first eight weeks it should be easier to resist the temptation to eat emotionally because you will need to document it in your log. If you are past the original eight weeks, then ask yourself, "Am I eating this because my body needs it or is it because I need it emotionally?" In cases like this, stop and think about what is most important for you. Is it the food or your fitness goals? You know what the right choice is. If it's late at night, just go to bed and rest assured that the cravings will have go away by the time the morning comes.

Protein Shakes

It's better to eat as much real food as possible, but if you are too busy to fix five to six real meals, you can substitute meals with a shake. You can have either a meal replacement packet mixed with water or a scoop of protein mixed in skim milk with a teaspoon of flaxseed oil. However, make sure that you eat at least two real meals a day, and keep in mind that the more real food you eat the better results you get, as real food increases your metabolism more than shakes.

For some healthy recipes, many created using protein powder, which you can incorporate into your meal plans, be sure to check APPENDIX D: RECIPES for some delicious Body Sculpting approved recipes designed by French Chef Marie-Annick Courtier!

SUPPLEMENTS

Many people incorrectly believe supplements are the most important part of a body sculpting program. However, supplements are simply additions to a good nutrition and training program. Supplements do not make up for improper training, or lack thereof, and a crappy diet. Supplements only work when your diet and your training program are optimized.

Nutritional supplements protect us from nutritional deficiencies. Your new exercise program's increased activity levels make your body require greater amounts of vitamins and minerals, and increase the chances that you will incur a nutritional deficiency without supplementation. Remember, even a slight nutrient deficiency can sabotage your body sculpting goals.

Unfortunately, we cannot rely solely on food to provide us with all the vitamins and minerals that our body requires. This is largely because the processing food goes through even before they arrive at the supermarket: cooking, air, and light have already robbed your foods of the vitamins that they normally offer. If you are deficient in one or more essential nutrients, your body may not be able to build muscle and burn fat properly.

However, not all supplements are equal. The use of supplements depends on both your goals and your budget. Below we describe the different categories of supplements and discuss the ones you will need to use at all times.

MULTIPLE VITAMIN AND MINERAL FORMULA

This type of supplement is essential to insure that our bodies operate at maximum efficiency. On a very simplistic level, without these vitamins and minerals, it is impossible to convert the food we eat into hormones, tissues and energy.

Vitamins are organic compounds produced by both animals and, which enhance the actions of proteins, causing and vegetables, which such as muscle building, fat burning and energy production. There are two types of vitamins:

- **Fat-soluble vitamins** are stored in fat and if taken in excessive amounts will become toxic. (Such as vitamins A, D, E, and K.)

- **Water-soluble vitamins** are not stored in the body. (Such as the B-Complex vitamins and Vitamin C.)

Minerals, inorganic compounds not produced by animals or vegetables, assure that your brain receives the correct signals from the body. They help with balance of fluids, muscular contractions and energy production as well as build muscle and bones. There are two types of minerals:

- **Bulk minerals** are called such because the body requires them in great quantities and often in the measure of grams. (Such as calcium, magnesium, potassium, sodium and phosphorus.)

- **Trace minerals** are required by the body in tiny amounts, usually in the order of micrograms. (Such as chromium, copper, cobalt, silicon, selenium, iron and zinc.)

SOURCES:

You must be very careful with the vitamin and

mineral formulas you choose. Some don't contain what the labels claim, and some come from such poor sources and are not absorbed very well by the body. For a list of reputable brands, please pass by www.BodySculptingBibles.com and download our FREE recommended supplements list.

QUANTITY:

Take as directed.

PROTEIN SUPPLEMENTS

Weight Gainers are protein shakes consisting mainly of whey proteins. Some also include milk or egg proteins. Characterized by their extremely high carbohydrate content, weight gainers were very popular back in the 90;s but their popularity has died mainly because many people do not have the metabolism of a hardgainer, and a high carbohydrate diet leads quickly to fat gains rather than muscle mass gains.

SOURCES:

For a list of reputable brands, please pass by www.BodySculptingBibles.com and download our FREE recommended supplements list.

QUANTITY:

The carbohydrate content is designed for a fast release, and is best in the mid-morning, mid-afternoon, and post workout meals. Weight gainers can be mixed with fruit juice or skim milk and, if you are trying to increase the calorie content, the use of flaxseed oil, fish oils, and fruits is useful. However, if you do not have the metabolism to support this, it's probably best to avoid these.

Meal Replacement Powders (MRPs) are lower in calories and have far less carbohydrates than weight gainers. Most powders are composed of whey proteins, but there are many new formulas now on the market that consist of a protein blend of whey and milk proteins. The carbohydrate component used to be maltodextrin, with 25-27 grams of carbohydrate per serving, but the new generation of formulas use slow-release carbohydrates like brown rice and oats to make the product lower in glycemic value. Essential fatty acids and a vitamin and mineral profile have also been added.

SOURCES:

Any health food store or drug store.

QUANTITY:

1 packet mixed with water per serving.
Protein Powders are powders that consist mainly of protein (typically whey protein, but you can also find blends). They typically contain no more than five grams of carbohydrates and 20-25 grams of protein per scoop. Calorie-wise, they could be anywhere from 100-125 calories.

SOURCES:

For a list of reputable brands, please pass by www.BodySculptingBibles.com and download our FREE recommended supplements list.

QUANTITY:

2 scoops mixed with 8 ounces of skim milk per serving.

Protein Bars are bars made out of any of the protein sources mentioned above. The carbohydrate mix usually is a combination of glycerin (sugar alcohol, and not really a carbohydrate) and sugars. Bars generally contain fats which are less than desirable. Use these bars only in cases of extreme emergency when there is nothing better available to eat.

SOURCES:

For a list of reputable brands, please pass by www.BodySculptingBibles.com and download our FREE recommended supplements list.

QUANTITY:

A serving is just one bar. For specific brand recommendations, please visit our Fan Page at www.facebook.com/bodysculptingbibles or our site at www.bodysculptingbibles.com.

GOOD OILS: FISH OILS, FLAX OIL, EXTRA-VIRGIN OLIVE OIL, AND PEANUT BUTTER

If you follow a very strict low-fat diet you'll find that you begin to start having trouble keeping your strength up and losing fat. It is really easy to incur a fat deficiency when your diet is really clean.

To fix this you should also be taking in good oil, or fat supplements.

- **Fish oils** are best obtained through a consumption of salmon a minimum of three times a week. Fish oil caps are good, but you need at least 10 per day in order to get even 10 grams of fish oil. Thus, if you are to supplement with fish oils, in lieu of consuming Wild Atlantic Salmon, please use a fish oil supplement like Carlson Fish Oils which is a very clean, toxic-free oil with lemon flavor.

- **Flax Oil** is best obtained from buying the whole ground flaxseed meal, which needs to be refrigerated at all times. Do not cook with this oil if you

choose to use it instead of the meal, as it is light and heat sensitive. It should appear to be a clear yellow. If you purchase oil with brown particles, it is rancid and should be returned or thrown out.

- Your **extra virgin olive oil** should preferably be canned in either Italy or Spain. It's best to purchase oil canned because light can reach the oil stored in a bottle and turn it rancid. Also remember that natural old-fashioned **peanut butter** is a great source of monounsaturated fats.

SOURCES:

For a list of reputable brands, please pass by www.BodySculptingBibles.com and download our FREE recommended supplements list.

QUANTITY:

Consume fats in the way recommended by the diet charts on page 83.

VITAMIN C

Vitamin C is a water-soluble vitamin that improves your immune system and assists in faster recovery from your workouts. It suppresses the amount of cortisol (a hormone that kills muscle and aids in the accumulation of fat) released by your body during a workout. This is the only vitamin we recommend taking in mega dose quantities. Because it is a water-soluble vitamin, it will not be stored by the body. If taken an hour before a workout (1000mg dose), research shows Vitamin C significantly reduces muscle soreness and speeds recovery.

Science has proven that in order for Vitamin C to reach the proper pathway and have an effect on the bones, where it's needed, it requires the addition of the supplement known as K-2. This supplement is being hailed as the missing nutrient and is behind something known as the "calcium paradox". Visit www.BodySculptingBibles.com for more information.

Important Note: Ensure that your water intake during the day is adequate (bodyweight X 0.66 = ounces of water per day). If you have a history of kidney stones, you should not take Vitamin C in these large quantities. As always, when in doubt, consult your doctor.

SOURCES:

For a list of reputable brands, please pass by www.BodySculptingBibles.com and download our FREE recommended supplements list.

QUANTITY:

We recommend a total of 3000 mg per day of Vitamin C. If your multiple vitamin pack already has 1000 mg, and you take this in the morning, then all you need is an extra 1000 mg at lunch and 1000 mg at dinner.

CHROMIUM PICOLINATE

There are many claims surrounding Chromium Picolinate, and most of them are as yet unproven. However, we suggest its use from our own experience with this mineral. Some of its benefits surround its enhanced effect on insulin, upgrading insulin's capability to produce muscle and energy. An insulin-boosting vitamin could potentially assist in gaining muscle and losing fat faster. Chromium can also keep blood sugar levels stable, thereby preventing insulin levels from going high enough to begin promoting fat storage. However, chromium only functions if a suitable diet is followed.

SOURCES:

All chromium picolinate produced in the market is manufactured by a company called Nutrition 21; it is sold at stores like GNC, Vitamin Shoppe, Walmart and Walgreens

QUANTITY:

200 mcg with the post-workout meal and with breakfast on days off.

SUPPLEMENT RECOMMENDATIONS SUMMARY

Essential to Take

- Multivitamin (taken with breakfast)

- Essential Oils and Monounsaturated Oils (as per nutrition guidelines)

- 1 gram Vitamin C (taken with breakfast, lunch, and dinner)

- Weight Gainer, Whey Protein Powder, or Meal Replacement Powder (to mix with skim milk or water for protein shakes)

- 200 mcg of Chromium Picolinate (post-workout with protein shake)

Fat Burning Stacks

- For a list of good fat burners, please pass by www.BodySculptingBibles.com and download our FREE recommended supplements list.

ALL ABOUT PROTEIN AND BIOLOGICAL VALUES (BV)

Each source of protein is measured by its quality, by Biological Value (BV). BV measures how well the body absorbs and uses the protein. The higher the BV, the more nitrogen your body can absorb, use, and retain. As a result, proteins with the highest BV promote the most lean muscle gains. Whey protein ranks with the highest BV value, a 104. Egg protein is second with 100, and milk proteins come in third at 91. Beef protein rates as 80 and soy proteins at 74. Because bean proteins are a plant-based protein, they rank a 49.

Whey Proteins Whey Concentrate/Whey Isolate are a great source. They have been recorded to improve sports performance by reducing stress and lowering cortisol levels, improving immunity by increasing glutathione (GSH) which also helps reduce overtraining, and improving liver functions in some forms of hepatitis. They also help reduce your blood pressure and fight HIV.

Whey Proteins are highly digestible and have an even better amino acid profile than egg whites. However, not all whey is created equal. The whey that gives you the benefits described above has to be micro-filtered at very low temperatures to allow production of high protein contents with no undenatured protein, and a minimum of fat, cholesterol, and lactose.

There are whey isolates and whey concentrates. Whey isolates are sub-fractions of whey absorbed rapidly into the system. While excellent for post-workout nutrition, whey isolate is a poor choice for supplementation during the day because if the body does not need all the amino acids released into the bloodstream, it will use them for energy production, not muscle building. Whey isolate also does not have many of the health enhancing properties, as the process required to produce whey isolate destroys many of the health/immune system enhancing sub-fractions. In conclusion, for during the day use, a product consisting mainly of whey concentrate is your best bet. After the workout, a whey isolate product will be a better choice.

Egg Protein is a super bio-available protein second only to whey. It is a slower released protein than whey, which makes it perfect for daytime use. We often mix egg and whey protein for one of the most bio-available protein shakes available.

Milk Proteins (Calcium Casseinate/Micellar Casein). Similar to egg proteins, this highly bioavailable protein source has slightly less BV, and is designed to slowly release into the blood stream. The natural, undenatured protein in milk is micellar casein which provides a steady release of amino acids, making this an excellent choice for a long-lasting muscle protecting protein.

Beef Proteins are slow released proteins that rate an 80 on the BV scale. While we are unaware of any protein supplement in powder form on the market that is derived from beef proteins, there are beef liver tablets. Beef proteins are abundant in blood-building iron and also B-vitamins, both factors that contribute to better nutrient use and energy production.

Soy Proteins have positive health benefits for both men and women. Studies show they may reduce the risk of hormone-dependent cancers (breast, prostate, etc), and possibly protect from other cancers as well. Soy has been well known to reduce high cholesterol and ease the symptoms of menopause. Soy also helps prevent osteoporosis by building up bone mass. Because of this, we recommend one serving of soy per day for women, but only for its health benefits. In the muscle-building department, soy is not useful; its BV value is 74, and because it has estrogen-like substances, it might reduce testosterone use, and for men, could be anti-constructive.

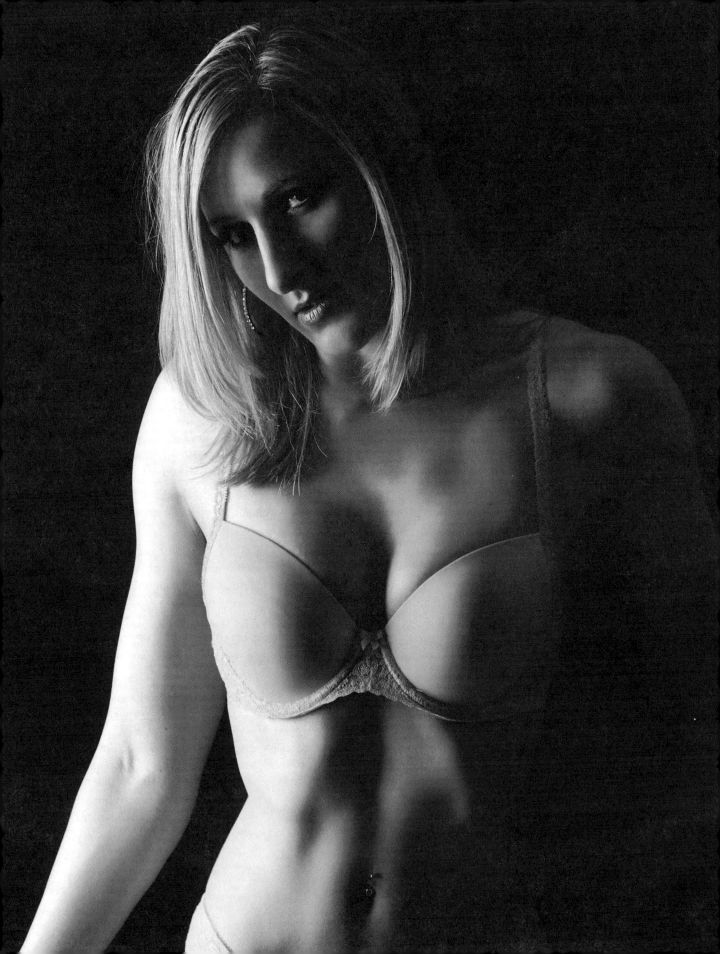

Chapter 5
Rest and Recovery

For immediate Body Sculpting Bible support & coaching directly from James & Hugo, please visit www.BodySculptingBibles.com

5

THE BODY
SCULPTING
BIBLE
FOR WOMEN

How much did you sleep last night; five, six maybe seven hours? Did you know that getting less than six hours a night can seriously affect your coordination, reaction time and judgment; not to mention your health?

Though the goal is to get in great shape, many of us are silently killing ourselves. With all of the stimulants now available such as high-octane coffee, ephedrine, "natural" fat burners and the like, why would we need sleep when we can simply get a "boost?" A recent segment on CNN discovered that "people who drove after being awake for 17 to 19 hours performed worse than those with a blood alcohol level of .05 percent. That's the legal limit for drunk driving in most western European countries, though most States in the U.S. set their blood alcohol limits at .1 percent and a few at .08 percent." The study revealed that 16 to 60 percent of all road accidents involved sleep deprivation.

Have you ever been in a situation where you needed to pull an "all-nighter" for school or work? We see it all the time; people bragging about not sleeping because they don't have enough time in a day. Not surprisingly, nearly half of all Americans have difficulty sleeping. A growing collection of research indicates that America's sleep problems have reached epidemic proportions and may be the country's number-one health problem. Would it change your mind if you knew that those who sleep fewer than six hours a night don't live as long as those who sleep seven hours or more?

Lack of sleep can be expensive: The National Commission on Sleep Disorders estimates that sleep deprivation costs $150 billion a year in higher stress and reduced workplace productivity. Yes, most of us truly enjoy staying up late, ready to dive into the night life. We are magnetized to late night movies and late night surfing on the internet, yet did you know that we are robbing ourselves of 338 hours—two full weeks—of rest per year?

New research indicates that rest and sleep may well be the third essential component of a long and healthy life, right up there with a good diet and regular exercise! "Society is being victimized by not getting enough sleep," says David Dinges, director of experimental psychiatry at the University of Pennsylvania School of Medicine. "Our productivity, our safety, our health are at risk." The findings are far from definitive but they strongly hint that long-term sleep debt could be a factor in the national epidemics of diabetes and obesity. Research is proving that sleep deprivation could weaken the immune system, leading to colds and other infections. There is even a bit of evidence proving how the increase in breast cancer, and perhaps other cancers, could have a link to decreased sleep.

THE SLEEP CYCLE

When we deprive ourselves of sleep, there is a delicate cycle that we disrupt.

Phase One: Phase one begins as soon as the sun sets, when the pineal gland starts to release melatonin, a hormone released in the absence of light and responsible for making us sleepy. When you lie down in your bed at this time, your muscles relax, heart rate and breathing slow down, and body temperature drops. The brain also relaxes but still remains alert. If you could look at the wave patterns being generated by the brain, you would see a change from the rapid beta waves of daytime to slower alpha waves. When the alpha waves disappear, replaced by theta waves, the sleeper has tumbled into the sensory void called stage one sleep. In this stage, the sleeper is unable to sense anything.

Phase Two: Phase two occurs a moment after phase one and in this stage the sleeper lays still for about 10 to 15 minutes.

Phase Three: After phase two is over, the sleeper falls into a deeper sleep. During this stage, the sleeper falls deeper into phase three which lasts about 5 to 15 minutes.

Phase Four: With a maximum of 15 minutes spent within the phase three cycle, the sleeper then falls into yet another relaxed stage called phase four, lasting a half hour or so. In stage four, the eyes move back and forth very quickly in what's called rapid eye movement, or REM. This is the point at which the first dream occurs. After this dream has ended, the sleeper goes back to phase two and starts the whole process over again. These processes repeat themselves about five times during the night.

Sleep research indicates that the average sleeper will sleep approximately eight hours and 15 minutes when uninterrupted. During this research, there were no alarm clocks or disturbing noises to interrupt normal sleep patterns. Eight hours and 15 minutes is believed to be the ideal physiological amount of time that the body requires for sleep.

MALADIES CAUSED BY SLEEP DEPRIVATION

The following are the maladies that, according to research, can result in consistent sleep deprivation:

- **Impaired glucose tolerance.** Without sleep, the central nervous system becomes more active, inhibiting the pancreas from producing adequate insulin, the hormone the body needs to digest glucose. "In healthy young men with no risk factor, in one week, we had them in a pre-diabetic state," says researcher Van Cauter when referring to a study that he conducted on the effects of sleep deprivation.

- **Possible link to obesity.** This is due to the fact that much of people's growth hormone is secreted during the first round of deep sleep. As both men and women age, they naturally spend less time in deep sleep, which reduces growth hormone secretion. Lack of sleep at a younger age, however, could drive down growth hormone prematurely, accelerating the fat-gaining process. In addition, research indicates a lowering of the hormone testosterone as well as fat gain and muscle loss.

- **Increased carbohydrate cravings.** Sleep deprivation negatively affects the production of a hormone called Leptin. This hormone is responsible for telling the body when it is full. However, with decreased production of this hormone, your body will crave calories (especially in the form of carbs) even though its requirements have been met. Not a good situation to be in for a dieter.

- **Weakened immune system.** Research indicates that sleep deprivation adversely affects the white blood cell count in humans as well as the body's ability to fight infections.

- **Increased risk of breast cancer.** Richard Stevens, a cancer researcher at the University of Connecticut Health Center, has speculated that there might be a connection between breast cancer and hormone cycles disrupted by late-night light. Melatonin, primarily secreted at night, may trigger a reduction in the body's production of estrogen. But light interferes with melatonin release (recall that the hormone is secreted in response to a lack of light), allowing estrogen levels to rise. Too much estrogen is known to promote the growth of breast cancers.

- **Decreased alertness and ability to focus.** A recent study showed that people who were awake for up to 19 hours scored worse on performance tests and alertness scales than those with a blood-alcohol level of .08 percent—legally drunk in some states.

- **Hardening of the arteries.** Some studies suggest that the stress imposed on the body due to lack of sleep causes a very sharp rise in cortisol levels. Such an imbalance can lead to hardening of the arteries, increasing the risk of heart attacks. In addition, we also know that very high cortisol levels lead to muscle loss, increased fat storage, loss of bone mass, depression, hypertension, insulin resistance (the cells in the body lose the ability to accept insulin), and lower growth hormone and testosterone production.

- **Depression and irritability.** Lack of sleep also causes depletion of neurotransmitters in the brain that are in charge of regulating mood. Because of this, sleep deprived people have a "shorter fuse" and also tend to get depressed more easily.

ARE YOU SLEEP DEPRIVED?

It's easy to tell if you're sleep-deprived. If you can lie down in the middle of the day and fall asleep within 10 minutes, you are sleep deprived. Catching up is basic math. For every hour, or fraction, under eight hours, you need an equal extra amount of time asleep soon after. But if you're hundreds of hours in debt, you may never pay it all off. According to recent research, 17 hours was all the catching up people could do, and it generally took three weeks. Most people probably need three times that amount of sleep!

FAQ:
I try to find time for seven to nine hours of sleep, but having a family and a full-time job just doesn't permit it.

ANSWER:
That's reality. The best case scenario is to get seven to nine hours per night. We're lucky if we get four to six sometimes! The key is not to feel bad or give up because you can't stick to every detail, but instead to become aware and do your best to stick to it. it's all about balance and doing your best to get back on track.

SLEEPING PILLS

Beware of sleeping pills! They not only tend to be addicting but people that use them find that they tend to wake up groggy. As far as melatonin supplementation, scientists are divided in opinion but most agree that the 3-milligram dose available in health food stores is too high, especially as the supplement has never been tested for safety in humans. Since we are very cautious when it comes to hormones, we would rather have you follow the guidelines below in order to ensure a good night's sleep:

- **Avoid activities that involve deep concentration** as these activities will increase adrenaline levels and will prevent the brain from achieving the state of relaxation required to achieve sleep.

- **Avoid watching disturbing shows at night on TV** as this may also increase your adrenaline levels thereby preventing you from a good night's sleep.

- **Avoid eating a large meal at night** since the digestion process will prevent you from falling asleep.

- **Attempt to totally relax at the same time each night.** By doing so you condition the body to relax itself once the specific time that you choose arrives. Ensure that at this time no thoughts other than relaxation and falling asleep come to your head. You need to really learn how to block all thoughts concerning work or other life issues that may be trying to get in your head. Listening to soothing music set at a low volume with the lights off can help you relax and achieve the state necessary to go to sleep.

CONCLUSION

You need seven to nine hours of sleep each night (eight being the ideal) in order for your body to run efficiently. Deprive your body of sleep and you'll have lousy fat loss and hinder your body's ability to increase lean muscle tone. Without enough sleep the body stops producing anabolic hormones (muscle producing/fat burning hormones; e.g. testosterone and growth hormone) and starts increasing the production of catabolic hormones (muscle destroying/fat depositing hormones; e.g. cortisol). So, to make matters worse, you'll also lose muscle, which lowers your metabolism. In addition, you will lack the energy and focus to get through your workouts, which will surely lead to overtraining. To top it off, research indicates that lack of sleep creates cravings and binges in addition to hardening of the arteries, which leads to heart attacks. In short: **turn off the TV, relax and hit the sack!**

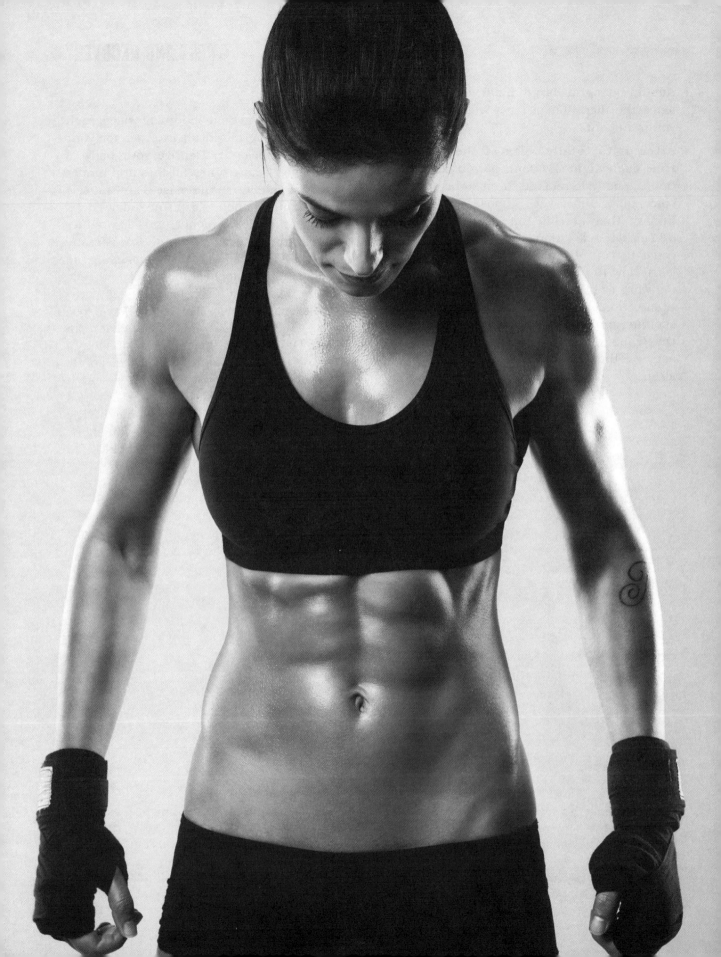

Part 3
Body Sculpting Exercises

Learning proper exercise technique is the backbone of every fitness program. If you train improperly you will not stimulate the intended muscle, and will risk major injury while receiving little or no results. When you learn to use proper exercise technique you will receive twice the results in half the time, guaranteed! We see people in the gym day in and day out who have no idea how to properly train their muscles. Some of them are professional bodybuilders, some are professional athletes, and some are even certified fitness trainers. Unfortunately, the ones who really suffer the most are people like you who rely on these role models for wisdom and guidance. We will show you the proper exercise technique to use for optimal results. Just remember to utilize your newfound knowledge. Like the old saying, "Feed a man a fish and he'll eat for a day, teach a man to fish and he'll eat for a lifetime." We expect the same of you. We don't want you to read the book once and then forget everything you've learned. We want you to learn and utilize that knowledge to achieve astounding results.

Applying proper exercise form and technique is, without doubt, the most important component of any fitness program. Without it, many, many setbacks will occur. First, the musculature you intend to exercise will not be stimulated as efficiently as possible. Exercise should not be focused around just lifting barbells and dumbbells. It shouldn't just be about how much weight you can lift. Optimum fitness is about the quality of exercise, the quality of your form and how you maintain that form, especially during heavier weight lifting. Proper exercise technique coupled with the Zone-Tone principle will bring you the most astonishing results with the minimum amount of sets. Why? Because as we have already discussed, one properly executed set is equivalent to five sets of "just going through the motions". It comes down to this; if you want to get the most out of your workout, keep the intensity high without sacrificing proper form.

As you read through each exercise introduction, you will notice that we discuss many of those "Hot Spot" areas that most women are concerned with targeting, plus we make suggestions to help make each exercise as productive as possible. If you ever feel confused and would like us to elaborate on any of the information we have discussed, please refer to the resource page in the back of the book for our contact information. We are always available to answer your questions and look forward to helping you make this experience free of confusion and nothing less than amazing!

Tip: Throughout this section, you will see questions answered about exercises that can cause pain and discomfort. Please remember that doing or not doing a specific exercise is not going to stop body sculpting results. Yes, the squat is the best exercise for your legs-but if you have a bad lower back, don't do it. If you can't do a specific exercise because it hurts you, there is always another one that will give you the same results. The primary reason to weight train should always be to improve your health and help you look and feel great. If you perform an exercise that you know will ultimately hurt you, we guarantee you'll be feeling really bad when you're laid up in bed. Follow your instincts and play it safe.

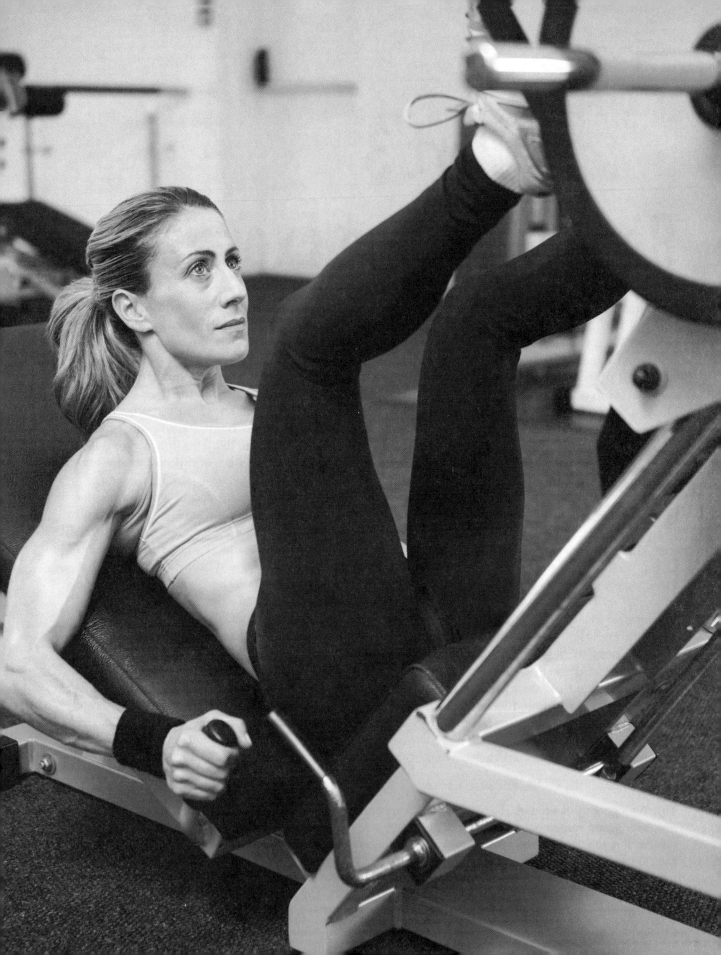

Chapter 6
Legs

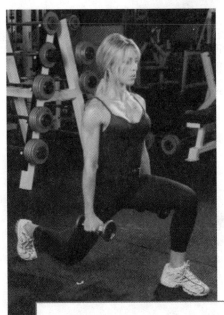

For immediate Body Sculpting Bible support & coaching directly from James & Hugo, please visit www.BodySculptingBibles.com

THE BODY SCULPTING BIBLE FOR WOMEN

6

Foot Stances and Quadriceps and Hamstring Development

To better target different areas of your legs, most specifically your quadriceps and your hamstrings, you need to pay attention to the stance in which you are standing. There are three main stances for each position (on the ground, and on a machine):

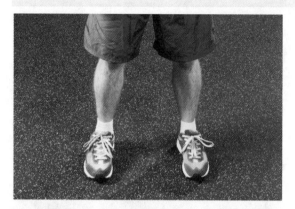

Shoulder-width stance with toes pointed slightly out: This stance works best for stimulating overall thigh development.

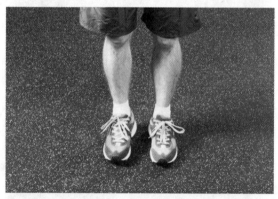

Close stance with toes pointed straight ahead: This stance works best for stimulating growth of the outer quadricep, better known as the vastus lateralis.

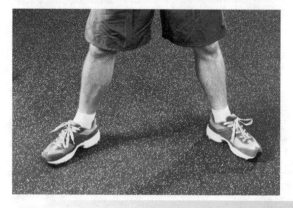

Wide stance with toes pointed out at least 45 degrees: This stance targets both the vastus medialis, which is the inside head of the quadriceps near the knee, and the inner thigh or adductor muscles.

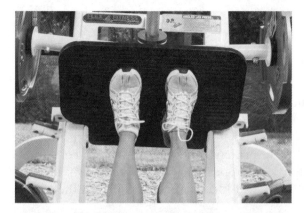

Toes straight: Good for overall development.

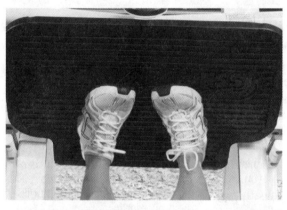

Toes in: Good for maximizing outer quadriceps and inner hamstring stimulation.

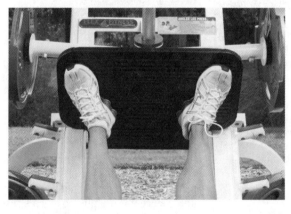

Toes out: Good for maximizing inner quad and outer hamstring stimulation.

It is important to mention that every time a quadriceps exercise is performed, it is imperative to push mainly with the toes, as that will emphasize quadriceps recruitment.

For hamstring exercises, you should push mainly with the heels, as that will emphasize hamstring/glute recruitment. In addition, there is only one main stance you should be concerned with for recruiting your hamstring, and that is the wide stance (toes pointed out at least 45 degrees).

Barbell Squat

This is one of the best exercises you can do to help sculpt beautifully toned and firm legs. The squat exercise is known to provide beneficial results to the whole body because you use several body muscles to synergistically join forces and execute the lift. Although you are focusing on your thighs, don't be surprised when you notice your butt suddenly beginning to firm up and look as if it has been lifted higher. This exercise will help primarily develop the quadriceps muscles (front of upper leg), the hamstring muscles (back of upper leg), the gluteal muscles (the butt), and the calves (back of lower leg). However, it also will incorporate virtually all the body's major muscle groups in one way or another.

PROPER ALIGNMENT

❶ Place a bar either on a squat safety rack or in a power cage, making sure you have the safety bars set just about even with the height of your thighs when the bar is parallel to the floor.

❷ Walk up to the bar and place your shoulders comfortably underneath it, making sure that the bar rests on the trapezoid muscles and not on the first and second cervical vertebrae. A shoulder pad is good to use. You can find them at most sporting good stores, or simply use a rolled up towel!

❸ Position your hands on the bar with a double shoulder width grip.

❹ Now, either assume a ready stance before lifting up the bar or step back into ready position with the weight already on your shoulders. We recommend the second option as it allows more room for the movement. If you are nervous about stepping backwards with the weight, you can always use the first option; or maybe you should re-evaluate how much weight you will be lifting. Whenever you feel nervous, be smart and consider either going a little lighter or having a qualified spotter assist you with the lift. Also, please don't take someone's word for being a good spotter. Either ask reliable sources for someone who is qualified, or look around for someone who you observe is a good spotter.

❺ Always align your body, starting from the bottom and moving to the top:

First, align your feet, making sure they are about shoulder width apart with a slight outward angle.

Next, slightly bend your knees to reduce undue stress from the lower back area.

Position your knees so that they are pointing directly in front of you.

Slightly contract the muscles of your lower back and the muscles of your abdominal section.

Stick out your chest while simultaneously squeezing your shoulder blades together. This helps to set the upper body in its proper position.

Finally, keep your head level at all times. Make sure your head and your eyes do not drop down or wander upward excessively as this is an easy way to lose your balance and fall.

TECHNIQUE AND FORM

Once you think you have properly aligned yourself, repeat the alignment steps starting from the bottom and moving up. Once you have secured your alignment, prepare to inhale as you begin your descent downward. As you execute the movement, keep the following points in mind:

❶ As you are squatting downward, it is very important that at no time throughout the movement do your knees go beyond your toes. This puts too much pressure on the knees, and can seriously damage them. Here is a technique that will help keep this from happening: As you begin your descent, mimic the motion and alignment of sitting in a chair. Make sure you keep your back as straight as possible. This motion will naturally help you utilize the proper form.

❷ Make sure you don't let your thighs go below horizontal as you could injure your lower back and knees.

❸ As you reach horizontal or just above it, begin to exhale and press off your feet, distributing the weight through the heel while pressing upward. You must concentrate on keeping and holding proper alignment throughout the movement.

❹ As you reach the top of the movement, make sure you do not lock your knees since this will put too much stress on the knee joint. If at any time during the movement you notice yourself getting sloppy or not retaining the proper alignment, stop immediately! Never jeopardize your safety with bad form.

❺ When you've done the desired amount of reps, walk the bar back into the rack and place it down.

Barbell Squat

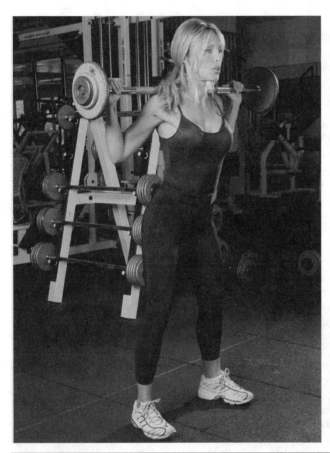
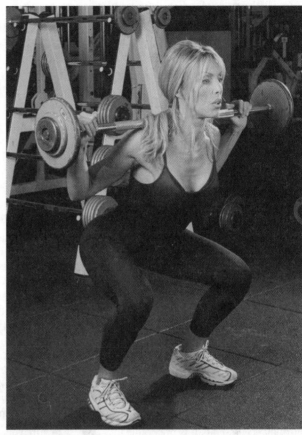

FAQ:

I have a bad back and I've heard that you can seriously injure your back performing this exercise.

ANSWER:

Squats are one of the greatest compound movements you can do for your entire body. When performed correctly, it will bring you great results. When done improperly, the squat will give you, well, squat! Here's the distinction: many people are injured when they try this with incorrect form or go overboard. Going overboard includes using too heavy of a weight, and not taking enough time or taking too much rest time between sets.

Recent research found that back injuries are often the result of poor lower back muscular endurance, in other words, the back's ability to hold and maintain a muscular contraction. To beef up your lower back's muscular endurance, perform exercises that concentrate on your balance and coordination, like the Lunge, Abdominal Crunch on the Ball, and other rotational exercises.

Dumbbell Squat

For a change of pace you might want to alternate between the barbell squat and the dumbbell squat. Both are very similar exercises in that they emphasize the same muscle groups, but each one has its benefits. With the barbell squat you can use more weight because you don't have to hold on to dumbbells. The dumbbells do make it easier to focus on your form, though, and once you begin to experience muscle fatigue, you can simply drop the dumbbells and still continue to squat without weight.

PROPER ALIGNMENT

❶ Hold a dumbbell in each hand with arms extended down and palms facing your body.

❷ Align your body from the bottom up by first taking a shoulder-width stance.

❸ Slightly bend your knees and avoid locking them during this exercise.

❹ Contract your abdominal muscles to help support and sustain your posture during the exercise.

❺ Stick your chest out and simultaneously bring your shoulder blades back, keeping them there throughout the movement.

❻ Keep your head level at all times, making sure your head or your eyes do not drop down, or excessively wander upward. This is an easy way to lose your balance and fall. It is preferable to look slightly above level rather than below because looking below level can greatly affect your equilibrium and jeopardize your safety.

❼ If you feel unstable, you may put small two pound plates under each heel for stability.

TECHNIQUE AND FORM

❶ When you think you have properly aligned yourself, repeat the alignment steps starting from the bottom and moving up. Once you have secured your alignment, prepare to inhale as you begin your descent.

❷ As you are squatting downward, it is very important that at no time throughout the movement do your knees go beyond your toes. This puts way too much pressure on the knees and can seriously damage them. Here is a technique that will help prevent this from happening: As you begin your descent, mimic the motion and alignment of sitting in a chair. Make sure you keep your back as straight as possible. This motion will naturally help you utilize the proper form.

❸ Make sure you don't let your thighs go below horizontal as you could injure your lower back; and this can also push the knees past the toes, once again leading to injury.

❹ As you reach horizontal or just above it, begin to exhale and press off your feet, distributing the weight through the heel while pressing

upward. Concentrate on keeping and holding proper alignment throughout the movement.

❺ As you reach the top of the movement, make sure you do not lock your knees since it will put too much stress on the knee joint. If at any time during the movement you should notice yourself getting sloppy or not retaining the proper alignment, stop immediately! Never jeopardize your safety with bad form!

❻ When you've done the desired amount of reps, squat down once again and place the dumbbells on the floor or place them back on the dumbbell rack. Never bend over to pick the dumbbells up or put them down. Doing this can injure your lower back area.

Dumbbell Squat

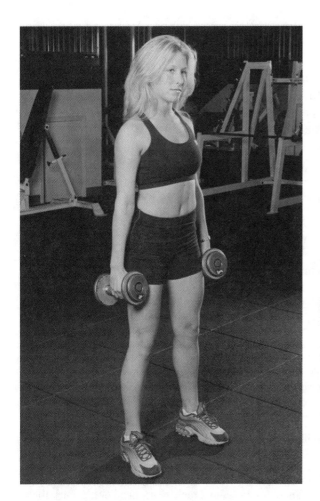
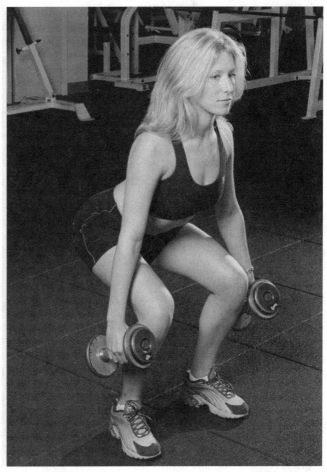

FAQ:

Because I don't have a barbell on my back, can I assume that the dumbbell squat will not bother my aching lower back?

Answer:

Whether you're doing squats with a barbell or a dumbbell, your back will be affected. Your objective must be to maintain proper form, anatomical alignment, and technique, from the beginning until the end of the exercise. if you get sloppy with any of these three elements, you risk the chance of injuring your lower back. The squat can be a very safe and effective exercise, so long as you are cautious enough to make it work.

Ballet Squat

This exercise is to be performed the same way as the barbell or dumbbell versions with the exception that your foot stance will be wider than shoulder-width. This variation will yield a stronger emphasis on the inner quads. Some women are afraid that a wide stance will give them a big butt and hips. This is not true. A wide-stance squat can actually help shape the quadriceps and the inner thighs. You must make sure, though, that you don't have too wide a stance. An overly wide stance can cause knee problems and possibly generate painful groin pulls. A good stance is about 1-1/2 times shoulder width with the toes pointed outward at a minimum of 25-30 degrees. No matter how wide your stance, your ankles should always remain in line with your knees. A good indication that a stance is too wide is when the ankles are outside of the knees in the bottom position of a squat. While you are discovering the width of stance best suited for you, don't worry about the amount of weight to use. Instead concentrate on your overall technique with your adjusted stance.

PROPER ALIGNMENT

❶ Hold a dumbbell in each hand with arms extended down and palms facing your body or a barbell on your back with your arms holding the barbell in place.

❷ Align your body from the bottom up by first taking a 1 1/2 shoulder-width stance.

❸ Slightly bend your knees and avoid locking them anytime during this exercise.

❹ Contract your abdominal muscles to help support and sustain your posture during exercise.

❺ Stick your chest out and simultaneously bring your shoulder blades back, keeping them there throughout the movement.

❻ Keep your head level at all times. Make sure your head and your eyes do not drop down or wander upward excessively as this is an easy way to lose your balance and fall. We would rather you look slightly above level, rather than below, as looking below level can greatly affect your equilibrium and jeopardize your safety

❼ If you feel unstable, you may put small two pound plates under each heel for stability.

TECHNIQUE AND FORM

❶ When you think you have properly aligned yourself, repeat the alignment steps, starting from the bottom and moving up. Once you have secured your alignment, prepare to inhale as you begin your descent.

❷ As you are squatting downward, it is very important that at no time throughout the movement do your knees go beyond your toes. This puts too much pressure on the knees, and can seriously damage them.

❸ Make sure you don't let your thighs go below horizontal since you could injure your lower back; and this can also push the knees past the toes, once again leading to injury.

❹ As you reach horizontal or just above it, begin to exhale and press off your feet distributing the weight throughout the heel while pressing upward. You must concentrate on

keeping and holding proper alignment throughout the movement.

❺ As you reach the top of the movement, make sure you do not lock your knees since it will put too much stress on the knee joint. If at any time during the movement you should feel or notice yourself getting sloppy or not retaining the proper alignment, stop immediately! Never jeopardize your safety with bad form!

❻ When you've done the desired amount of reps, simply walk the bar back to the rack. Or, if using dumbbells, squat down once again and place them on the floor or back on the dumbbell rack. Never bend over to pick the dumbbells up or put them down. Doing this can definitely injure your lower back area.

Ballet Squat

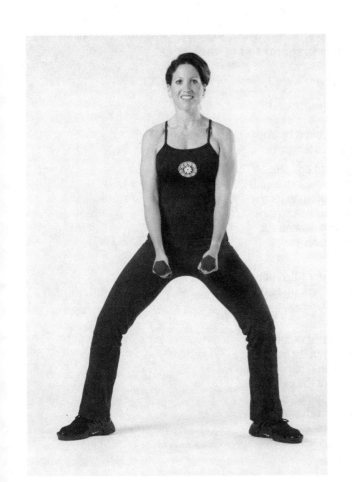 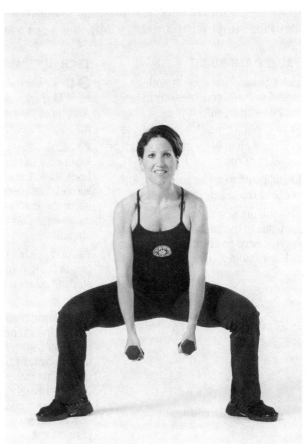

Sissy Squat

This exercise is a great way to squat, using your own bodyweight as resistance. You can perform this practically anywhere, and it's especially useful when you're on the road. You shouldn't try this exercise if you suffer from knee problems, however, as it stresses the knee. Once you've got the basics down, target your quads differently by trying a variation. For example, use just one arm for support, and use the opposite arm to hold a plate on top of your chest.

PROPER ALIGNMENT

❶ Make sure that there is nothing behind you so if you lose your balance and fall nothing will hit you.

❷ Stand upright with feel shoulder-width apart and heels raised an inch or two off the floor.

❸ Hold onto a stationary object such as one of the beams of a squat rack.

❹ If you are new to the exercise, it's a good idea to use two arms for support-so you'll need two beams of the squat rack in front of you.

TECHNIQUE AND FORM

❶ Using your arms to hold yourself, bend at the knees and slowly lower your torso toward the ground by bringing your pelvis and knees forward.

❷ Inhale as you go down and stop when your buttocks almost touch your heels. Hold the stretch position for a second. Ensure that your hamstrings touch the calves at the bottom of the movement. This emphasizes the stretch!

❸ After the hold, use your thigh muscles to bring your torso back up to the starting position and exhale as you go up.

❹ Perform the determined number of repetitions after coming all the way up to the starting position and pausing momentarily at the top of the movement. This makes sure you do not bounce up and down, which would place more stress on your knees, and it also ensures the squat is done with perfect form.

Sissy Squat

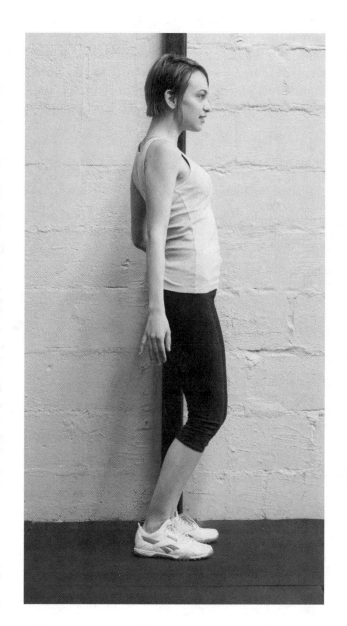
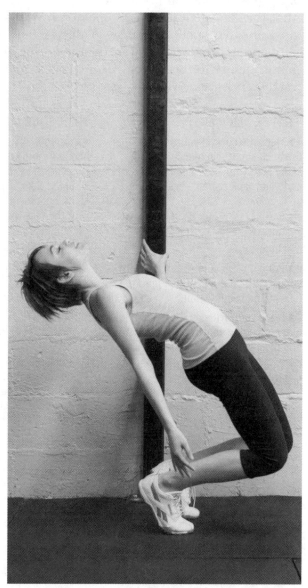

Hack Squat

While free weights (like dumbbells and barbells) will help to target your body in motion, machines are also a great addition to your workout routine. The best thing about machines is that they isolate a body part, making it very safe to use them when recovering from an injury in an unrelated spot. Of course, if this is the case, you should be consulting your doctor before attempting any exercises. Form is still crucial when using machines. It's a myth that you automatically are in the correct form when seated at a machine. Be careful to position yourself correctly. Try varying your foot position to target different parts of your quads.

PROPER ALIGNMENT

❶ Place the back of your torso against the hack squat machine back pad. Make sure your head is up at all times and your back remains against the pad.

❷ Position your shoulders under the shoulder pads provided on the machine.

❸ Put your legs in a shoulder-width stance with your feet on the platform, toes pointed slightly out.

❹ Place your arms on the side handles of the machine above your shoulders and disengage the safety bars.

❺ Your legs should be straight without locking your knees.

TECHNIQUE AND FORM

❶ Begin to slowly lower the unit by bending your knees. Inhale and continue down until your thighs are parallel to the floor. The fronts of the knees should make an imaginary straight line with the toes that is perpendicular to the thighs.

❷ During the movement, your back will move along the pad (but the pad win stay in one place).

❸ Exhale and begin to raise the unit by pushing the platform with your toes, straightening your legs, and returning to the starting position.

❹ Remember to pause slightly at the top of the movement, making sure that your lowering is as measured as possible, in order to remain in perfect form.

Hack Squat

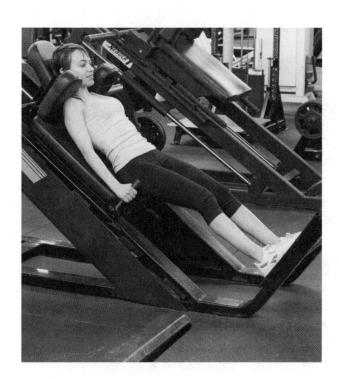

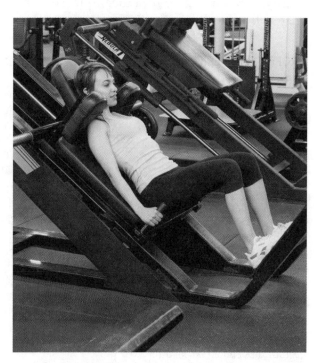

Front Squat

If you are new to this exercise, use less weight. The squat is very safe, but only if performed properly, and this particular squat may be best suited for advanced athletes. If you have back problems, substitute the dumbbell squat variation or a leg press for the front squats. If you do perform this exercise, maintain perfect form and never slouch forward because this can cause injury. Try varying your stance to target a different muscle group in your quadriceps. This exercise is best performed inside a squat rack for safety.

PROPER ALIGNMENT

❶ Set the bar on a squat rack that best matches your height. A small block can be placed under the heels to improve balance.

❷ Bring your arms up under the bar, keeping your elbows high and your upper arms slightly above parallel to the floor.

❸ Rest the bar on top of the deltoids and cross your arms while grasping the bar for full control.

❹ Lift the bar off the rack by pushing with you legs while straightening your torso.

❺ Step away from he rack and position your legs with a shoulder-width stance.

❻ Your toes should be pointing slightly out and your head should be up at all times to keep your back straight.

TECHNIQUE AND FORM

❶ Inhale and bend your knees slowly and continue down until your thighs are slightly parallel to the floor. The fronts of your knees should not be past your toes. If you do this, you are placing undue stress on the knee and doing the exercise incorrectly

❷ Raise the bar again, exhale and push the floor with your toes to straighten your legs and return to the starting position.

❸ Pause for a second at the top of the movement before performing the rest of the repetitions required. This allows you to ensure you are not using momentum to continue from one repetition to the next.

Front Squat

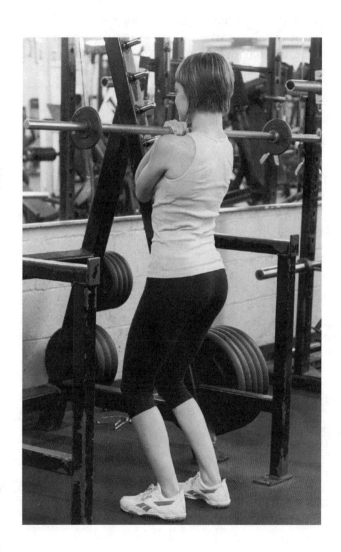
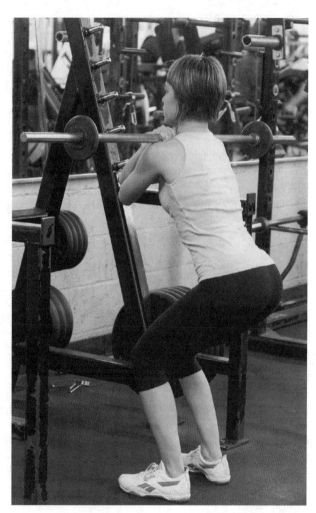

Dumbbell Lunge

This exercise is an excellent movement for all of the muscles in the legs. It primarily stresses the quads, buttocks and hamstring muscles with a secondary emphasis on the calf muscles. This exercise can also be performed with a barbell on the back. The barbell variation can place more stress on the lower back, but because you do not have to hold the dumbbells you might be able to concentrate better on your form. If you do choose to use a barbell, please make sure to first practice the dumbbell version for superior balance and coordination of the movement. Use the same steps described below and start out with no weight, until you feel capable and confident about using heavier weights.

PROPER ALIGNMENT

❶ Hold a dumbbell in each hand with arms extended down and palms facing your body.

❷ Align your body from the bottom up, first taking a stance with the feet together and the toes pointing straight ahead.

❸ Keep your knees slightly bent to avoid any stress from locking the knee joint.

❹ Slightly contract the abdominal muscles.

❺ Stick the chest out while simultaneously bringing the shoulder blades back, keeping them there throughout the movement.

❻ Keep your head level at all times, making sure your head and your eyes do not drop down or excessively wander upward.

TECHNIQUE AND FORM

❶ Step forward with your right foot.

❷ Bend at the knee making sure you descend slowly and in control.

❸ As your knee bends and your hips descend, only lower yourself until your left knee is about two inches from the ground and then stop.

❹ When you step forward at the beginning of the movement, make sure to position yourself so that the knee does not go past the toes when you are in the bent-knee position with your left knee two inches from the ground.

❺ Begin to reverse the movement by pressing off the right foot only. You may naturally want to use the left knee to assist in pushing back up, but do not let this happen. The objective is to fully isolate the right leg muscles and use the left leg only as a balancing tool, sort of like the rudder on a boat.

❻ Make sure you do not use momentum as you push off with the right leg to return. This will totally inhibit the stimulation of the leg muscles.

❼ Return to the start position but do not rest. Switch legs and repeat the same movement making sure to maintain the alignment and posture throughout the movement.

FAQ:
Isn't the lunge nothing more than a fancy second-rate exercise?

ANSWER:
When done correctly, lunges are actually one of the best leg exercises you can do to both build and strengthen the entirety of your leg muscles.

Dumbbell Lunge

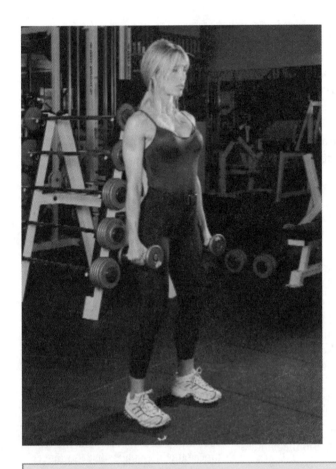

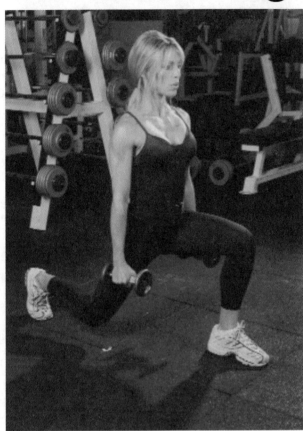

FAQ:
If squats can be dangerous, what about lunges?

ANSWER:
Any exercise can be dangerous if you don't pay attention to proper form, anatomical alignment, and exercise technique. with squats, because both feet are planted on the ground, both areas of the lower back become vulnerable. Also, because the lower back muscles (Errector Spinae) are working to hold your lumbar curve, they can become considerably exhausted during the exercise.

Lunges, on the other hand, work one leg at a time. This independent work also affects the lower back muscles-but differently than the squat. In other words, while one leg is working, the other side of your body is actually being guarded from exhaustion. Remember, muscular endurance is just how long a muscle can endure under tension. With squats, it's all or nothing. With lunges, you can pace yourself.

Lunges also really emphasize the negative (lengthening) phase of the exercise. The range of motion required to perform a lunge correctly is also usually much greater than with squats. Make sure to step in slowly with the lunge; going too quickly can be very dangerous to your lower back, knees, and many other areas of the body.

Leg Press

The leg press machine is a great exercise for all of the leg muscles. It can be used in place of the traditional barbell squat or to supplement your leg routine. If you are in a rush to get through your workout, this would be an opportune time to use the leg press exercise over the squat, due to the decreased set up time for the leg press exercise.

There are two ways to perform this exercise: One leg at a time or both legs at the same time. In this book we will discuss the more common two-legged version. However, the execution for the exercise remains the same for both versions. The leg press can also be performed on a plate-loaded machine. Note: Please make sure not to attempt to use very heavy weights if you decide to try the one-legged version of the exercise.

PROPER ALIGNMENT

❶ Sit on the machine with your back on the padded support and align your feet evenly on the platform. The height placement of your feet on the platform will zone in on different areas of the quadriceps. The higher your foot placement on the platform the less intense the quad contraction and the less knee involvement.

The lower your foot placement on the platform, the more intense the quad contraction will be; but you will put a lot of stress and shear force on the knees.

❷ Make sure that your back and head are kept flush against the back pad and that you are seated securely in the seat.

❸ Take hold of the release lever handles and disengage the lock pins.

TECHNIQUE & FORM

❶ Immediately take hold of the secured handles, which are usually located to the sides of you. If the handles are placed in an awkward position, you can also take hold of the seat edge. This can help take some stress off the lower back.

❷ With the feet spaced evenly apart and flat upon the platform, slowly lower the sled towards you.

❸ Once again, do not grip the handles too tightly.

❹ Let the sled come down to a point just before your thighs would touch your chest. Depending on your condition, you might not want to bring the sled this low. Monitor your individual situation. Too many trainees don't allow the sled to go deep enough to sustain any type of quad muscle involvement, and they'll pack on the weights. Lighten the weight and tone!

❺ When you have reached the bottom portion of the exercise, return back to the starting position by slowly pushing the platform evenly with both feet. Do not lock your knees! This could injure your knees and will also take the resistance off of the quads, distributing it directly to the knee joints.

FAQ:

If I have a lower back injury, is the leg press a good choice for a leg exercise? I assume this is the case because it's a seated exercise.

ANSWER:

Actually, the leg press can be much more harmful than any other leg exercise, when you have an injured lower back. This doesn't have to be the case, so you must follow some advice to avoid further injury. One of the best exercises you can do on the leg press, if you are concerned with your lower back, is the one-legged press. Working just one leg at a time prevents you from lifting your back from its correct position. While one leg is working, the other is planted and supporting correct form. You must be careful, though-don't go too heavy. Make sure to stay steady during the movement; any jerking can disrupt your form and possibly injure your lower back.

Leg Press

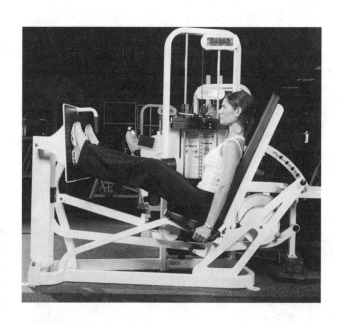 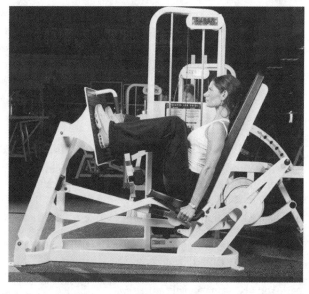

VARIATION

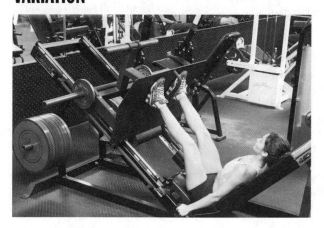 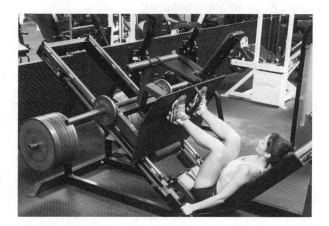

Leg Extension

This exercise can be a miracle when it comes to really zoning in on the quadriceps muscles, located right on the front of the upper leg area. This exercise also helps strengthen the knees, which are a commonly injured area. The leg extension is recommended by most physical therapists as a good exercise for knee rehabilitation. Please take note: The key to the effectiveness and safety of this exercise is to choose a machine whose starting position allows your toes to be right in front of your knees. A machine in which your toes start behind your knees (with the upper leg and the lower leg at an angle of below 90-degrees) can cause injury to the knee.

There are two ways to perform this exercise: one leg at a time or both legs at the same time. In this book we will discuss the more common two-legged version. However, the execution for the exercise remains the same for both versions. Note: Please make sure not to attempt to use very heavy weights if you decide to try the one-legged version of the exercise.

PROPER ALIGNMENT

❶ Seat yourself on the machine and position the back pad so that you are sitting totally upright.

❷ The back of your knees must be pressed flush against the front of the seat, which will help you avoid a potential knee injury caused by allowing the knee to hang over the seat without support. You also want to make sure that the axis of the knees are in line with the machine axis, helping to set up the proper alignment (biomechanics) of the knee and direct the maximum resistance to the quadriceps. In addition, ensure that the starting position allows the toes to be in front of the knees and that the upper leg and lower leg create a 90-degree angle.

❸ Adjust the shin roller pad against the lowest point of the shin to help optimize the shin as a lever and the knee as the fulcrum. This will again help to direct the majority of the resistance to the thigh muscles. Before you begin the exercise, lightly grip the handles provided or grab the front of the seat on each side of your legs.

TECHNIQUE AND FORM

❶ Begin the exercise with your legs totally relaxed and your shins behind the roller pad positioned at the bottom.

❷ Isometrically contract the quad muscles and slowly begin to lift the weight by lifting the roller pad with the shins.

❸ As you extend upward, stay in control by allowing the quad muscles to lift the weight. Do not use momentum or leverage. This is a very easy exercise to cheat on by using quick bursts of momentum at the bottom of the movement, or by leaning back and using leverage to lift the weight.

❹ As you reach the point of full extension, when the part of your leg below your knee is extended and as close as possible to being in a direct line with your upper thigh, focus only on fully contracting the quad muscles. Sometimes people have the tendency to go through the exercise motions without consciously contracting the muscles that are supposed to be lifting the weight. As long as you make a great

effort to contract the quad muscle fully at the top of full extension, you will be taking full advantage of the exercise.

❺ Make sure that once you get to the fully extended position of the exercise, you don't just let the leg drop but slowly return back to the beginning of the movement.

❻ As you reach the bottom, do not rest! Slowly and smoothly lift the roller pad with your shins back to full extension. Always make sure that you are going through the full range of motion for these exercises as doing so will provide the maximum muscular development.

Leg Extension

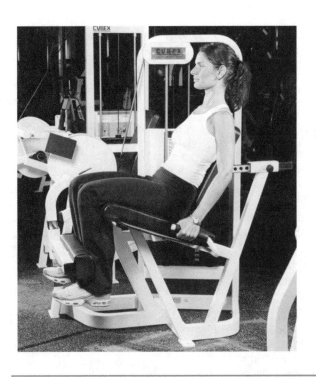

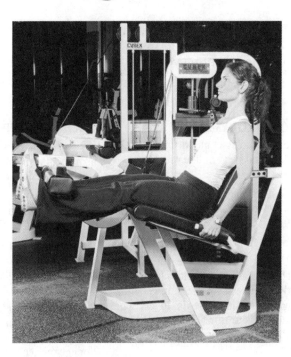

FAQ:

I've seen people using lots of momentum when they do this exercise. Should I move as much weight as possible, even if I don't feel my quads being stimulated?

ANSWER:

The purpose for doing any exercise is to stimulate the muscles you are working. In other words, if you don't feel the muscle really contract (especially at the top of the movement), and you instead feel your joints taking the brunt of the exercise, you are doing more harm than good to your body.

The point of this exercise is to put full emphasis on the front of your thighs (quadriceps). If you don't feel these muscles working, you're either going too heavy or you may not be a good fit for that machine. Some are built for a different shape of body. Make certain that your lower back is supported by the back pad and that the backs of your knees lie flush against the seat pad. Adjust the shin pad so that it is between the top of your foot and your shin.

If that doesn't work, try another leg extension machine and go just heavy enough so that it is a challenge, but not where you need momentum and joint support to move the weight. You should not be using momentum. If you are, the weight you are using is too heavy.

Adductor Machine

The Adductor Machine is a great isolator for the inner thigh muscle group. Make sure you do not set the machine to too wide of a position. To increase the challenge of this exercise, sit straight up without resting your back against the back pad as you perform your repetitions.

PROPER ALIGNMENT

1 Sit on the machine with your back straight and head in line with your spine.

2 Position the pads on either side so that they rest against your inner thighs.

3 Select the weight you choose to use.

4 Use the handles at the side of the machine to adjust the width (range of motion) between your legs. In general, he width should cause you to feel some tension in your inner thighs in the start position but not place great strain on them.

TECHNIQUE AND FORM

1 Once you arc in the proper position, exhale as you bring your legs towards each other, maintaining tension throughout the movement.

2 Pause for a moment at the top of the movement to eliminate momentum.

3 Inhale as you separate your legs and return to the starting position. Repeat for the suggested number of repetitions.

4 If you have to exert a lot of effort to bring your legs together, or begin to compensate by using your back or torso, you need to either lighten the weight or reduce your range of motion (the width between the pads).

Adductor Machine

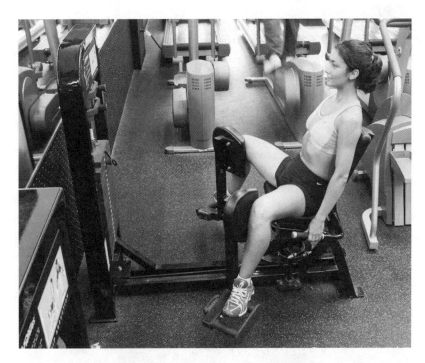

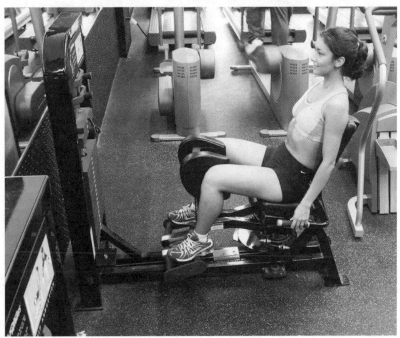

Abductor Machine

The Abductor Machine is a great isolator for the outer thigh muscle group. Machines are extremely useful when you need to work around an injury to prevent further harm.

PROPER ALIGNMENT

❶ Sit on the machine with your back straight and your head in line with your spine.

❷ Use the handles at the sides of the machine to bring your legs to where they are nearly touching.

❸ Position the pads on either side of your legs so that they rest against your outer thighs. This is your starting position.

TECHNIQUE AND FORM

❶ Once you are in the proper position, exhale as you separate your legs, maintaining tension throughout. the movement.

❷ Pause for a moment at the top of the movement to eliminate momentum.

❸ Inhale as you bring your legs closer together, returning to the starting position. Repeat for the suggested number of repetitions.

❹ To increase the challenge of this exercise, sit straight up without resting your back against the back pad as you perform your repetitions.

Abductor Machine

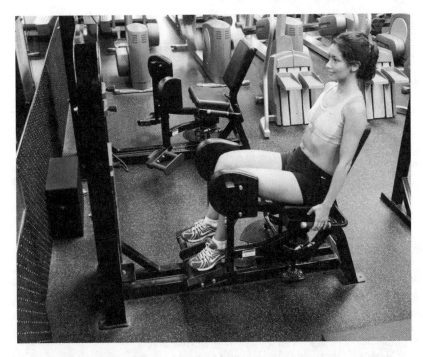

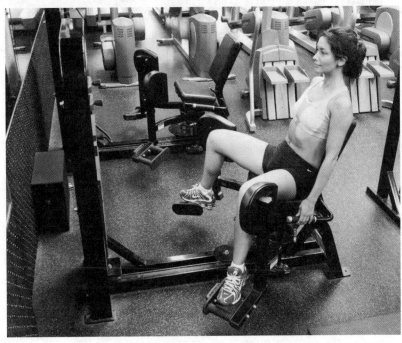

Butt Blaster

This machine hones the gluteal muscles by isolating them one leg at a time. A freeweight alternative that works in much the same fashion is the squat.

PROPER ALIGNMENT

❶ Select the weight with the machine's pins.

❷ Get on your hands and knees. holding on to the handles at the front of the machine.

❸ Lift your right leg up behind you, keeping it bent at a 90-degree angle. If the machine has a platform, place the sole of the right foot against the platform.

❹ Keep your abdominals pulled in and your back flat it's important that you keep your bark as flat as a table throughout the entire range of motion to avoid injuring your lower back.

TECHNIQUE AND FORM

❶ Once you are in the starting position, exhale and press your right leg up as you simultaneously squeeze your gluteal muscles.

❷ When you reach the top position, hold for a count or two before lowering almost to the start position.

❸ Do not allow the platform to come entirely down to the starting position. This makes sure you are maintaining tension in your muscles as you begin your next repetition.

❹ If you feel any pain in your lower back, lighten up on the weight or select a different exercise for the gluteals.

❺ Repeat for the recommended number of repetitions, then switch the working leg and repeat.

Butt Blaster

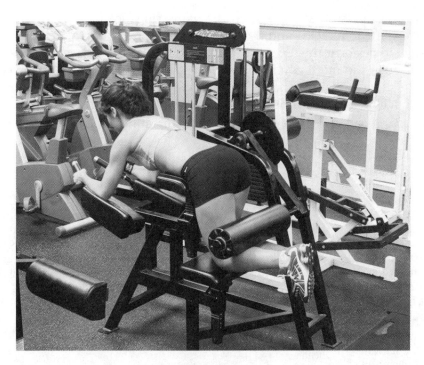

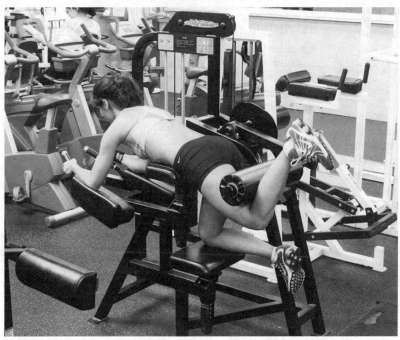

Lying Leg Curl

The lying leg curl is an exercise that focuses on the hamstrings located on the back of the upper leg. It also affects the gluteal muscles and the muscles of the lower back (erector spinae).

There are two ways to perform this exercise: one leg at a time or both legs at the same time. In this book we will discuss the more common two-legged version. However, the execution for the exercise remains the same for both versions. Note: Please make sure not to attempt to use very heavy weights if you decide to try the one-legged version of the exercise.

VARIATION: Some gyms will not have a lying leg curl machine, but they do have a seated leg curl machine. You can use this machine instead.

PROPER ALIGNMENT

There are several machines for training the hamstring muscles, but we recommend the lying leg curl machine. If you prefer, you may use the seated leg curl machine instead. Both are good; however, we believe the lying machine is superior. No matter which machine you choose, the alignment will basically be the same.

1 Position yourself on the machine and, as always, begin the alignment of your body starting with your feet.

2 Lock your pelvis into place by contracting your abdominal muscles.

3 Try to focus only on the hamstring muscles.

4 When you're lying down, relax your upper body. (Allowing your body to stay tense during the exercise will only negatively affect hamstring stimulation.) If you like, you can hold on to the set of handles, which are usually supplied. Just make sure you do so with a very light grip. Squeezing too hard can change the focus of resistance in the hamstring muscles, causing this exercise to be less beneficial. Holding too tight can also cause leverage to do the work for you instead of working the muscle. Remember, don't sell yourself short trying to find the easy way of exercising. You are here to work, not to

make things easy. Besides, work is what produces results.

5 Relax your neck and head. If you choose the seated leg curl machine, you should follow the same form; that is, space your feet evenly.

6 Keep your knees pointed directly in front of you throughout the movement.

7 Contract your abdominal muscles and relax your upper body, neck and head.

TECHNIQUE AND FORM

1 As you begin the movement, contract the hamstrings before actually moving as this will help to focus the resistance on the hamstring muscles and better stimulate the muscles.

2 Drive your heels to your butt, while pointing (this is very important) your toes toward your knees ("flexing your feet"). It will be the same whether sitting or lying down. Pointing your toes towards your knees helps to better isolate the hamstring muscles. Refer to the pictures labeled "relaxed" and "flexed".

3 When you reach your butt, try to hold that position for a count of two seconds. This will help increase the intensity of the exercise; and, once again, better stimulate the hamstring muscles.

4 As you descend, do so with a slow, controlled movement. When you reach the starting position, without rest, slowly and smoothly change directions, moving upward once again. Following these guidelines will ensure your safety and greater results.

FAQ:

This is the only exercise I've been doing for my hamstrings. is it enough?

ANSWER:

You should be doing a variety of exercises that stimulate the hamstrings. While the lying leg curl machine is a great isolation exercise, there are plenty of other exercises that will incorporate parts of the hamstrings and help to fully develop this muscle. They include, but are not limited to: stiff-legged deadlift, standing leg curl, seated leg curl, glute-ham raise, and step-up.

Lying Leg Curl

FLEXED

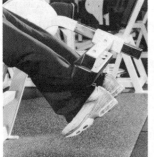
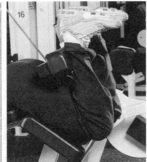

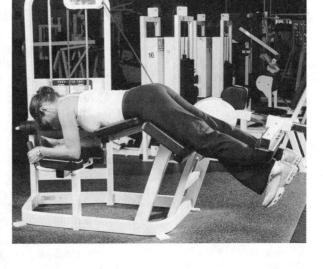

RELAXED

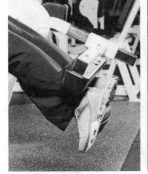
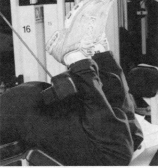

VARIATION

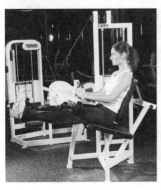
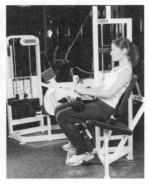

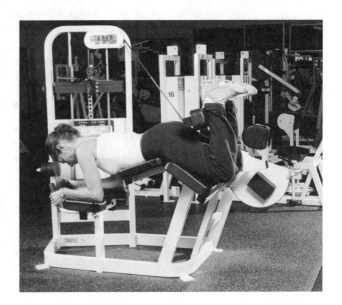

135

Standing Hamstring Curl

This version of the hamstring curl isolates the hamstring muscles and, because you are working just one leg at a time, helps you to address any imbalances you may have in your legs.

PROPER ALIGNMENT

❶ Stand next to the lever arm of the machine so that it is to the right of your leg.

❷ Hook your right heel under the roller pad. Depending on the machine you use, you will either be kneeling on a kneel rest with your left leg, or standing with your left leg on a platform.

TECHNIQUE AND FORM

❶ Keeping your upper right leg (from the knee to the hip) in place, exhale and curl your right foot up as high as it can go.

❷ At the top of the movement, squeeze the hamstring muscles hard and hold for one to two seconds. Tie sure you are using muscular contraction and not momentum to curl your leg.

❸ Lower your right foot in a controlled motion, inhaling as you do so.

❹ Repeat for the recommended number of repetitions for one leg, then switch sides to work the other leg.

❺ If you find you are arching your back or using your shoulders to help you to contract, you are using momentum. If this is the case, you should reduce the weight you are using.

Standing Hamstring Curl

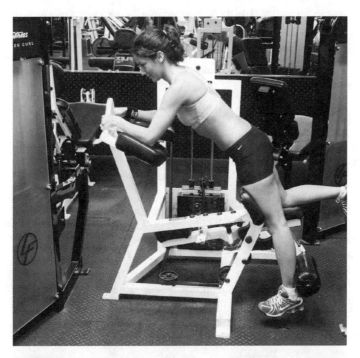

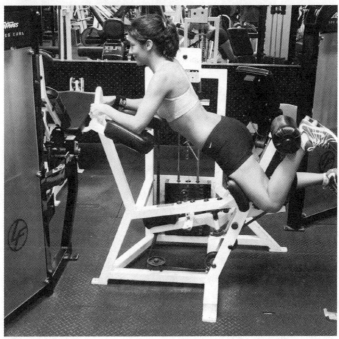

Step-Up

There are a couple of variations to this basic exercise. You can try performing all repetitions on one leg at a time, as well as using a barbell instead of dumbbells. Once again, using a barbell instead of dumbbells protects your wrists from injury caused by twisting.

PROPER ALIGNMENT

❶ Choose a weight appropriate to your skill level. If you are just starting out, try this exercise with just your body weight.

❷ Position your feet shoulder-width apart, pointing your toes forward. You will be approximately half a foot behind an elevated platform like a step or flat 10 pound weights on the ground.

❸ Hold the dumbbells at your sides, palms facing each other.

❹ Stand up straight, your knees straight but not locked, with your chest out, shoulders back, and eyes forward.

TECHNIQUE AND FORM

❶ Begin the movement by placing your right foot on the elevated platform, making sure that your heel and toe make solid contact, and neither are off the edge.

❷ Step up fully onto the platform by extending the hip and the knee of your right leg.

❸ Use the heel to lift the rest of your body up and place the foot of the left leg on the platform as well. Exhale as you push up.

❹ Inhale and step down with your left leg by flexing the hip and knee of the right leg.

❺ Return to the original standing position by placing the right foot next to the left foot.

❻ Repeat this exercise, alternating legs, until you have performed the number of repetitions required.

Step-Up

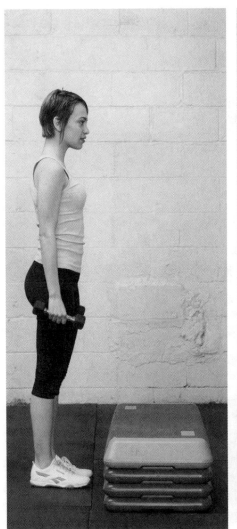 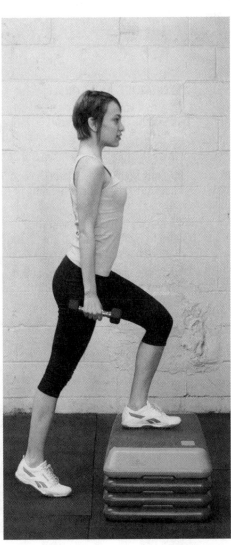 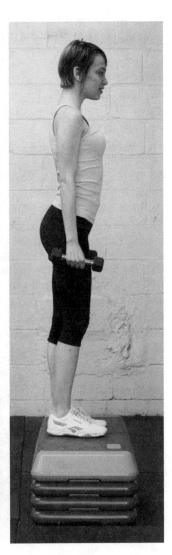

Glute-Ham Raise

The glute-ham raise is a great way to work your hamstrings, although it can be dangerous if you are a beginner. It's crucial to have a spotter if you are new to this exercise. It can also be hard on your lower back, so be careful if you have injuries. To make this easier, have your spotter assist you in getting to the upright position. If you are looking for a way to increase resistance, add weight by holding a plate to your chest.

PROPER ALIGNMENT

❶ You will need to use a pull-down machine for this exercise. First, adjust the padded supports of the machine as far down as possible.

❷ Kneel upright on the seat of the machine, facing away from it. Use a partner's support if necessary.

❸ Place your ankles between the padded supports and your feet flat against the platform where typically your thighs would sit. There should be a 90 degree angle created by the upper and lower leg.

❹ Hold your arms down by your sides, and keep your shoulders back and your chest up.

TECHNIQUE AND FORM

❶ Bring your torso forward slowly. You should be thrusting your hips forward and straightening your knees slightly.

❷ As the torso comes down, inhale.

❸ Only your knees should be bending. Make sure you are not bending at the waist.

❹ As you exhale, pull your body upright by flexing at the knees until you are back In the original position.

❺ Pause slightly at the top of the movement, then resume with the next repetition.

Glute-Ham Raise

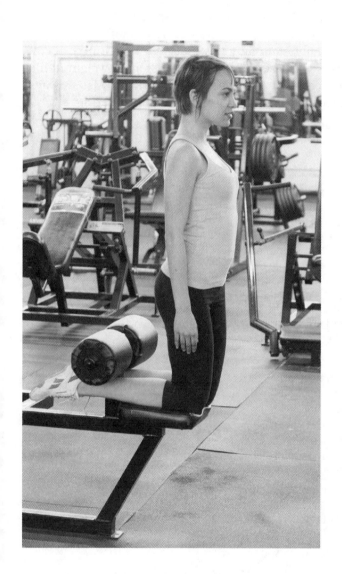 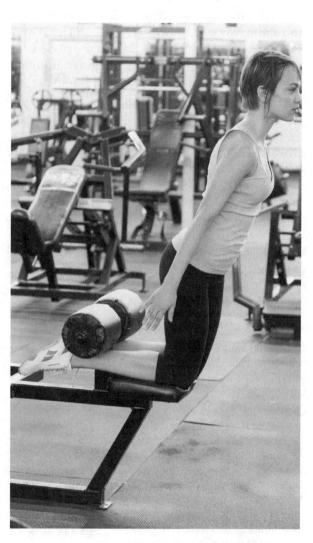

Stiff-Legged Deadlift

The stiff-legged deadlift is a very good exercise for the hamstring muscles located between your butt and knees. This is also a great exercise for the lower back muscles also known as the 'erectors'. If you have a lower back injury, we advise that you don't do this exercise. Although it is a fantastic exercise to help strengthen the lower back, if you already have a lower back injury, it can do more harm than good. If you do decide to try this exercise, first start out using no weight at all. By simply going through the exercise motion, you can feel the hamstrings working. Also, always make sure that you have warmed the muscles of the lower back thoroughly before starting.

VARIATION: Try this exercise with a barbell to best support your wrists.

PROPER ALIGNMENT

❶ Choose a weight for your barbell or dumbbells, making sure that it is light enough to practice perfect form.

❷ Position your feet shoulder-width apart, pointing straight ahead at all times during the movement.

❸ Position your hands on the barbell with a grip wider than your feet position. Your hands positioned slightly outside your foot stance should be adequate.

❹ Stand up straight and hold the barbell across your thighs or the dumbbells at your side with your palms facing toward your legs.

❺ The object here is to keep your legs completely straight, staying locked at the knee joints and bending forward at the waist. It is very, very important to make sure you keep your back completely straight while bending forward. We recommend that as you bend down, you keep your head and eyes looking straight ahead and level. If you look down at the ground, you will be very likely to hyper-flex your spine and cause a lower back injury.

TECHNIQUE AND FORM

Before you begin the exercise and throughout the execution, you must direct all of your focus to the hamstring muscles of the rear thigh, to help activate them even more. "Put your mind in the muscle!" When you return to the starting top position of the exercise, focus on the erector muscles of the lower back by slightly arching the spine and sticking the chest out, contracting those lower back muscles.

❶ With your body straight, legs locked and arms hanging down, begin the exercise by bending over at the waist.

❷ Remember to look straight ahead as you bend over. Your eyes must be looking level with your body as you reach parallel to the floor.

❸ As you bend over, concentrate on the hamstring muscles of the thigh and make sure your back is straight as you lower yourself.

❹ As you reach a point where your torso is parallel to the floor and the bar or dumbbells are fairly close to touching the floor, slowly and without rest begin lifting your body back up from the waist, concentrating on focusing all of the work to the hamstring muscles of the thigh. Do not use any momentum during this movement, especially at this position! You will really feel the hamstring muscles contract in the lower position as you slowly change directions and begin your way upward.

❺ Keep your head and eyes looking straight ahead as you return to the standing position.

❻ As you return to the start position, really contract your hamstring muscles, but don't stop there. As you stand straight up, stick your chest way out and slightly arch your spine while you contract the muscles of the lower back.

❼ Hold that position for only one second, then slowly and smoothly begin lowering your body again, maintaining the same exact form as when you began the exercise.

Stiff-Legged Deadlift

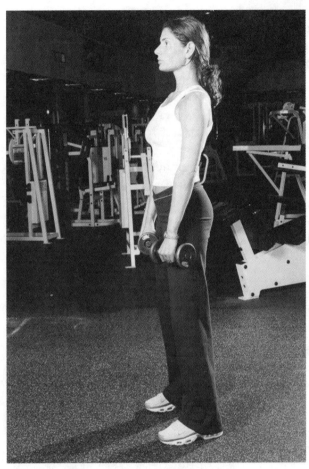

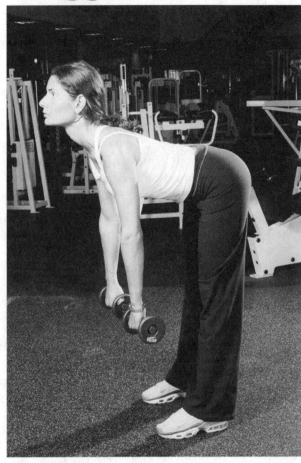

VARIATION

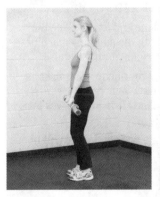

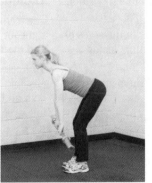

FAQ:
I see many people doing this exercise and they are looking down at the ground while doing it.

ANSWER:
Looking at the ground while doing this or any exercise in a similar stance (for example, squats, lunges, dead-lifts, etc.), can be detrimental to your safety and could even "hamstring" your results. Looking down at the ground while doing this exercise round out your lower back and puts your lower back muscles in a very vulnerable state. When you round the low back instead of maintaining a lumbar curve, you have a very good chance of straining the lower back muscles.

Standing Calf Raise

The standing calf raise is a great tool for building quality calves. By using a pair of dumbbells to hold at your sides, you can create beautifully sculpted calves in the privacy of your home. Of course, you'll want to get yourself a pair of dumbbells that you can add extra weight to. I would recommend a pair of dumbbells which are made to hold heavier weights.

There are two ways to perform this exercise: One leg at a time or both legs at the same time. In this book we will discuss the more common two-legged version. However, the execution for the exercise remains the same for both versions. Note: Please make sure not to attempt to use very heavy weights if you decide to try the one-legged version of the exercise.

If your gym mops frequently, please make sure to dry the area or machine pad before doing calf raises. You could be seriously injured if your feet slip off the platform.

VARIATION: A variation of the standing calf raise is using just one leg. For this, you should make sure to have a fixed object nearby as support, like the beam of a squat rack. Simply work one leg at a time by holding the other behind you, bending its knee.

PROPER ALIGNMENT

For the machine:

❶ Set the weight to a resistance you can handle while practicing perfect form.

❷ Step on the platform and take hold of the grip bars on the sides of the shoulder harness.

❸ With your feet pointing straight ahead, place your toes and the balls of your feet on the platform.

❹ Set the shoulder pads so they will be slightly lower than your shoulders while you are in this position.

❺ Bend at the knees and position your shoulders underneath the shoulder pads comfortably.

❻ Stand up straight so that your shoulders lift the shoulder pads, which will lift the weight plates up.

❼ Keep your knees pointing straight ahead and keep them bent very slightly during the exercise. The bent-knee position can help stretch the calves in the lower position and will save your lower back in the upper position.

❽ Make sure to keep your body straight during the exercise. Be careful not to bend at the waist during any portion of the movement or hyperextend your back at the top of the movement. Doing either of these can injure your back.

❾ Stick your chest out and keep your shoulders squared at all times during the exercise.

❿ Keep your head straight and level and look straight ahead at all times.

For dumbbells:

❶ First, pick up the dumbbells and stand in front of a platform, which should be about 1 inch high.

❷ Step onto the platform and position your feet a couple of inches apart.

❸ Bring the dumbbells to the sides of your body, with your palms facing each other.

❹ Place your toes and the balls of your feet on the platform.

❺ Keep your knees pointing straight ahead and keep them bent very slightly during the exercise as the bent knee position can help stretch the calves in

the lower position and will save your lower back in the upper position.

❻ You must make sure to keep your body straight during the exercise. Be careful not to bend at the waist during any portion of the movement or hyperextend your back at the top of the movement. Doing either of these can injure your back.

❼ Stick your chest out and keep your shoulders squared at all times during the exercise.

❽ Keep your head straight and level and look straight ahead at all times.

TECHNIQUE AND FORM

The technique and form will be the same for both the standing machine and the standing dumbbell raise.

❶ Keeping your body as straight as possible, lower your heels toward the floor and slowly bring the calves to a full stretch.

❷ Hold this position for a count of one second.

Standing Calf Raise

❸ From this position, without momentum, push off the balls of your feet and come up onto your tiptoes, pushing as high off the toes as possible. Contract the calves as hard as you possibly can and concentrate all of your efforts on doing so. Hold this position for a one second count.

❹ Slowly begin lowering your body to the stretch position, making sure you make the calf muscles endure the negative portion of the resistance.

❺ As you reach the bottom position, with the heels pointing to the floor, make sure you do not allow your heels to drop too fast. Go slow and focus on the stretching of the calf muscles.

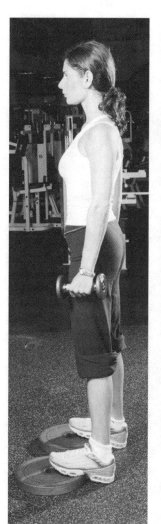
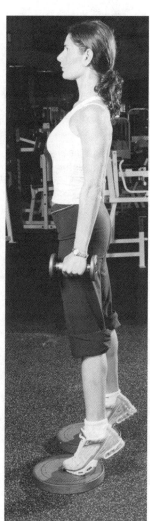

VARIATION

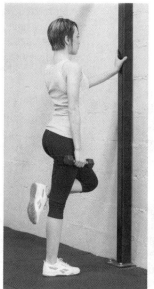
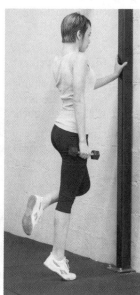

Multi-Directional Calf Raise

By performing a series of calf raises at different angles, you target all the muscle fibers involved in providing your calves with complete definition. For this exercise you won't be able to achieve a full stretch at the bottom unless you are on some kind of platform, but it is effective even without one.

PROPER ALIGNMENT

❶ Stand with your torso upright, holding two dumbbells in your hands by your side.

❷ Keep your abdomen pulled in and your shoulders back. Look straight ahead.

TECHNIQUE AND FORM

❶ With your toes pointing straight ahead, raise your heels off of the floor as you exhale by contracting the calves.

❷ Hold the top of the contraction for a second, then inhale while lowering your heels slowly to the starting position.

❸ Repeat for the desired number of repetitions.

❹ Move your feet into position for the next set of repetitions by pointing your toes towards each other, making about a six-inch gap between your heels. Raise your heels off of the floor as you exhale by contracting the calves.

❺ Hold the top of the contraction for a second, then inhale while lowering your heels slowly to the starting position.

❻ Repeat for the desired number of repetitions.

❼ Move your feet into position for the next set of repetitions by touching your heels together and pointing your toes out to the sides. There should be about a six-inch gap between your toes. Raise your heels off of the floor as you exhale by contracting the calves.

❽ .Hold the top of the contraction for a second, then inhale while lowering your heels slowly to the starting position.

❾ Repeat for the desired number of repetitions.

Multi-Directional Calf Raise

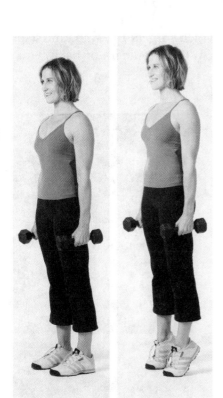
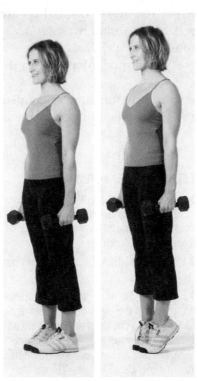
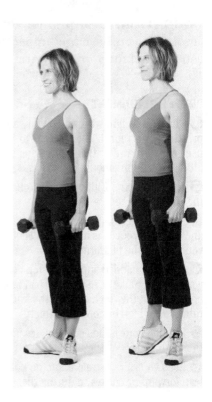

Seated Machine Calf Raise

This exercise primarily targets the muscle located underneath the gastrocnemius. This movement is an excellent tool for shaping the calves. But, although you might think that this exercise alone will develop the calves, it won't. You must train the calves over different angles to truly develop the calf muscles into a work of art. Some women are concerned that direct training of their calves will make them look masculine. Don't worry, it won't! Your calves will always look feminine, but they will now have a sexy and muscular tone to their appearance.

VARIATION: As a variation. try the standing machine calf raise, which targets the same muscle group. If you have any upper body weakness or injuries, especialy in the shoulders or back, you should not attempt this variation.

PROPER ALIGNMENT

❶ Choose a weight with which you can practice perfect form. The object is to use good form rather than just trying to lift a gargantuan amount of weight.

❷ Sit down and position your feet on the platform.

❸ With your feet pointing straight ahead, place your toes and the balls of your feet on the platform.

❹ Place the padded support on top of your thighs. Make sure that the pad fits snug against the thigh close to the knee rather than high on top of the thigh.

❺ Position your hands on the sides of the thigh pad.

❻ Keep your torso straight and do not lean forward or backward during the exercise.

❼ Keep your head straight and level and look straight ahead at all times.

TECHNIQUE AND FORM

❶ Once you are in position and ready to begin the exercise, lower your heels toward the floor and slowly bring the calves to a full stretch.

❷ Hold this position for a count of one to two seconds.

❸ From this position, without momentum, push off the balls of your feet and come up on to your tiptoes, pushing as high off the toes as possible. Contract the calves as hard as you possibly can and concentrate all of your efforts on doing so. Hold this position for a one to two second count.

❹ Slowly begin lowering your body back once again to the stretch position, making sure you make the calf muscles endure the negative portion of the resistance.

❺ As you reach the bottom position, with the heels pointing to the floor, make sure you do not allow your heels to drop too fast. Go slow and focus on the stretching of the calf muscles.

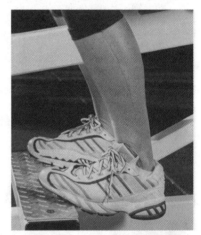

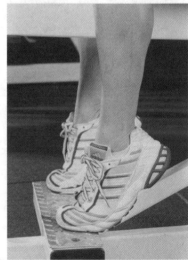

Seated Machine Calf Raise

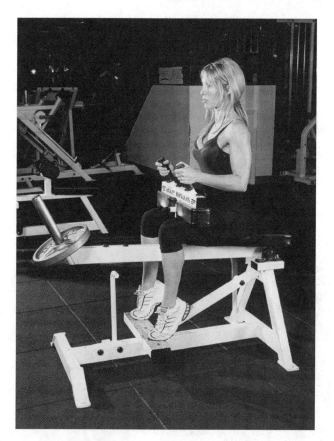 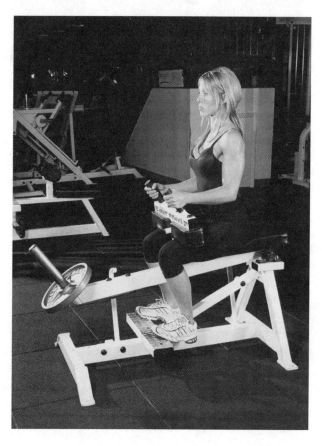

VARIATION

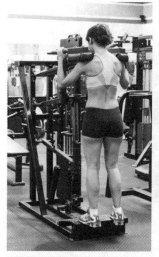 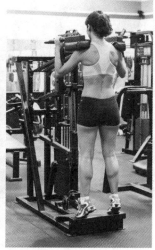

Donkey Calf Raise

This is a great exercise for the calves because it helps to develop the entire calf musculature. You have the option of performing this exercise in a few different ways. One way is with the use of a specially designed machine called the donkey calf press. Another way, is to use the assistance of another person. The form and technique are virtually identical except that your assistant actually sits on you!

We have also come up with our own variation of the donkey calf raise. Most of the gyms you frequent will have a piece of fitness gear called the "Dip Belt". It is a leather belt with an attached chain, allowing you to add weight plates. Look at the picture below to see how it looks and how it is used. Instead of using a machine or an assistant, you simply strap the belt to your waist, add weight and begin. Follow the same steps listed below with the exception of step #4 in proper alignment.

PROPER ALIGNMENT

❶ Take a firm grip on a bar or the rail of a staircase.

❷ Bend over at the hips, so that your torso is parallel to the floor.

❸ Place a four to five inch platform or piece of wood beneath your feet.

❹ Have your assistant sit upon the lumbar region of your lower back, making sure that he or she is secure. Your assistant must be sure not to move around or one of you could be seriously injured.

TECHNIQUE AND FORM

❶ Make sure that you are secure and in stable alignment.

❷ Begin by pressing up onto the tips of your toes, focusing on the entire calf area.

❸ Press up as high as you can and briefly hold the contraction.

❹ Slowly lower yourself, bringing the heels down towards the ground for a deep stretch. Do not go too deep.

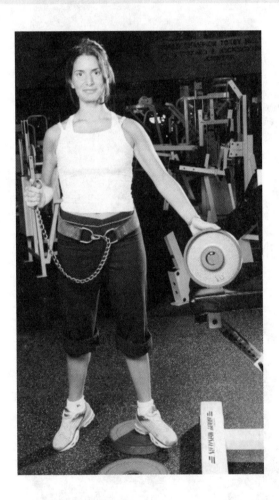

Donkey Calf Raise

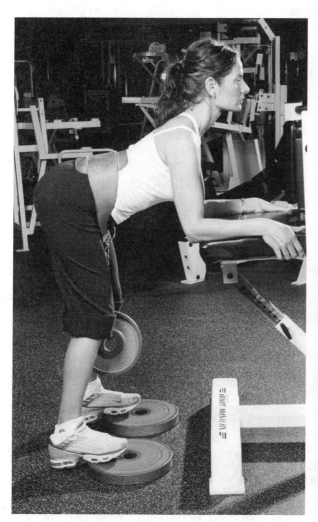 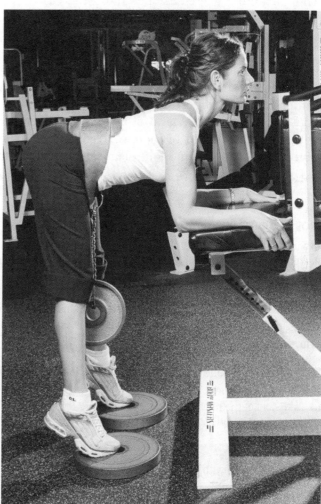

Calf Press

This particular exercise zones in on the gastrocnemius muscles of the calves. It is performed on the same machine you use for leg presses. This is an excellent alternative to standing calf raises and for people with lower back injuries.

At the top of the movement, make sure to really squeeze. The next time you're in the gym, look at how the average person performs a calf press or raise. You'll notice that their range of motion is extremely shallow. This might be because they are using too much weight or they simply don't understand the importance of getting a full range of motion. If you do use a full range of motion, you can do less work and still see much better results than someone doing much more work with a limited range of motion. Please note: If you do have an injury that prevents you from using a full range of motion, please go according to what works better for you.

VARIATION: The calf press may also be accomplished on a plate-loaded machine.

PROPER ALIGNMENT

❶ Step on to the platform of the machine and place your feet about 3-5 inches apart.

❷ Load the machine with the desired resistance.

❸ Position your feet on the platform so only the upper edge of your feet rests on the platform. The other half will hang off the platform.

❹ Take hold of the handles, usually located to the sides of the machine.

❺ Try to keep the legs straight during the exercise with your knees slightly bent.

TECHNIQUE AND FORM

❶ Maintaining your form, raise up onto the tips of your toes as high as you can and hold.

❷ Focus on contracting the calf muscles at this point. It is one thing to just do the movement, it is another to intensely participate in it!

❸ Slowly lower yourself, bringing the heels towards you for a deep stretch. Do not go too deep.

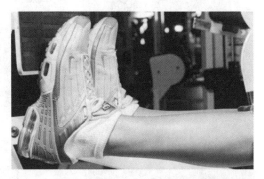

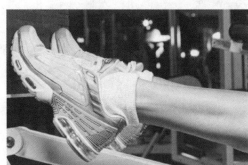

FAQ:

When I perform the calf press should I keep my knees locked?

ANSWER:

Locking out your knees can not only damage your knees, but actually takes away from stimulating your calf muscles. You may think that locking out your knees helps you to fully contract the calves, but you will actually be able to get a better range of motion by keeping a slight bend in both knees.

Calf Press

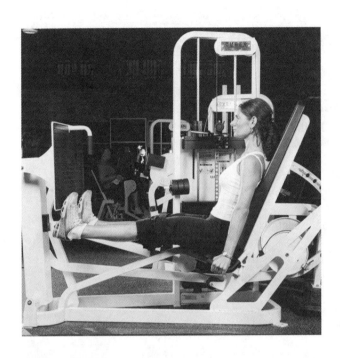 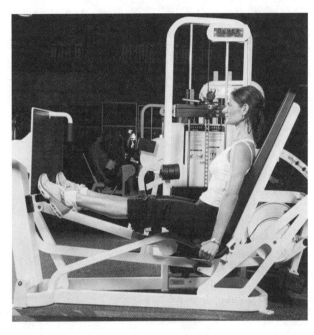

VARIATION

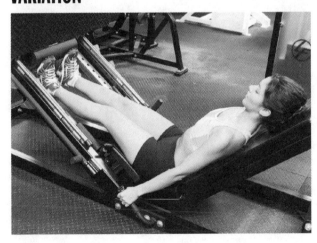 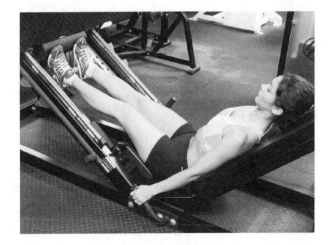

Tibia Raise

This exercise works the front of your calves, and depends on your body weight as resistance. If you're interested in making it more difficult and need to add resistance, you can hold a dumbbell between your feet (squeezing your feet together to grip the dumbbell securely).

PROPER ALIGNMENT

❶ Pull a calf block or other type of raised platform up to a fixed object that can support your weight (like a squat rack).

❷ Step up onto the calf block, placing your heels on the forward edge. Your feet should be facing straight ahead, with toes pointing down and your legs slightly less than shoulder-width apart.

❸ Reach out with one arm to hold onto the fixed object to keep your torso in balance. You should not be using the object to take away from the resistance of the exercise.

TECHNIQUE AND FORM

❶ Lower your toes until they are at a comfortable position with your heels solidly on the calf block.

❷ Now exhale, and raise your toes towards you. Point them up as high as possible.

❸ Hold one second in the contracted position.

❹ Inhale while lowering your toes back to the original position.

❺ Pause for a moment at the bottom of the movement, then repeat for the recommended number of repetitions.

Tibia Raise

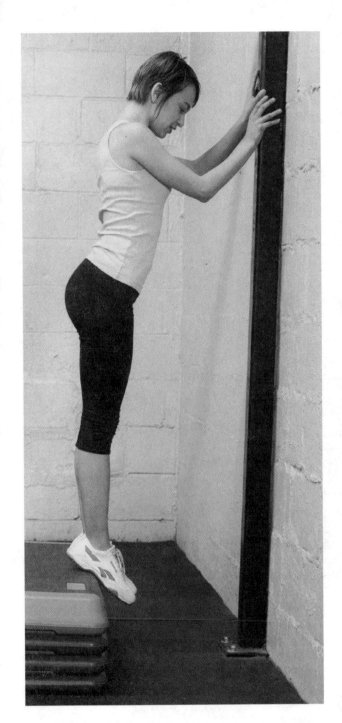
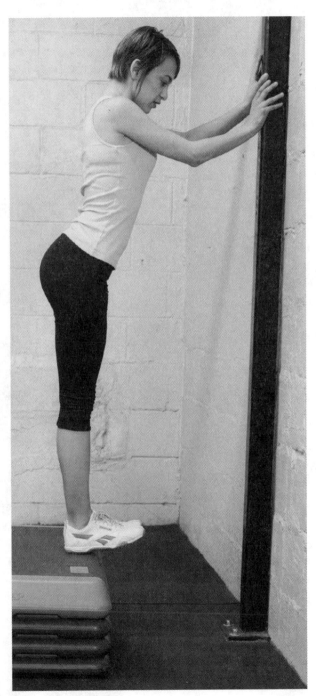

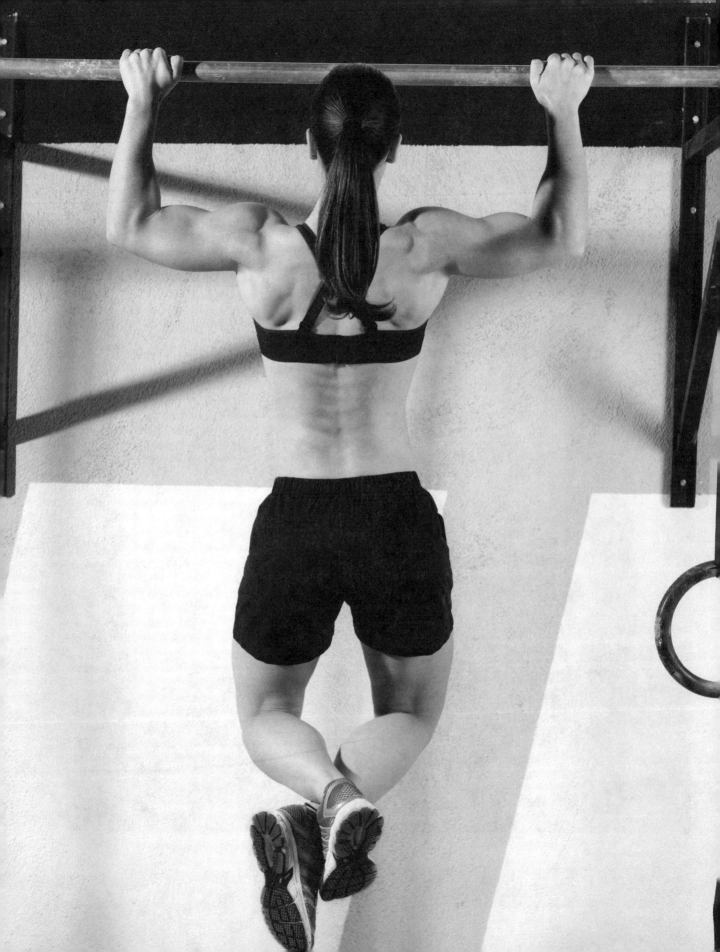

Chapter 7
Back

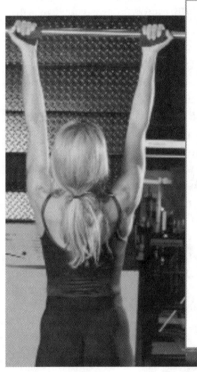

The back is composed of several different muscles. We will focus on the very best exercises for development of the back region. A toned and firm back makes your waist seem smaller and helps to keep your postural alignment nice and straight. Do not worry about that V-Taper look that some men are obsessed with achieving. These exercises and the outlined program will not put slabs of muscle on your body, unless of course your objective is to attain that look. By the end of the program, what you will see is your body, the way you expected to see it, beautiful! Pay attention to the proper alignment, technique and form principles as this will help to ensure your success.

For immediate Body Sculpting Bible support & coaching directly from James & Hugo, please visit www.BodySculptingBibles.com

7

THE **BODY**
SCULPTING
BIBLE
FOR**WOMEN**

EXERCISES THAT UTILIZE VARIOUS HAND POSITIONS AND HOW EACH VARIATION CAN AFFECT DIFFERENT MUSCLE GROUPS

Most people do not realize just how powerful a slight variation in your handgrip and hand position on the exercise bar can be. Even in virtually identical exercises, variation of your hand placement can stimulate completely different areas of muscle concentration.

Whether you choose a wide-grip or a narrow-grip, an overhand-grip or an underhand-grip, the area of muscle concentration will in some way be different. The enormous variety of exercise bar attachments available to us further enables us to attach many diversely shaped attachment bars to a pulley cable system. (If you are unaware of the large assortments of attachment bars available to you and how each works, refer to the web site resource page in the back of this book for further information).

You can perform exercise movements that are almost identical to one another, but a difference in exercise bars, hand placement, grip position and the mechanics of the body, can result in the stimulation of many different muscle groups.

Let's take pull-ups as an example. If you look at the differences between the wide-grip pull-up and the narrow-grip pull-up, you will notice that the wide-grip pull-up utilizes a wide and overhand grip placement. The narrow-grip pull-up utilizes a narrow and underhand grip placement. Now take a moment and think about what muscles are primarily working when you perform a wide-grip pull-up or a wide-grip pull-down. Because of the overhand-grip you take with these particular exercises, muscles such as the forearm muscles (extensor muscles), shoulder muscles (deltoids), and the back muscles (latissimus dorsi and erector spinae) will take a majority of the work efforts necessary to carry out these movements.

During the underhand narrow-grip pull-up, because of your underhand grip placement, the biceps muscles take the role of prime muscles involved during exercise execution. Although your focus should be to keep the biceps from becoming involved too much during this exercise and to instead concentrate on stimulation of the back muscles, it can be extremely difficult, if not impossible to completely avoid the participation of the biceps muscles.

In order to further increase your focus on specific muscle groups, you should practice the mind/muscle connection and muscle control techniques found within the Zone-Tone method.

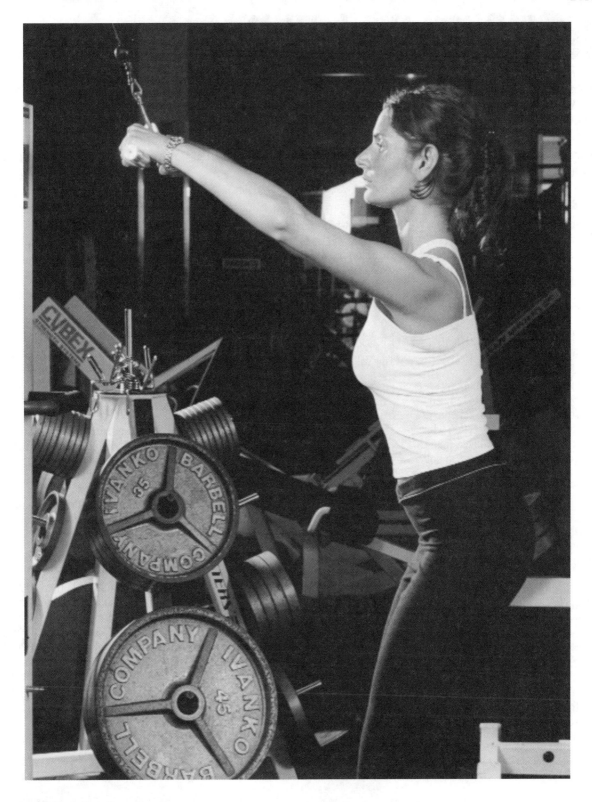

Bent-Over Barbell Row

The bent-over barbell row is an excellent exercise for the muscles of the mid back. It places primary emphasis on the mid back muscles and the outer back muscles (latissimus dorsi) with a secondary emphasis on the on the lower back, rear deltoids and biceps muscles. Please don't rush into using weights that are too heavy, which minimizes results and can give you a serious lower back injury. If you use proper form with lighter weights, your results will be terrific and you'll be lifting more weight in no time!

PROPER ALIGNMENT

❶ Place a bar in front of you on the ground, or on a rack level with your hips. Placing the bar any higher will just make it harder for you to lift it when the weights are increased.

❷ Align your feet about shoulder width apart.

❸ Make sure your knees are pointing directly in front of you throughout the movement.

❹ Bend over at the hips, making sure that your lower back is not slumped over. To make sure of this, squeeze or contract your abdominal section while slightly arching your low back, mimicking yourself sitting in a chair. Do not bend over all the way as this can injure the lower back. Bending at the hips to a position where your upper arm (triceps) can still follow directly towards the ceiling is sufficient for back muscle stimulation. If you stand too upright, this positioning will not sufficiently activate the back muscles. You can recognize this mistake by noticing that the back of your arms (triceps) are not following directly towards the ceiling and the focus of muscle activation in this case will most likely be the trapezoid muscles. You must be bent over to a degree where the elbows will naturally remain close to the body. At the same time, the back of the arms (triceps) follow a row-like movement, directly towards the ceiling.

❺ Pick up the bar using either a palms-down or a palms-up grip. The palms-down grip is recommended for beginners as with this grip there tends to be less biceps involvement. Advanced trainees can benefit from a palms-up grip as it stresses the "lats" in a more direct manner.

❻ Stick out your chest while slightly squeezing your shoulder blades together. This will position and keep your body in the proper alignment throughout the movement. Holding these alignment positions throughout the exercise will help make sure that stimulation remains in the back muscles.

❼ Keep your head up and looking straight ahead throughout the movement. This will help you keep your balance and make it easier to maintain the described position.

TECHNIQUE AND FORM

As you pick up the bar, think about what muscles you are about to exercise. The latissimus dorsi, also known as the "lats," are located on the outermost side of the back and are a good point focus.

❶ Align your body in the correct postural alignment.

❷ Let the bar hang down.

❸ Keep the elbows slightly wider than shoulder-width.

❹ Slightly squeeze the shoulder blades together.

❺ Begin rowing the elbows up toward the ceiling, allowing the back of the arms (triceps) to lead the motion.

❻ Drive the elbows and back of the arms upward until the barbell is touching your lower belly and you are able to fully contract the back muscles. Imagine that there is an egg in the middle of your back. Your objective for each repetition, when the bar is being pulled to your belly, is to crack the egg with your back muscles.

❼ Try to squeeze and hold that position for a 2-second count, focusing on an intense contraction of the back muscles. When you consciously squeeze the muscles at the top of the movement, you isolate specific muscles, increase their involvement, and optimize your workout.

❽ Begin your descent downward with a slow and controlled movement.

❾ As you reach the bottom, slowly and smoothly begin the movement upward again without resting. Make sure that no momentum is involved while changing over from the bottom position to the upward movement. Once again, when your form starts to get sloppy, STOP! Either reduce the weight or take a rest in preparation for the next set.

Bent-Over Barbell Row

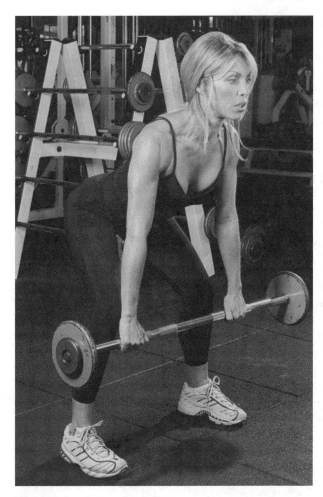
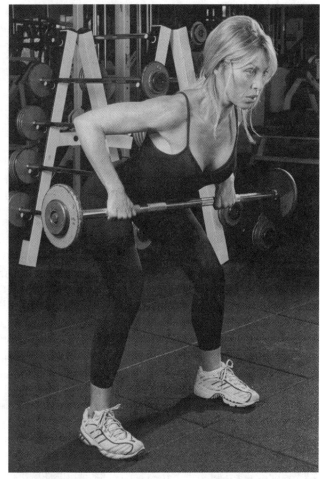

FAQ:

I sometimes see people bent over to a degree where their torso is completely parallel to the floor. Is this safe?

ANSWER:

No. When you bend over that much, you are more likely to injure your lower back. It is very important to maintain a lumbar curve in your lower back during this type of exercise. If you end to where your torso is parallel to the floor, it is not going to make the exercise any more effective-and is far more dangerous.

Dumbbell One-Arm Row

The dumbbell row emphasizes the same set of muscles as the bent-over barbell row with the added benefit of less lower back involvement. In addition, this exercise allows you to focus more on the back muscles because you will be doing one side at a time.

There are two ways to perform this exercise: one arm at a time or both arms at the same time (in which case the exercise will be identical to barbell rows except for the fact that the palms of the hands will be facing you). In this book we will discuss the more common one-arm version. This exercise variation is great if you have back problems or are concerned that you have not yet mastered the bent-over row exercise.

PROPER ALIGNMENT

This exercise is very similar to the bent-over row. You will be exercising the same muscle group, the back muscle; however, with the dumbbell row your position will be different and you will be exercising one limb at a time as opposed to two.

❶ To start, pick up a dumbbell that is light enough to focus primarily on form. Many people find that practicing perfect form with a light weight is much easier than practicing with no weight. The reason for this is because the resistance helps you to feel the desired muscle being exercised, making it easier to isolate and stimulate that muscle.

❷ Find a bench and set the dumbbell at the right side of it.

❸ Position your right foot on the floor while positioning your left knee on the bench. Your left hand should be positioned slightly in front of your body on the bench. Lean slightly into your left hand to help support your body weight. Here you will be training the right side of your back.

❹ Pick up the dumbbell with your right hand while remembering to support your body weight with your left hand.

❺ Your back should be parallel to the floor. The back should be flat as you lean over from the hips and you should be looking straight ahead to help maintain balance and form. Do not look down or up during the exercise.

TECHNIQUE AND FORM

As you pick up the dumbbell, think about the muscle you are about to exercise; the right side of the back called the latissimus dorsi, or the "lats."

❶ Align your body in the exercise's correct postural alignment.

❷ Let the dumbbell hang down.

❸ Slightly lift the right shoulder blade, making sure that it maintains a level position.

❹ Begin rowing the right elbow up toward the ceiling, allowing the back of the arms (triceps) to lead the motion.

❺ Row the right elbow and back of the right arm up towards the ceiling, and row as far as you can until the back of the arm and elbow reach the level of the torso. Make sure that you are fully contracting the right side of the back muscles. Imagine that there is an egg in the middle of your mid-back. Your objective, when the dumbbell is being rowed, is to squeeze the right side of the back muscles to the left and crack the egg with your back muscles.

❻ Try to squeeze and hold that position for a two-second count, focusing on an intense contraction of the back muscles.

❼ Begin your descent with a slow and controlled movement.

❽ As you reach the bottom, slowly and smoothly begin the movement upward again without resting. Make sure that no momentum is involved when changing over from the bottom position back to the upward movement. Again, when your form starts to get sloppy, STOP! Either reduce the weight, or take a rest in preparation for the next set.

Dumbbell One-Arm Row

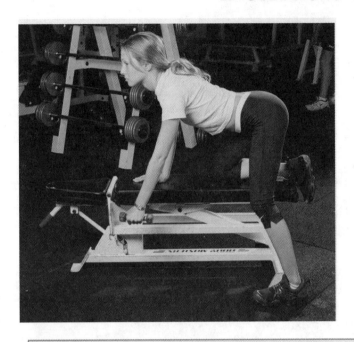 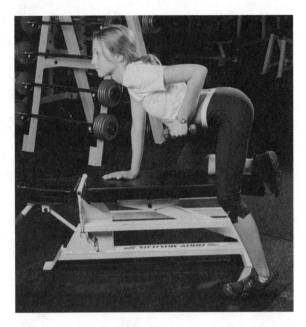

FAQ:

I always see guys using big weights during this exercise. I want a powerful back. How heavy should I go?

ANSWER:

Have you ever paid close attention to the people using those huge amounts of weight for this exercise? Often, the person is barely bent over and is using more momentum than a sling shot. The objective of this exercise is to stimulate the back muscles. Let the muscles you intend to stimulate do the work, not your ego! That will get you your sculpted back.

Two-Arm Row

This is a great exercise for your back, but improper form could lead to injury. This exercise is not recommended for people with back problems. Instead, try a seated low-pulley row with a v-bar. Make sure you maintain perfect form for this exercise and never slouch the back forward as this can cause back injury. If you are new to this exercise, begin using a small amount of weight.

PROPER ALIGNMENT

❶ Hold a dumbbell in each hand with your palms facing your torso.

❷ Your knees should be bent slightly, head up, and your shoulders back. The weights should hang with your arms perpendicular to the floor.

❸ Now, push your torso forward by bending at the waist, keeping your back straight until it is almost parallel to the floor.

TECHNIQUE AND FORM

❶ While holding your torso stationary, exhale and life the dumbbells to your ribs. Keep your elbows close to your body. You should not be using your forearms for anything but positioning.

❷ At the top of the contraction, squeeze your back muscles and hold for one second.

❸ Slowly lower the weights to the starting position, inhaling as you do so.

Two-Arm Row

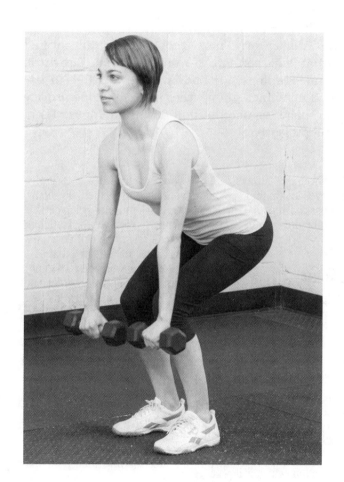
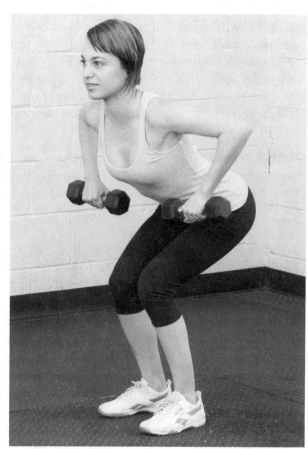

Wide Grip Pull-Up to Front

The pull-up is a very challenging back exercise. However, its ability to deliver quick results and functional upper body strength makes it well worth its weight in gold. Its main emphasis is on the "lats" and the mid-back muscles. There is no involvement of the lower back muscles in this exercise. Secondary muscles involved are the rear deltoids and the biceps.

Note: If you cannot pull up your own body weight, don't worry, most people can't (and not just women, but men too!). There are two things that you can do. If your gym has Gravitron machines (machines that assist you in pulling and pushing your body weight) feel free to use those. If your health club is not equipped with such machines, then either have someone provide the assistance (as in the pictures on the following page) or use the pull-down machines. Then, when you get strong enough, feel free to start doing pull-ups.

PROPER ALIGNMENT

The pull-up focuses on the natural resistance and mechanics of the body. Too many people perform this exercise incorrectly. They use too much momentum, do not use a full range of motion, or simply do not know the proper technique and form to follow for optimum results.

❶ To start, take hold of an overhead bar with an overhand grip.

❷ Align your body by spacing your hands about shoulder-width apart. It's important to realize that different hand spacing will sometimes focus on one muscle more than another. We recommend a grip 1 1/2 times your shoulder width since it will help keep the biceps from being stimulated and is a great position for back muscle stimulation.

❸ Contract your abdominal section to help sustain your postural alignment throughout the movement.

❹ Stick your chest out while depressing your shoulders (downward), which will help sustain the intended musculature of the back.

❺ Throughout the movement, always keep your head and eyes looking up. Knowing that you must reach your target position at the top adds that extra push.

TECHNIQUE AND FORM

❶ Holding onto the bar with an overhand grip 1 1/2 times your shoulder width, let your body hang while bending your knees and crossing your feet.

❷ Keep your elbows as wide as you can while you push your body up.

❸ As you are pulling up, make sure your chest is sticking out as much as possible. Your shoulders should be depressed (downward) and as relaxed as possible.

❹ When you reach the top (which will be when you can no longer move upward while maintaining the proper alignment), consciously focus on squeezing and contracting the back muscles as hard as you can. Try to hold that contraction for at least one to two seconds to help isolate the back muscles.

❺ As you begin your descent, slowly lower your body while mentally focusing on the back muscles being activated. When you feel yourself fatiguing or losing control on the way down, try to pull back up. You'll notice that as you get tired, even your best attempt to pull yourself back up will not stop your descent. This technique will add some additional intensity and overall stimulation of the back muscles.

❻ For a full range of motion, let your arms straighten completely at the bottom of the movement. Most people only come down two-thirds of the way and leave out perhaps the most important portion of the exercise—the fully stretched position. Next, slowly and smoothly begin the transition upward once again without using any momentum.

Wide Grip Pull-Up to Front

WIDE GRIP PULL-UP WITH ASSISTANCE

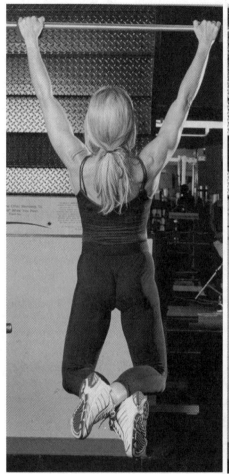
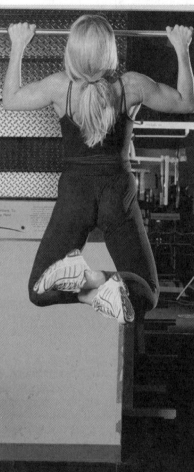
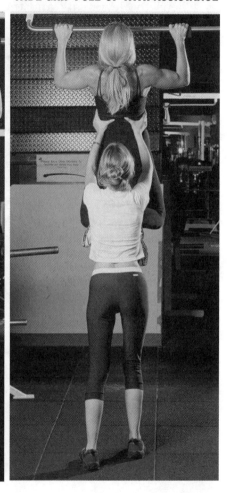

FAQ:
In the exercise description, you mention depressing the shoulders downward. How do I do this and why?

ANSWER:
Depressing the shoulders downward helps to take some of the initial stimulus away from the trapezoid, rhomboid, and teres muscles of the upper back. these muscles are naturally stimulated during a pull-up. When you lower your shoulders, you will help block the assistive muscles and force the lats to become the primary working muscles.

Neutral Grip Pull-Up

The pull-up is a difficult exercise that requires a lot of upper body strength. This version widens the lower lats and the small serratus muscles on the lower outside of the pecs. The pull-up can deliver fast results and functional upper body strength. It focuses on the natural resistance and mechanics of the body. It is easy to perform it incorrectly. Do not use momentum: it is necessary to perform a full range of motion in order to see results. Always use proper technique and form.

If you do not have the strength to do this exercise, use a pull-up assist machine if available. These machines use weight to help you push your body up. Another option is to have a spotter hold your legs. If neither of these two options is available, substitute a pull-down using the V-bar attachment.

If you are looking to add weight to this exercise, try using a weight belt.

PROPER ALIGNMENT

❶ Reach up to grasp a pull-up bar with a palms-facing grip. Hold your body steady; keep your head and eyes looking up the entire movement. Knowing that you must reach your target position at the top adds that extra push.

❷ Stick your chest out and lean back slightly in order to better engage your lat muscles.

❸ Contract your abs--this helps you sustain your postural alignment throughout the movement.

TECHNIQUE AND FORM

❶ Pull your torso up, using your lats, and contract your abs while leaning your head back slightly so that you do not hit your head on the chin-up bar. Stick your chest out as much as possible. Your shoulders should be as relaxed and depressed as possible.

❷ Exhale and continue until your chest nearly touches the V-bar.

❸ Hold for a second or two, at least, in this contracted position-consciously focusing on squeezing and contracting the back muscles as much as possible. Holding the contraction helps to isolate the back muscles. Then slowly lower back to the starting position as you inhale and focus on your back muscles being activated. When you feel yourself fatiguing or losing control on the way down, try to pull back up. You will notice that as you get tired, even your best attempt to pull yourself back up will not stop your descent. This will add to the overall intensity and stimulation of the back muscles.

❹ For a full range of motion, let your arms straighten out completely at the bottom of the movement. The fully stretched position is perhaps the most important segment of the exercise. Lowering slowly and with control is essential. It enables you to reap the muscle-building benefits of the negative or eccentric phase of an exercise [the phase during which you elongate your working muscles).

❺ Without resting or using momentum, repeat this exercise slowly and smoothly for the recommended number of repetitions.

Neutral Grip Pull-Up

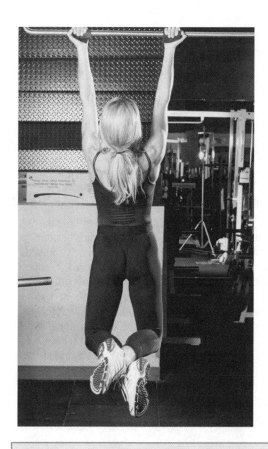 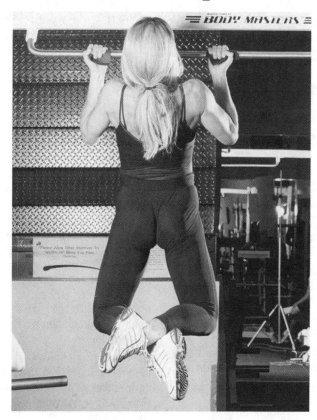

FAQ:

I rarely ever see anyone doing pull-ups. Aren't pull-downs a more effective back exercise?

ANSWER:

The reason why you probably don't see many people doing pull-ups in your gym is either your gym doesn't have pull-up bars or, more likely, the exercise is too difficult for most people to do. This doesn't mean that because pull-ups are difficult, you should shy away from them. Yes, pull-ups take some practice to perfect, but once you get the hang of them, they can quickly become one of the most productive and challenging upper body exercises.

The only way you can progress at doing pull-ups is to practice. By practicing consistently and challenging yourself to always exceed the level and performance of your previous workout session, you will inevitably get to the point where pull-ups become easier and easier to do.

When you get to the point where you can do 8-12 pull-ups, using a full range of motion and no momentum, it will be time to further challenge yourself by adding additional weight (using a weight belt or weight plate held between your thighs).

Wide-Grip Pull-Down

If you are not able to pull up your own body weight, you can use the lat pull-down machine to help increase your strength. Although the pull-up is a much better exercise for back muscle development because it works with the body's natural mechanics and range of motion, the pull-down can be a great primer to help get you ready for the pull-up. You also have a greater ability here to practice your Zone-Tone techniques, making sure to isolate the specific muscles of the back.

PROPER ALIGNMENT

❶ Position the thigh support so that you are in a snug position with your feet placed flat on the floor.

❷ Choose your desired weight and take a grip equal to twice your shoulder length.

❸ Lean back slightly from the hips while contracting the abdominal muscles for support.

❹ As you prepare to pull down, stick your chest out while keeping your elbows wide.

❺ With a slight lean backwards at the hips, your chest pushed out and your elbows wide, you are ready to begin the exercise.

TECHNIQUE AND FORM

❶ Once in position and focused on the muscles of the back, pull the bar down to your collar bone while maintaining your postural alignment.

❷ Make sure that you pull the bar down in a smooth, controlled manner, letting the muscles of the back do the work and not your biceps or momentum. If you don't know the difference between controlled form and momentum already, you will feel the difference in muscle stimulation when you use controlled form.

❸ As you reach the bottom of the movement, make sure to squeeze the back muscles for a count of 1 1/2 seconds with the bar close to or touching the collar bone.

❹ Slowly begin moving the bar upward and allow it to return to the start position.

❺ When you reach the top, do not rest! Immediately begin pulling down making sure you do so slowly while maintaining the correct form and postural alignment. Remember the "time under tension" principle of continued motion and no rest. You are here to work, not rest. You will accomplish a great deal more by keeping constant tension in the muscle throughout the entire set as opposed to resting at every transition of the top and bottom positions.

Wide-Grip Pull-Down

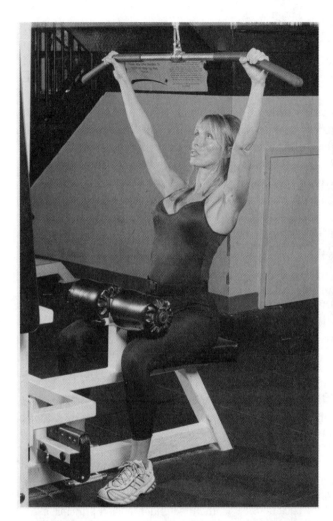

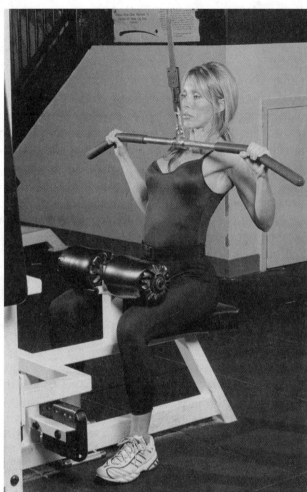

FAQ:
In the pull-up exercise, you request that you depress the shoulders to help isolate the lats. Would it make sense to do that here, as well?

ANSWER:
Yes! There are many things to remember and if you can remember to include the depression of the shoulders maneuver, in addition to the other variables of the pull-down exercise, it will only help to enhance the results.

Close-Grip Pull-Down

During the narrow-grip pull-down exercise, the positioning of your hands will take a different hand position and grip placement when compared to the narrow-grip pull-up. The narrow-grip attachment as you can see in the pictures on the next page has two handles that are structured parallel to one another. When you take your hand position, the palms of your hands will be closely facing each other.

As you can clearly see, your whole arm position has now changed in comparison to the narrow underhand-grip pull-up. Notice how close the arms are to one another. You can see how the arms remain close to the body from the beginning of the exercise to the finish position. If you perform the narrow-grip exercise and immediately follow with the wide-grip pull-down exercise, you will feel a major difference in the muscles that are stimulated. This is evidence of how the variation in bar attachments and your hand placement can dramatically stimulate different muscles.

The same way you have the option of using the lat pull-down machine to help those women who are not able to do a wide-grip pull-up, the same applies for women who cannot yet do a narrow-grip underhand pull-up.

VARIATION: One variation you can try are close-grip pull-downs. In this variation, you will install a wide bar instead of a V-bar, and grasp the bar with palms facing your torso and a narrower than shoulder-width grip.

PROPER ALIGNMENT

❶ Position the thigh support so that you are in a snug position with your feet placed flat on the floor.

❷ Choose your desired weight and take the narrow grip that you have chosen.

❸ Lean back slightly from the hips while slightly contracting the abdominal muscles for support.

❹ As you prepare to pull down, stick your chest out while keeping your elbows narrow and close to your body.

❺ With a slight lean backwards at the hips, your chest pushed out and your elbows staying close to your body, you are ready to begin the exercise.

TECHNIQUE AND FORM

❶ Once in position and focused on the muscles of the back, pull the bar down to your upper chest region, maintaining your postural alignment.

❷ Make sure that you pull the bar down in a smooth, controlled manner, letting the muscles of the back do the work, keeping your biceps and momentum from becoming involved. If you don't know the difference between controlled form and momentum already, you will surely feel the difference in muscle stimulation when you use correct, controlled form.

❸ As you reach the bottom of the movement, make sure to squeeze the back muscles for a count of 1 1/2 seconds with the bar close to or touching the upper chest region.

❹ Slowly allow the bar to move upward until it is in the start position.

❺ When you reach the top, do not rest! Immediately begin pulling back down, making sure you do so slowly while maintaining the correct form and postural alignment. Remember the time under tension principle of continued motion and no rest. You are here to work, not rest. You will accomplish a great deal more by keeping constant tension on the muscles, throughout the entire set as opposed to resting at every transition of the top and bottom positions.

Close-Grip Pull-Down

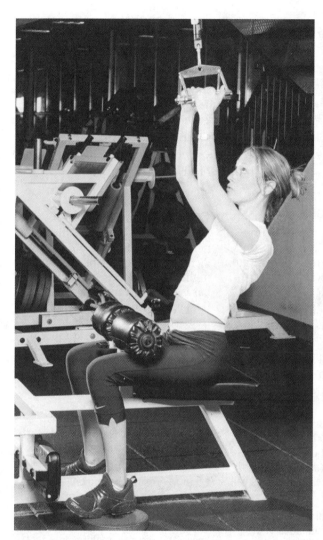
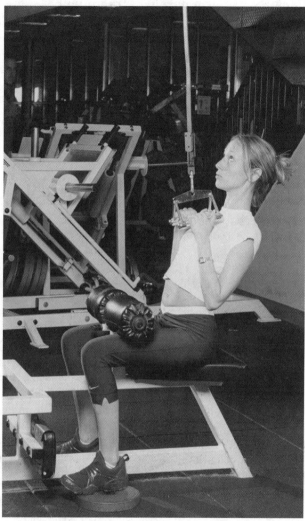

FAQ:
When I do this exercise, it hurts my shoulders.

ANSWER:
If you experience pain with any exercise, stop! It doesn't make sense to continue doing an exercise if it is hurting you. Try variations of this exercise until you find a pain-free version. Some variations you can try to include similar movements, hand grips, bar attachments, or machines. A simple modification can make all the difference in the world.

Seated Low-Pulley Row

Using a close-grip parallel attachment

The low-pulley row, which exercises the lower lats and mid-back muscles, is an exercise that most people perform incorrectly. They either lean too far forward in the beginning of the movement or too far backward when they squeeze the bar to their stomachs (peak contraction position), thus taking the stress right off the lat muscles. Many people also use only momentum instead of muscle to move the weight—especially if they are trying to lift too much.

Throughout your training, you will notice how you can choose between a variety of handles to use for this exercise and many others. Each one hits a slightly different area of the back, which provides a great variety for an exciting and never stale back routine. The description of technique and form below assumes that you will be using a close-grip parallel bar attachment.

PROPER ALIGNMENT

❶ Once you attach the bar to the pulley system, take a seat on the machine bench.

❷ Choose a weight that will allow you to practice perfect form while also providing enough weight to stimulate the back muscles. Using too light a weight will keep you from feeling the desired muscle stimulation.

❸ Take hold of the bar, either leaning forward or having someone hand it to you.

❹ Sit straight up while you bend at the knees.

❺ Plant your feet evenly on each side of the platform and point them straight ahead.

❻ Slightly contract the abdominal muscles.

❼ Stick your chest out and retract the scapula and shoulder blades.

❽ Keep your elbows close to your body and hands down by your lower abdominals.

❾ Keep your head level and look straight ahead throughout the movement.

TECHNIQUE AND FORM

❶ First, to avoid lower-back injury, make sure that your knees are bent and that you don't lean too far forward. A very slight lean forward is okay.

❷ With the arms fully stretched forward, retract the scapula from this position. This will pre-isolate the lat muscles of the back.

❸ Your objective will be to pull the bar back to your lower-to-mid abdominal section, making sure you adhere to the following steps.

❹ You will want to keep the elbows riding close to the body, helping to stimulate the back muscles. The farther you bring the arms away from the body, the less the desired muscles will be stimulated.

❺ As you begin pulling the bar toward your abdominal section, stick your chest out as far as it will go while you strive to sit straight up. Do not lean backwards.

❻ Concentrate completely on the lat muscles of the back so they do most of the work.

❼ When the bar reaches your abdominal section squeeze the back muscles as hard as you possibly can. Picture having an egg planted square in the middle of your back. While the bar is touching your abdominal section, your main objective, while contracting the muscles of the back as hard as you can, will be to squeeze your shoulder blades together so hard that the egg breaks.

❽ Hold the contracted position for a count of two seconds.

❾ From the contracted position, slowly begin your return to the starting position with a slow and controlled movement.

❿ As you reach the starting position, slowly and smoothly begin pulling the bar towards you without resting. Maintain the same form as when you began the exercise, making sure that no momentum is involved while changing over from the contracted position to the starting position.

Seated Low-Pulley Row

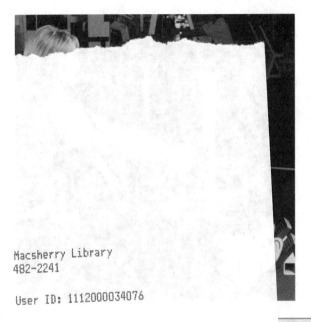

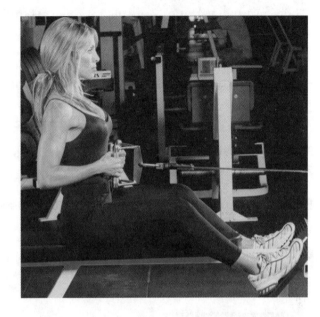

c.

v back injury. This is especially true if you're going very heavy.
rward while your lower back muscles hold you in place. When
of this pull, it can strain your lower back muscles. Your best
r lower back, keep your abdominals contracted to help secure
l at the hips, and avoid momentum at all costs. These four
the lower back.

Dumbbell Pullover

There are two variations of this exercise. There is one that focuses mostly on the chest muscles and one that focuses more on the back muscles. What will enable you to focus on the two different muscle groups is the alignment, technique and form of your body and the exercise. Please pay attention to the exercise description steps below to help differentiate between the two exercise variations. This particular exercise variation is for the back muscles. Not only will this exercise help to create a beautifully toned and tight back region, but it will also benefit the triceps muscles located on the back of the upper arms.

PROPER ALIGNMENT

❶ Lie with your body across a flat bench.

❷ Ensure that your neck and your upper back are the only body parts resting on the bench.

❸ Lift a dumbbell overhead and hold it at arm's length right in front of your face. (Please ensure that the dumbbells

you are using have their weights properly secured).

TECHNIQUE AND FORM

❶ Slowly lower the dumbbell over your head in an arc.

❷ Ensure that your hips are not being raised as you lower the weight.

❸ When you reach the fully stretched position, hold the stretch for a second and start raising the weight back up in an arc until you reach the starting position once again.

CHEST VARIATION

A variation of the pullover exercise is for the chest muscles. You will notice how the bent arm technique, along with the lowering of the torso help to bring concentration to the chest muscles rather than the back muscles. This is NOT an alternate exercise to stimulate back muscle growth.

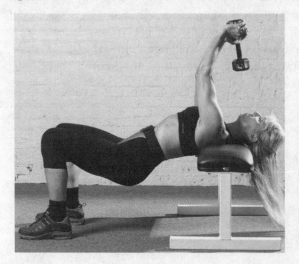
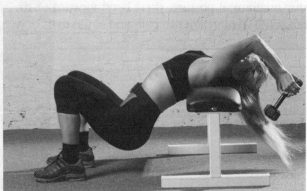

Dumbbell Pullover

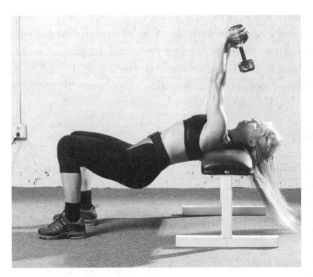 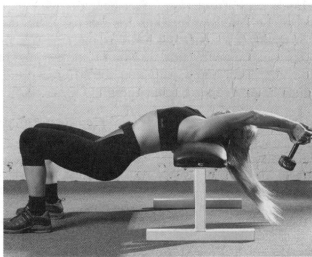

FAQ:
In your exercise pictures, I see very little difference between the chest and back versions of this exercise. What are they?

ANSWER:
With the chest variation, your objective is to sink the torso down as low as you can while simultaneously bringing your arms as low as possible, resulting in a workout that functions from the shoulder joint only. Remember to keep those elbows locked in place and don't allow them to lower the dumbbell.

With the back variation, your objective is to keep the torso up and maintain the level throughout, while keeping your arms and elbows much straighter than in the chest variation.

Straight Arm Pull-Down

This is a great isolation exercise for the back as it allows you to work without the involvement of secondary muscles such as the biceps. In addition, you get the bonus of working the abs indirectly as you will need to contract them in order to maintain the position required to perform the exercise. This will without a doubt become one of your favorite exercises. It gives you the ability to really learn how to isolate those stubborn back muscles. Just make sure to follow the correct steps listed below for optimal results.

PROPER ALIGNMENT

❶ Stand in front of a pull-down bar with your arms extended in front of you holding on to the bar at shoulder width using a palms down grip.

❷ In order to gain stability, bend your legs slightly at the knees, contract your abdominals and keep your weight at the heels.

❸ Keep the elbows slightly bent and the wrists straight and in a locked position.

❹ Maintain a comfortable and forward tilt of the upper body in order to maintain stability throughout the movement.

TECHNIQUE AND FORM

❶ Push the bar down towards the body in an arc like motion, making sure that you are only moving from the shoulder joint and not extending at the elbow. There must be no movement at the elbow joint. It must be locked securely in place.

❷ Contract your lats as you lower the bar towards your thighs.

❸ As soon as the bar touches your thighs, hold the position for a second or two and then slowly go back to the starting position.

FAQ:
I've seen people using wider than a shoulder-width grip. Why?

ANSWER:
A shoulder-width grip usually makes for a great position to engage the back muscles, but what works for most might no work for you. If you don't think you are fully getting the benefit from the shoulder-width grip, by all means try another grip width. Try both narrower and wider grips and see what works best for you and your particular body mechanics.

Straight Arm Pull-Down

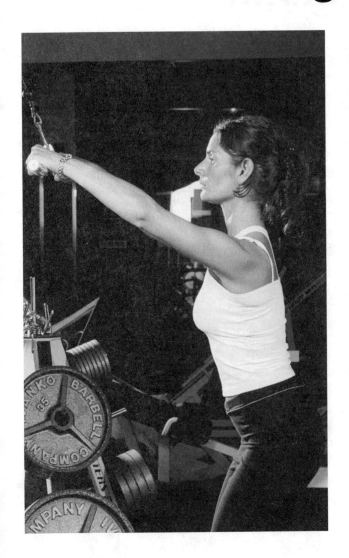
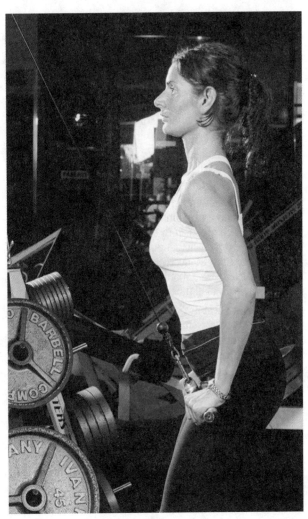

TWO-ARM ROW MACHINE

This machine targets the mid-back muscles along with the latissimus dorsi. Secondary emphasis is placed on the trapezius, rhomboids, and biceps brachii muscles. For a similar dumbbell exercise, try the One-Arm Row with either grip.

TECHNIQUE AND FORM

❶ Sit on the machine and adjust the seat of the machine so that your upper chest is placed just above the handle bars provided by the lever.

❷ Select the desired resistance and grasp the handle bars with an overhand grip (palms facing down, and thumbs pointing towards each other). Your elbows should be placed out to the sides. The torso, shoulders, and upper arms should be elevated, creating a 90-degree angle between the torso and the upper arms. There should be a straight imaginary line between the bottom of the neck and the elbow.

❸ Using your chest muscles and not your arms, push the machine lever away from you until your arms are fully extended in front of you. Hold the contracted position for a second. Breathe out as you perform this movement.

❹ Return to the starting position as you breathe in.

TRAINER'S TIPS

❶ The only body parts moving should be the arms as they move the lever forward. The back and head should always remain on the seat. Many people bring the head forward as they perform the movement but this can hyperextend the neck muscles.

❷ Keep control of the machine at all times and concentrate on using the chest muscles as opposed to the arms.

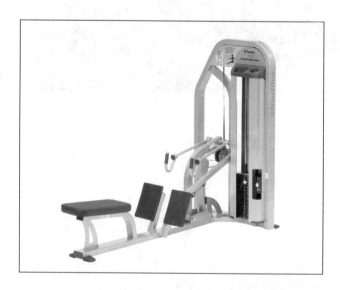

Chapter 8
Chest

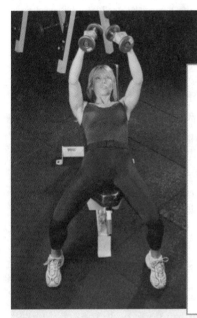

There are many misconceptions when it comes to women and chest training. While chest training will not increase your cup size, you can tone and firm the surrounding muscles of the breast bone, which will prevent your breasts from drooping. Having a healthy, muscular chest can also give a more balanced, symmetrical look to your physical appearance.

For immediate Body Sculpting Bible support & coaching directly from James & Hugo, please visit www.BodySculptingBibles.com

8

THE BODY SCULPTING BIBLE FOR WOMEN

There are four areas of the chest that women should emphasize:

a) Upper Chest Area with exercises such as the Incline Dumbbell Press.

b) Overall Pec Area that attaches to the breasts, giving them support, with exercises such as the dumbbell press, Chest Dips and Push-ups.

c) Outer Chest Upper Area with exercises such as the Incline Dumbbell Flys.

d) Inner Upper Chest Area with exercises such as the Incline Cable Crossovers.

We will mostly recommend dumbbells for the performance of chest exercises for several reasons:

1. They allow for a greater range of motion and a deeper stretch at the bottom of the movements.

2. They allow for better isolation and muscle contraction at the top of the movements, helping to recruit more muscle fibers within the chest and surrounding musculature.

3. They are harder to control and hold than a barbell, helping to strengthen and develop the extremely important antagonistic and synergistic muscles of the chest and shoulders. Overall, the benefits you'll receive from using dumbbells outweigh the barbell by a long shot.

PROPER ALIGNMENT

The postural alignment is basically the same for all of the following chest exercises. However, you will notice differences in some of the following positions, techniques and forms. The most important thing to remember is to always consciously focus and contract the muscles of the chest while maintaining the postural alignment and form during all of the exercises. This will help to stimulate the chest muscles during exercise.

The following sequence of movements will ensure that you learn how to properly lift a dumbbell off the ground and into position to start many of the exercises we describe. It will also demonstrate how to bring the dumbbells back to the start position of an exercise when you have completed it from a lying position. This is an invaluable technique to learn and can prevent many injuries.

1. When you pick up dumbbells, make sure to bend at the knees while you lift the weight with your legs.

2. Lift with your legs, not with your back! You can easily injure your lower back by bending over to pick up the weight.

3. While standing, place the bottom plate of the dumbbells against your thighs and keep them there as you sit on the bench seat. You will find that by keeping the dumbbells against your thighs as you sit, you will be able to easily manipulate them to the top of your thighs.

4. Begin positioning your body into the correct postural alignment, starting from the bottom of your body and moving to the top.

5. Space your feet about shoulder width apart.

6. Make sure your knees are pointing straight ahead throughout the movement.

7. As you raise the dumbbells to the starting position on top of your thighs, do not try to muscle them up with your arm muscles. This will only drain your strength and can easily cause an injury. You need 100 percent of your strength for the exercise itself and cannot afford to

waste it on something that you can easily avoid. To properly raise the dumbbells from your thighs into exercise position, follow these guidelines; you will be using your leg muscles and momentum to help place you and the dumbbells into position. While sitting in an upright position, with the dumbbells on your thighs, thrust one leg up, leveraging one dumbbell up to around your chest level.

8. Immediately thrust the second dumbbell upward, while simultaneously allowing momentum and the dumbbells to guide you back into the lying position while your abdominal muscles help safely ease you into that position. The reason for lying back immediately when the second dumbbell is thrust upward is so you do not injure your shoulder joints or lower back from having to hold the dumbbells in that otherwise awkward position. Lying back immediately following the dumbbell's momentum while allowing the abdominal muscles to ease you into position will help ensure your safety and keep your strength at its peak for the exercise. This may sound difficult, but it's not. It is the safest and easiest way of getting the dumbbells into position (especially if you're using heavy dumbbells).

9. Once you've gotten the dumbbells up, lay back, until your back touches the bench.

10. The dumbbells should now be in position at the sides of your chest.

11. Again make sure your feet are shoulder width apart, and that they are flat on the ground at all times.

12. Make sure your knees are straight.

13. Your lower back should be flat against the bench at all times, with no excessive arch in the lower lumbar region (small of the back).

14. Make sure your back is flat against the bench, with the arms and elbows out to the sides and the forearms perpendicular to the floor. When you're correctly positioned, retract or squeeze the shoulder blades together. At first it may seem uncomfortable or odd, but do not underestimate the significance of this technique. You must learn to hold this position throughout the movement, and consistent practice will ensure this. By squeezing the shoulder blades together and keeping your entire back in constant contact with the bench, you will actually be taking the anterior shoulder out of the exercise. The chest muscles will now be the primary muscles lifting the weight.

15. Relax your head throughout the move ment, and make sure you do not twist it or lift it from the bench while engaged in the exercise. Alignment is generally the same for all of the exercises.

FAQ:
In the exercise description, you mention depressing the shoulders downward. How do I do this and why?

ANSWER:
Depressing the shoulders downward helps to take some of the initial stimulus away from the trapezoid, rhomboid, and teres muscles of the upper back. These muscles are naturally stimulated during a pull-up. When you lower your shoulders, you will help block the assistive muscles and force the lats to become the primary working muscles.

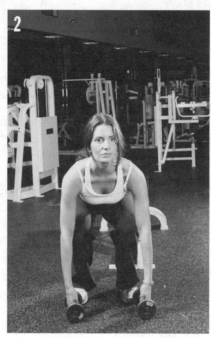

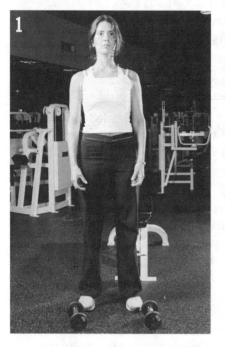

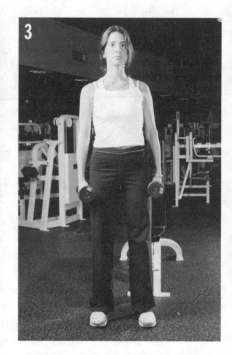

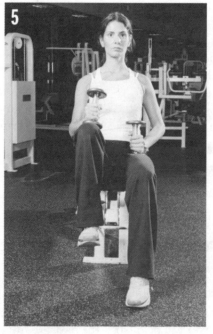

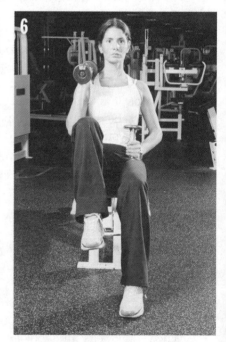

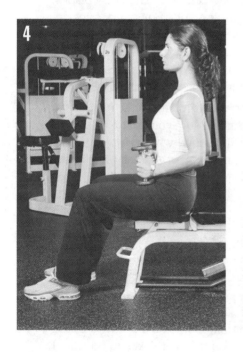

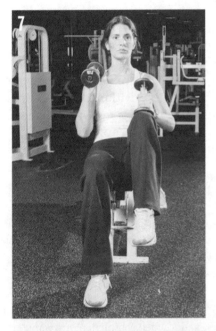

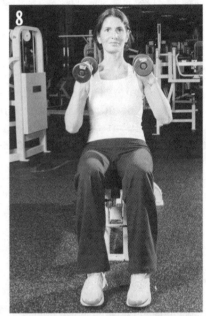

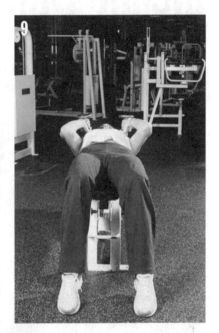

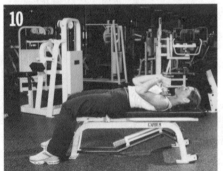

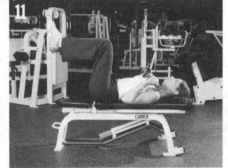

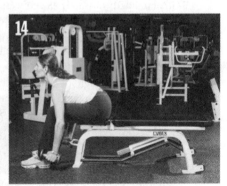

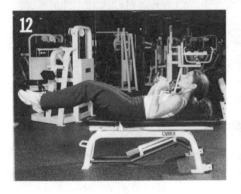

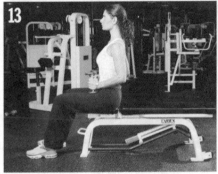

Incline Dumbbell Press

This is an excellent exercise for the upper pectoral muscles. The dumbbells are more challenging than the barbells as they involve stabilizer muscles needed in order to keep the weights in balance. The exercise can be performed in two manners for variety: with palms facing away or palms facing each other. For both variations, the only difference is the position of the palms throughout the movement. The movement itself remains the same. You will notice how you have the option of either touching the dumbbells at the top of the movement or keeping them separated when you reach the top of the movement. Some people feel the ability to get a better muscular contraction in the chest muscles when they touch them at the top, while others feel like it is a waste of valuable time and strength. Try both, and see what works better for you.

TECHNIQUE AND FORM

❶ With the dumbbells on your thighs, thrust one leg up, leveraging one dumbbell up to about your chest level.

❷ Immediately thrust the second dumbbell upward while simultaneously allowing momentum and the dumbbells to guide you back into the angled, incline position. Use your abdominal muscles to help safely ease you into that position.

❸ As you are lying on the inclined bench, align your body as you were instructed above.

❹ Position the dumbbells out to the side of your chest, keeping your elbows wide and your forearms perpendicular to the floor throughout the exercise movement. Find a position that is wide enough to be comfortable and not so wide as to redirect the force to the shoulders. Some trainers believe that bringing the arms out excessively to the sides of the body will help to better isolate the chest muscles. This is a misconception that can actually inhibit chest development and, worse, cause injury. The wider you go beyond a comfortable position, the more likely you are to redirect the force of the weight on to the shoulders rather than the pecs. Even worse, when you widen your arms excessively and then proceed to press a heavy or even moderate weight,

you are actually causing the outer pectoral muscle to tear. Once again, bring your arms out to the side of your body to a point where they are still positioned wide, but not excessively!

❺ Because the incline dumbbell press positions you on an inclined angle, your shoulder muscles are more likely to move the weight rather than the chest muscles. To avoid this, not only will you want to retract the shoulder blades back or together against the bench; but you must also depress or press the shoulders downward. This slight variation will take the shoulders out of the chest movement, allowing the chest to be the primary area worked during the exercise.

❻ With the chest in its elevated position, the elbows out and wide, and the forearms perpendicular to the floor, press the dumbbells up toward the ceiling.

❼ As you reach the top of the exercise, you can either touch the dumbbells together or press them straight up like a bench press. You can play around with different positions at the top of the movement as you may get a better muscle contraction varying the dumbbell positions. Two people may use two different dumbbell variations in order to fully stimulate their chest muscles. The most important thing you are concerned with is getting the most intense contraction possible! There are a couple of different ways to do this. You can simply touch the dumbbells together and squeeze, or you can turn the dumbbells slightly inward at the top of the movement, allowing for a controlled and isolated contraction. Are you starting to see how you can apply the many new tools of this program to any and all facets of your training regimen?

❽ Begin lowering the weight while holding your proper postural alignment throughout the exercise.

❾ As your elbows and the back of your arms are lowered, bring the dumbbells to a level that is comfortable, making sure that the chest muscles hold the majority of the resistance. If you don't have any type of shoulder injuries or muscle impingement, you may allow the dumbbells to lower to a comfortable stretch where the dumbbells are parallel with your chest. Always make sure that you stay in control of the dumbbells and maintain this control throughout the exercise.

❿ Once you reach the bottom position, slowly begin to press the dumbbells up again in a controlled, smooth and fluid motion without using any momentum.

Incline Dumbbell Press

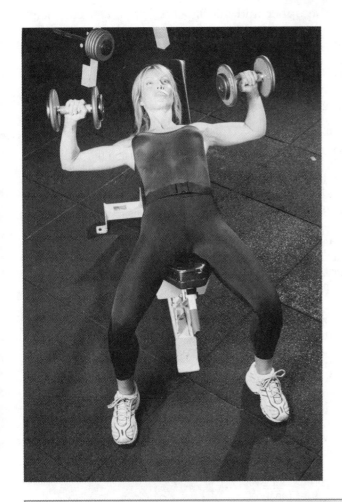
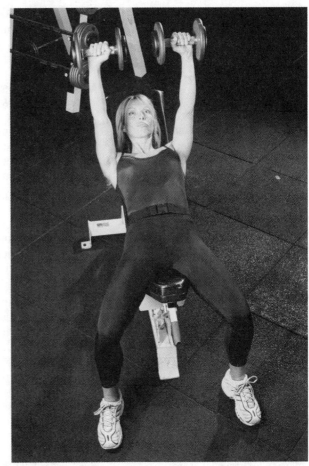

FAQ:
Because I am now sitting on an incline versus a flat surface, does the shoulder maneuver still involve retraction of the shoulder blades?

ANSWER:
Great question! Now that you are on an incline bench, simultaneously retract (bring straight back) and depress (pull down) your shoulders to help isolate the upper chest muscles as much as possible.

Flat Dumbbell Press

This is a great exercise for toning the muscles of the upper and middle chest region. It can help create cleavage and gives the breasts a natural lift. Once again, try the two variations we spoke of in the last exercise. Try touching the dumbbells at the top of the movement and also try pressing them straight up, as you would do with a traditional barbell bench press exercise.

TECHNIQUE AND FORM

This exercise requires you to use the same technique as the incline dumbbell press, but there will be some slight variations in your postural alignment. You will align your body the same way you did before, but now you will obviously be in a flat position. You'll want to focus more on retracting the shoulder blades rather than depressing them. Otherwise, follow the same technique and form for this exercise as you learned for the incline press.

❶ With the dumbbells on your thighs, thrust one leg up, leveraging one dumbbell up to about your chest level. Immediately thrust the second dumbbell upward while simultaneously allowing momentum and the dumbbells to guide you back into the lying, supine position (flat, with your body facing the ceiling). Use your abdominal muscles to safely ease you into that position.

❷ Lay back and align your body as you were instructed above.

❸ Position the dumbbells to the outside of your chest, keeping the elbows wide and the forearms perpendicular to the floor throughout the exercise movement.

❹ Because your shoulder muscles are more likely to move the weight than your chest muscles, you must retract the shoulder blades back or together against the flat bench. This slight variation will take the shoulders out of the chest movement, allowing the chest to be the primary area working during the exercise.

❺ With the chest in its elevated position, the elbows out and wide and the forearms perpendicular to the floor, press the dumbbells up toward the ceiling.

❻ As you reach the top of the exercise, you can either touch the dumbbells together (as shown in picture C) or press them straight up (as shown in Picture B) like a bench press. You can play around with different positions at the top of the movement as you may get a better muscle contraction varying the dumbbell positions. Two people may use two different dumbbell variations in order to fully stimulate their chest muscles. The most important thing you are concerned with is getting the most intense contraction possible! There are a couple of different ways to do this. You can simply touch the dumbbells together and squeeze, or you can turn the dumbbells slightly inward at the top of the movement, allowing for a more controlled and isolated contraction.

❼ Begin lowering the weight while holding your proper postural alignment throughout the exercise.

❽ As your elbows and the back of your arms reach parallel or bench level, slowly begin to press the dumbbells up again in a controlled, smooth, fluid motion, without using any momentum.

Flat Dumbbell Press

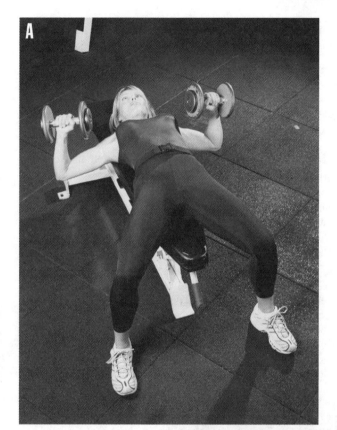

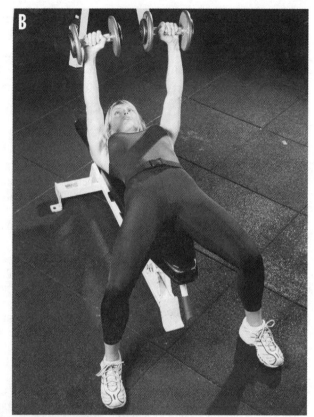

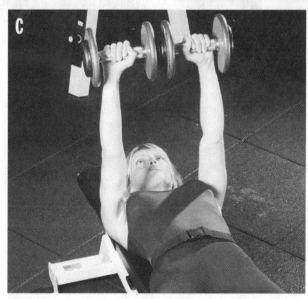

Flat Dumbbell Fly

This exercise is truly a great one. It might seem a bit hard to master, but once you do, it will be a pleasure to perform. It might look as if this exercise is identical to the dumbbell bench press, but it is not. With the dumbbell press, you are extending at the elbow joint and utilizing something called horizontal adduction (a movement together) of the shoulder joints. The flat dumbbell fly focuses on the mid-chest muscles and incorporates only the shoulder joints—not the elbow joint—in the movement. The elbows must be locked into place to allow the true magic to begin.

TECHNIQUE AND FORM

For this exercise, your postural alignment will be very similar to the other two chest exercises, but your technique and form will be very different. You will retract the shoulder blades just as you did in the flat and incline dumbbell press, but the angle of the movement is changed. Instead of using the combination of horizontal shoulder adduction (when the shoulders move inward), and elbow extension (when the elbows flex and extend during pressing), for this exercise you'll lock the elbow joint in place. You will set up the arms just as you would for the flat dumbbell press with the arms wide and forearms perpendicular to the floor, but having the elbows locked will prevent any elbows extension or flexion. This technique will exclude the triceps from being involved in the exercise while focusing the resistance completely within the chest muscles.

❶ You'll want to align your body exactly as you did with the flat dumbbell press, but now you will have the palms of your hands facing each other instead of facing the wall in front of you. Your forearms will be facing the ceiling, rather than the wall in front of you.

❷ This time you'll be using a visualization technique while engaged in the movement of the exercise. As you begin to squeeze the dumbbells towards each other, you will be following an arch-shaped movement. As you follow this arch, I want you to picture yourself hugging a tree. In other words, make believe there is a tree between you and the dumbbells; you will be mimicking the exact motion of hugging it. This visualization technique will help keep you in the correct position to follow the arch movement. All of this will ensure that your chest muscles receive the most intense stimulation and contraction possible.

❸ As you reach the top of the movement, be sure to consciously contract the chest muscles as hard as you possibly can for maximum muscle stimulation!

❹ Begin lowering the weight while holding the proper alignment, technique and form throughout the movement. As you reach the bottom of the movement, be sure not to let the back of the arms go too far below the level of the flat bench as this could cause injury to the shoulders' rotator cuff. When you do reach the bottom of the movement, slowly begin squeezing the dumbbells upward in an arch again with a smooth, controlled, fluid motion, making sure that you avoid using momentum!

Flat Dumbbell Fly

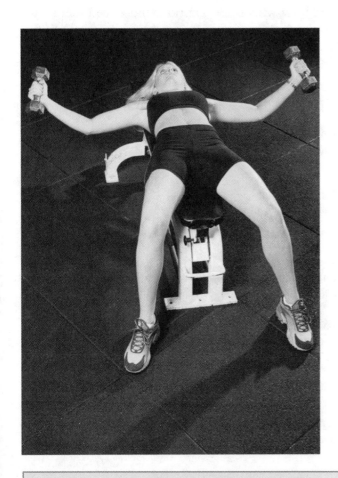
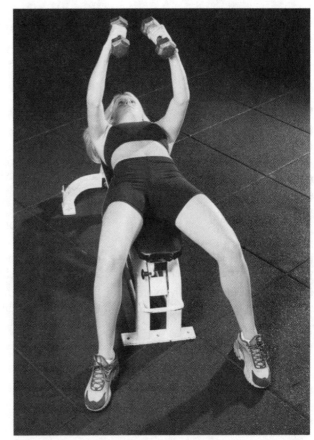

FAQ:
How does the chest maneuver work with this exercise?

ANSWER:
Because your anterior deltoids are in direct alignment with the line of movement, it is pretty difficult to take them out of this movement. The positive thing about this exercise is the fact that the triceps are not involved. When you take the triceps out of the movement, it becomes a very powerful way of helping to isolate stimulation in the chest muscles.

Incline Dumbbell Fly

This exercise is virtually identical to the flat dumbbell fly with the exception that it will focus on the upper chest muscles. Remember that no matter what anyone tells you, it is impossible to avoid hitting muscles located in the same muscle groups. For example, if you are focusing on you upper chest muscles, you will inevitably be stimulating the mid-chest muscles as well. It is great to zone in on the exact muscles you desire to train, but don't be surprised when nearby muscles are also feeling the work.

PROPER ALIGNMENT

❶ Sit back on an incline bench with your feet wider than shoulder-width apart and flat on the floor.

❷ Make sure your shoulders are flat against the pad and your chest is out.

❸ Using your thighs to help you get the dumbbells up to your arms, clean the dumbbells one at a time and hold them at shoulder width. Your back of your hands will be facing behind you.

❹ Bend your elbows slightly to prevent stress at the biceps tendon.

TECHNIQUE AND FORM

❶ Inhale while you lower your arms together in a wide arc. You should go until you feel a stretch in your chest. Your elbow joints will remain stationary, as the movement occurs solely at the shoulder joints.

❷ Pause for a moment at the bottom of the movement.

❸ Now, exhale and return your arms to the starting position, using the same arc of movement.

❹ Hold the upright position for a second and repeat for the desired number of repetitions.

Incline Dumbbell Fly

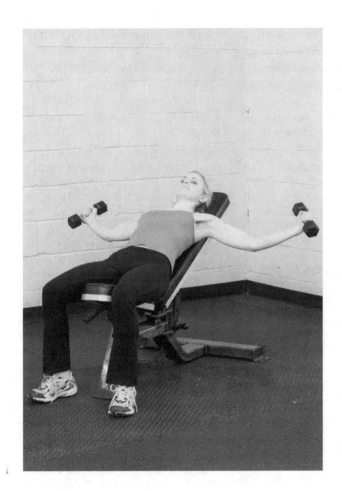
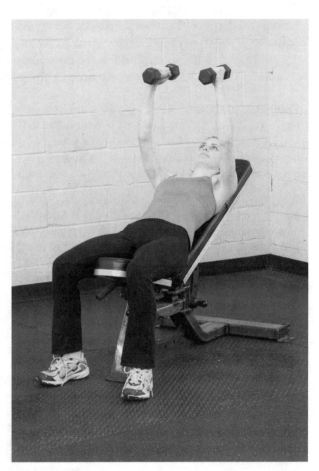

Chest Dip

The chest dip is a great muscle-enhancing exercise that focuses on the lower chest and serratus muscles. Unlike the triceps dip, where you keep your body in a straight vertical line, the chest dip requires that you bend forward to isolate the chest muscles.

Don't worry if you can't do a dip on your own—most people can't. Our model in the pictures on the next page is using a Gravitron to help support her weight.

PROPER ALIGNMENT

With this exercise, you'll want to bend at the knees, lock your feet and bend forward as you lower yourself. You must stay bent over to keep the focus of resistance in the chest muscles. These three steps will help transfer most of the resistance to the chest muscles and avoid triceps muscle recruitment. To do this, you will need a dip station or machine. If you are working out in your home, we suggest you purchase an inexpensive dip unit from one of the sports-related retail chains or a wholesale fitness supply store. In a wholesale store, you can usually negotiate a lower price and the quality of the apparatus is usually much better. Look in your local yellow pages for a store nearest you.

❶ Place your hands on the parallel bars as you position yourself for postural alignment.

❷ The best way to align yourself is to raise yourself up onto the dip bars by locking out your arms. You will then align your body, starting with your head and moving down to your feet.

❸ While suspended in the top position of the exercise, your head will at first be level and looking straight ahead. You may find that bending your head slightly forward as you lower yourself will help you lean forward for increased muscle stimulation in the chest. You must constantly focus all of your attention on the chest muscles during this exercise as this will help increase the involvement of the chest muscles and keep you in the proper alignment.

❹ Bend your legs at the knees and hook your feet over one another. This will help keep your back arched forward for the ultimate involvement of the chest muscles. Your arms and elbows will ride away from your body as you lower yourself and when pushing upward to the lockout position. This will help keep the triceps muscles from becoming involved with the exercise.

TECHNIQUE AND FORM

❶ Make sure that you have correct postural alignment. Begin the exercise once you are in position with your arms locked out (only in the beginning and end) and your body suspended from the floor.

❷ As you lower yourself from the lockout position immediately begin to lean forward. The farther you lean forward, the more your chest muscles will work.

❸ Lower yourself slowly while resisting your body weight all the way to the bottom position.

❹ Keep the elbows and arms away from your body, helping to better isolate the chest muscles and avoid recruiting the triceps muscles.

❺ Lower yourself until the backs of your arms are parallel or slightly beyond parallel to the floor. Remember, you should never go so low that you feel any chest or shoulder pain, or you could seriously injure yourself. Go to a point where you are comfortable and increase a little more the next session if needed.

❻ When you reach the bottom position, do not rest! Slowly, with a smooth transition, begin to press your body upward without using any momentum. Make sure that you maintain your postural alignment.

❼ As you begin pressing upward, make sure that all of your focus is once again directed to your chest muscles. This alone will help stimulate the triceps through increased muscle control. As you near the top of the motion, your goal is not to lock out the joint, but to contract and squeeze the chest muscles as hard as you possibly can for a one-second count. It is important for the chest muscles to hold you in this position rather than lock out with the triceps or the elbow joints.

❽ Remember that there should be no rest at the top of the exercise after the contraction period. From that lock out position, once again slowly lower yourself as you resist the weight of your body back to the bottom position. If you get to a point where your body weight is too light for the exercise, you may use a dip belt to hook some additional weight to your body, thus increasing the resistance. Please make sure that if you do use additional weight, you do so in small incremental stages.

Chest Dip

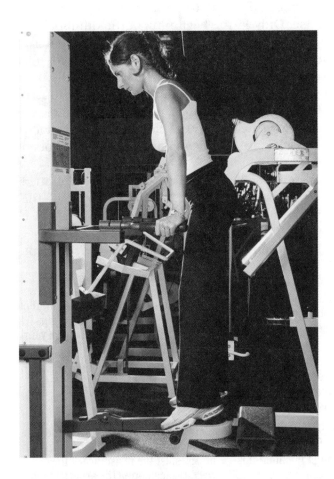
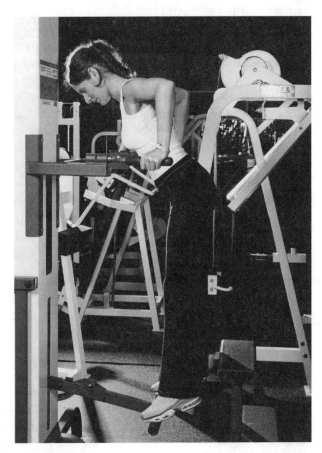

FAQ:

When I do chest dips, I feel a lot of pressure and pain in my shoulders. Why?

ANSWER:

The chest dip can be a very powerful and productive exercise. You do, however, need to make sure that you protect yourself from injury. Keep a few things in mind when doing the chest dip. Don't go too heavy, unless you know your muscles, joints, and connective tissue can handle it. Although you may be very strong and feel that your flexibility is great, you still may not be as strong as necessary to do this exercise at its full capacity. Don't go to low in your descent. To a degree, going low is great for training the chest through its full range of motion, but going too low defeats that purpose as eventually the chest will minimally be involved and the brunt of the stimulus will be directed to the shoulder.

Incline Cable Crossover

Incline cable crossovers are very similar to the dumbbell fly, but there is a major advantage when you perform the incline cable crossover exercise. Only in the beginning of the dumbbell fly exercise is the majority of the resistance placed upon the chest muscles. This soon changes when the dumbbells are brought vertical (arms and dumbbells extended over the chest). At this point, instead of the pecs being responsible for sustaining the resistance of the dumbbells, the elbow joints and shoulder joints are. The force of gravity disappears when the arms are brought to this vertical position. Cable crossovers don't have this disadvantage. In fact, the degree of resistance remains constant throughout the entire movement. In the pictures of our model demonstrating the exercise, notice how her chest muscles are still being stimulated in the open arms position.

Performing incline cable crossovers provides even greater benefits than the results obtained from doing regular cable crossovers. Incline cable crossovers add to the development of the upper chest muscles, and give you the appearance of a much larger chest overall. This exercise develops the pectoralis major and minor.

Common mistakes during this exercise include an uneven grip position and allowing the arms (elbows) to flex and extend during the movement.

PROPER ALIGNMENT

❶ Set the pin to the desired resistance and attach the handles to the cables.

❷ If possible, set the pulley level to a height just below your upper chest. This will allow for a more focused contraction in the upper pecs. If you are not able to adjust the pulley height, this is fine, but make sure to keep the focus on the upper pecs.

❸ Take hold of the handles with an overhand grip and position yourself so that you are in the middle of the pulley machine (in order to position yourself in the middle of the machine, you must pull each of the handles closer to you, thus lifting both weight stacks simultaneously.)

❹ Make sure that both weight stacks are even on the right and left sides. Do not allow the weight stacks to become uneven or you will create a muscle imbalance when you begin the exercise.

❺ With the handles in hand, palms facing each other and standing in the middle of the machine, bend your elbows slightly and lock them there throughout the exercise.

❻ You will begin this exercise in the extended position (arms opened up as if about to give a hug) as opposed to the dumbbell fly where you started in a flexed (contracted) position.

❼ Keep a slight bend in the knees to prevent lower-back strain.

❽ Remember, you must maintain this perfect alignment, so select a weight light enough so you can maintain form throughout the movement.

TECHNIQUE AND FORM

❶ You should be positioned in the middle of the cable crossover and parallel to the weight stacks with the hand grips in hand and arms extended out to the sides of your body. The resistance will provide a nice stretch to the pec muscles.

❷ To begin the exercise, keep the arms slightly bent and contract the chest muscles.

❸ Bring the cables across and in front of the body until the two hand grips touch at the level of or just above your upper chest.

❹ Make sure to contract the chest muscles as hard as possible in this position and hold for a one second count.

❺ Once the two hands touch and you have forcefully contracted the chest muscles, let the resistance of the weight stacks bring the arms back to the starting position in a slow controlled manner.

❻ Repeat the movement.

Incline Cable Crossover

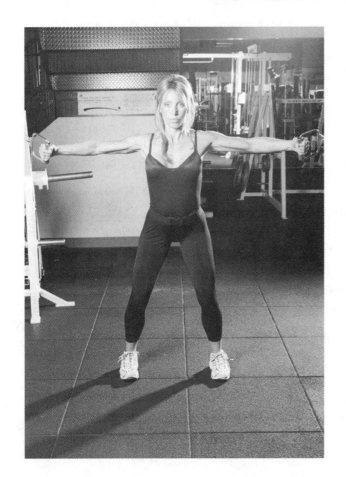
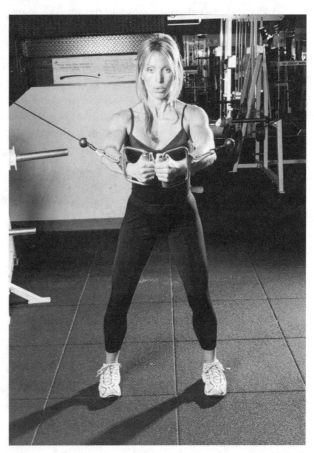

Push-Up

The push-up has become a neglected exercise that hasn't received the acclaim it warrants. The push-up is a very powerful exercise for developing the chest muscles, triceps and anterior deltoid muscles. It allows the trainee to utilize the proper biomechanics, which can better help isolate the chest muscles. Push-ups work beautifully in a super-set protocol, helping to fully exhaust the chest muscles for total recruitment of the muscle fibers in the chest.

Please notice the variation of hand widths that you can play with here. The wider the hand width, the more focus on the outer chest muscles. The closer the hand width, as shown in the diamond hand position, the more focus on the inner chest muscles and the triceps muscles of the arms. It is truly remarkable how you can customize your exercises according to what feels right and what doesn't.

PROPER ALIGNMENT

❶ Align your body face down with your arms extended in an elevated position. Keep your elbows slightly bent.

❷ Your hands should be flat on the floor directly underneath and a little wider than your shoulders.

❸ Keep the legs completely straight and your toes on the floor.

❹ Throughout the exercise, keep your head looking down in a neutral position.

TECHNIQUE AND FORM

❶ With your body properly aligned, lower yourself to within one inch of the floor. Ensure that your elbows travel out away from your body. Push-ups performed with the elbows traveling close to your body mainly target the triceps muscles.

❷ Make sure to inhale through your nose on the way down and exhale through the mouth on your way up.

❸ Focus on your chest muscles (feel them working here) and push your body off the floor using your toes as a pivot point.

❹ Make sure to keep your back straight, stomach muscles tightened and keep your head in line with your body. Maintaining the proper alignment is crucial.

❺ When you reach the top of the movement, make sure to contract the chest muscles as hard as you can. Try to avoid hyper-extending the elbow joints!

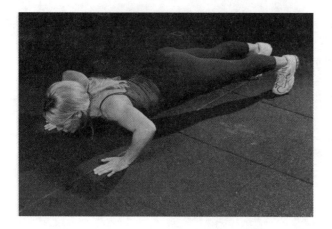
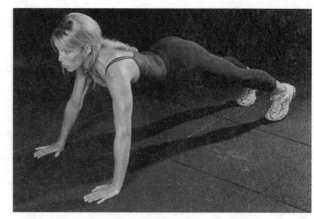

Push-Up

Narrow hand width will hit more of the inner chest and triceps muscles.

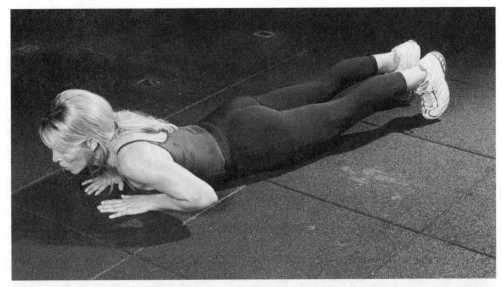

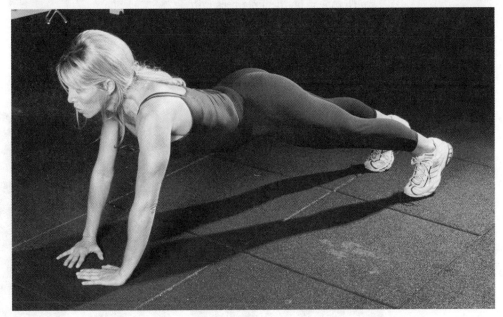

Assisted Push-Up

If you need to, you may use this modified push-up exercise until you have gained enough strength to do the regular push-up. This version is also an invaluable technique used when you have reached a level of experience that will allow you to push towards maximum muscular failure. Eventually, you will want to get to a level that will allow you to push out a couple of more repetitions when you can no longer do so on your own. These extra reps can be great for creating superb results in your physique.

Another option—shown in the photograph on the next page—is to have an assistant support part of your weight as you push up.

TECHNIQUE AND FORM

1 Take the same position and maintain the same form and technique as you would with the regular push-up. However, let your knees stay in contact with the floor.

2 You will find this exercise much easier because you will only be pushing up about half of your body weight.

3 Follow the same procedure as the regular push-up.

4 If you can still not perform push-ups by using the modified position described above, then perform them standing up at an angle against the wall.

MODIFICATIONS

Just like using various hand placement widths during the bench press exercise to focus in on specific areas of the chest, you can vary hand placement with the push-up.

• The wider your hand width, the more you'll zone in on the outer pecs with less triceps involvement.

• The closer the hand width, the more you'll zone in on the inner pecs with more triceps involvement.

• A medium hand width placement will be about 65 percent chest and 35 percent triceps.

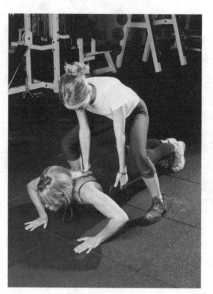
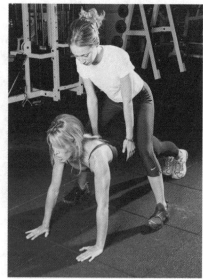

Bench Press Machine

This machine targets the pectoralis major (the mid-chest portion). Secondary emphasis is placed on the clavicular portion of the pectoralis major (upper chest), anterior deltoids, and triceps. For a similar dumbbell exercise, try either a Flat or Incline Dumbbell Bench Press.

TECHNIQUE AND FORM

❶ Sit on the machine and adjust the seat of the machine so that your upper chest is placed just above the handle bars provided by the lever.

❷ Select the desired resistance and grasp the handle bars with an overhand grip (palms facing down, and thumbs pointing towards each other). Your elbows should be placed out to the sides. The torso, shoulders, and upper arms should be elevated, creating a 90-degree angle between the torso and the upper arms. There should be a straight imaginary line between the bottom of the neck and the elbow.

❸ Using your chest muscles and not your arms, push the machine lever away from you until your arms are fully extended in front of you. Hold the contracted position for a second. Breathe out as you perform this movement.

❹ Return to the starting position as you breathe in.

TRAINER'S TIPS

❶ The only body parts moving should be the arms as they move the lever forward. The back and head should always remain on the seat. Many people bring the head forward as they perform the movement but this can hyperextend the neck muscles.

❷ Keep control of the machine at all times and concentrate on using the chest muscles as opposed to the arms.

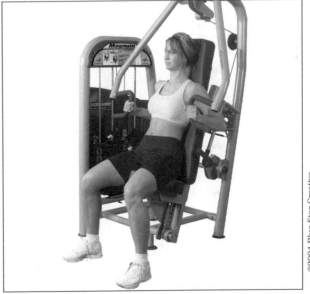

Peck Deck Machine

This machine targets the pectoralis major (the mid chest portion). Secondary emphasis is placed on the clavicular portion of the pectoralis major (upper chest) and anterior deltoids.

TECHNIQUE AND FORM

1 Sit on the machine and adjust the seat so that your upper chest is placed just above the handle bars provided by the lever.

2 Select the desired resistance and grasp the handle bars with a neutral grip (palms facing each other).

3 Position your upper arms in front of you, hands close to each other and upper arms parallel to the floor. This will be your starting position.

4 Move the levers back to the stretched position in which the arms are in line with your torso. Breathe in as you perform this movement.

5 Bring the levers back to the starting position as you exhale and contract the chest muscles. Hold for a second.

TRAINER'S TIPS

1 Keep a slight bend to your elbows in order to prevent stress at the biceps tendon.

2 Keep your back and the head on the back pad to avoid undue stress on the neck.

3 Some machines have handles instead of pads. If this is the case, perform the same movement but with your entire arm parallel to the floor.

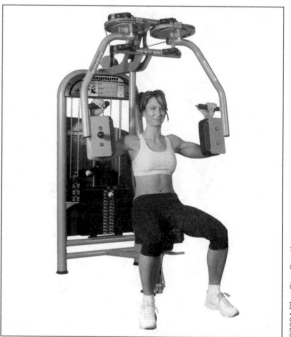

©2004 Blue Star Creative

Chapter 9
Shoulders

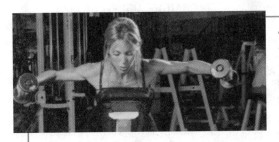

The shoulders can be a very stubborn body part, especially if you don't know how to train them correctly. Even a slight variation in an exercise's proper form can mean the difference between no results and major results. Some women have the ability to train incorrectly and still create beautiful looking results. There are usually many reasons for this occurrence, including genetics: some people have a body part or two that simply don't need isolation or intense exercises to allow them to develop. In most cases, however, the shoulders have a tendency to lag behind other muscle groups. Understand that most upper body exercises include the shoulders as a secondary muscle group, which could inhibit results for the shoulders because of overtraining. What it comes down to is this: If you don't learn how to train the shoulders correctly, you will not get the results you desire. If you learn what we teach and implement the material into your shoulder training, you can definitely expect to receive the results you've desired.

For immediate Body Sculpting Bible support & coaching directly from James & Hugo, please visit www.BodySculptingBibles.com

9

THE BODY
SCULPTING
BIBLE
FOR WOMEN

Dumbbell Shoulder Press

This exercise is a wonderful exercise for developing the shapely, lean shoulders many women strive for. Strong and toned shoulders make you look confident and secure. What good are toned triceps if the attached shoulder areas are flabby? No good at all. Work on creating muscle symmetry and your entire body will look completely balanced. The dumbbell shoulder press will focus on all of the muscles of the shoulder for complete shoulder muscle development.

PROPER ALIGNMENT

❶ Set your bench setting to a 90-degree angle (fully upright position), unless of course you already have access to a 90-degree angle seat.

❷ Pick up your dumbbells and place them on your thighs.

❸ Align your body from the bottom up.

❹ Make sure that your feet are flat on the floor facing straight ahead throughout the exercise. Your knees should also be facing straight ahead.

❺ Make sure that your whole back region is flush against the upright bench's back support. You must also concentrate on letting your chest relax. When you sit upright, it is natural that your chest will rise and move into the same upright position. This is bad because your chest muscles become the primary muscles working during the exercise and will take the focus away from the shoulders. You want to focus on keeping your back straight against the back pad while completely relaxing your chest. This will help direct all of the stimulation onto the shoulder muscles. If you see your chest rise or feel your chest muscles handling the majority of the work or helping to lift the weights, stop and correct yourself. You are either going too heavy or

you just need to practice your form without weight.

❻ Once you are seated in a fully upright position with the dumbbells on your thighs, thrust up one leg at a time. Let momentum help to lift the dumbbells into your starting position.

❼ Make sure that both dumbbells are held with your palms facing in front of you and level with the top of the shoulders.

❽ Relax your chest while keeping your back totally upright and your head and neck as relaxed as possible. Please note that you must never turn your head while doing any of these exercises. Position your body into the proper alignment, keeping your head straight, and stay that way throughout the exercise. If you don't, you could end up seriously injured!

❾ Keep your elbows as wide as possible as if you were trying to touch your elbows behind your back.

❿ Keep your upper arm horizontal to the floor; don't let the biceps and triceps sink below your shoulder height—this is the ideal level for a full range of motion for this exercise.

⓫ Keep your forearms in a perpendicular position while keeping your forearms pointed directly towards the ceiling at all times.

TECHNIQUE AND FORM

❶ After you've set yourself up in proper alignment, slowly begin pressing the dumbbells up towards the ceiling in a smooth, controlled, fluid motion, making sure that you do not use any momentum. I advise that you do not touch the dumbbells at the top and instead press the weights in a straight-line overhead. Touching the dumbbells at the top of the movement may put some undue stress onto the rotator cuff muscles.

❷ When you reach the top of the movement, do not lock out the elbow joint. When you lock out the elbow joint, you distribute all of the weight from the shoulders to the elbow joint, thus interrupting muscle stimulation. This can hurt the elbow joint and limit shoulder muscle stimulation.

❸ Without resting, slowly bring the dumbbells back down, making sure that your arms are wide, your head is level and that you maintain an upright position with your chest relaxed.

Dumbbell Shoulder Press

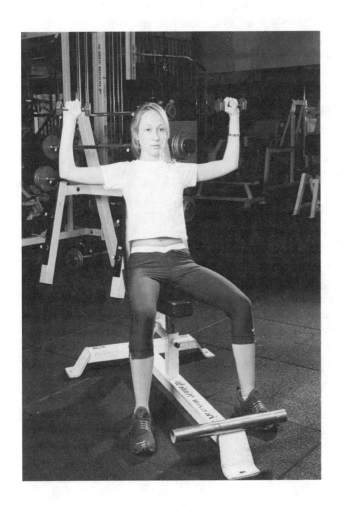 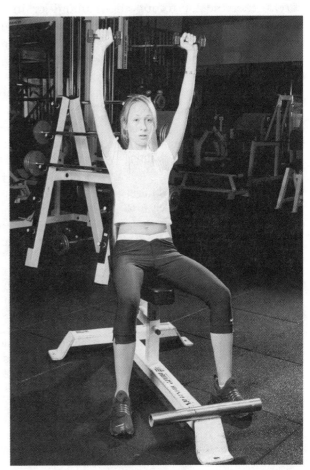

Dumbbell Lateral Raise

The shoulders have a tendency to be stubborn and are not necessarily easy to develop. This is a great exercise for toning those shoulder muscles located on the outside of the upper arms. Developing these muscles can give you the appearance of having a smaller waist. Pay attention to the description below as this exercise is often performed incorrectly. This will make the difference between no results and the results you want.

PROPER ALIGNMENT

❶ Take a standing position with a shoulder-width stance. Align the body from the bottom up, beginning with the feet. Make sure the feet are pointing straight ahead.

❷ Keep the knees pointing straight ahead and slightly bent to help avoid any unnecessary back strain.

❸ Hold a dumbbell in each hand with arms down at your sides. Your palms should be pointed toward your body.

❹ It is important to remember that as you lift the dumbbells, your palms should be facing downward, so your shoulder muscles rather than the biceps muscles do the work.

TECHNIQUE AND FORM

❶ Keeping your arms straight and at the sides of your body, lift the weights directly out to the sides until they reach the level of your cheeks.

❷ Hold the weights there for a one-second count.

❸ While maintaining your posture and body alignment, slowly lower the dumbbells in a controlled fashion back to the starting point. Make sure you pick a dumbbell weight that allows you to practice perfect form. If you pick a weight that is too heavy, momentum will force muscles other than the shoulder to do the work. Some people have the tendency to bend at the elbows. Keeping the arms straight allows for better isolation of the medial deltoid.

Dumbbell Lateral Raise

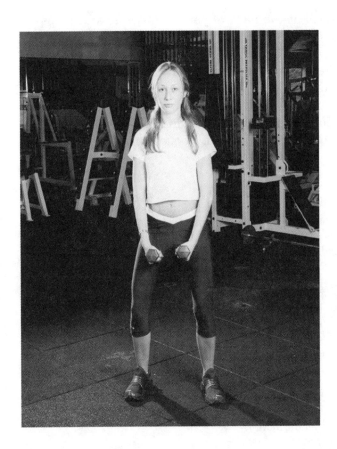 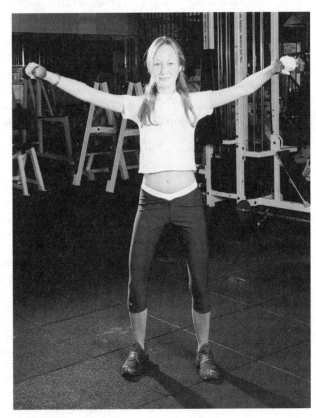

FAQ:

When I see people doing this exercise in my gym, they often bend their knees and heave the weights up. What is this doing?

ANSWER:

It's doing more harm than good. Using your knees to create momentum and lift the weights up and out to your sides does not benefit you at all. As you see in the exercise description picture, you life the weight by focusing on lifting the elbows straight out to the sides of your body. keeping the arms completely straight can be difficult and tough on the shoulder joints, which is why keeping a slight bend in your elbows will take some stress off of them.

Seated Bent-Over Lateral Raise

This exercise develops the rear deltoids, the muscles at the back of your shoulders, and helps to give your shoulders a three-dimensional appearance.

VARIATION: This exercise can also be done standing, but those with lower back problems are better off performing it seated. If you choose to stand, select a neutral position with a shoulder-width stance. Align, your body from the bottom up, beginning with the feet. Make sure your feet are pointing straight ahead. Keep your knees pointing straight ahead and slightly bent to help avoid any unnecessary back strain. Hold a dumbbell in each hand. Look straight ahead. Bend over at your hips

PROPER ALIGNMENT

❶ Place a couple of dumbbells parallel to and in front of a flat bench.

❷ Sit on the end of the bench with your legs together and the dumbbells behind your calves.

❸ Bend at the waist while keeping your back straight in order to pick up the dumbbells. The palms of your hands should be facing each other as you pick them up.

❹ Make sure your abdominals are pulled in throughout this exercise.

TECHNIQUE AND FORM

❶ Keeping your torso forward and stationary. and the arms slightly bent at the elbows, slowly and without momentum, lift the dumbbells straight out to the sides of the body until both arms are parallel to the floor-about shoulder height. Exhale as you lift the weights. Avoid swinging the torso or bringing the arms back instead of to the side. This is very important for rear deltoid isolation. Your elbows should be leading the exercise. Many people doing this and similar exercises lead with the dumbbells and take all the focus off the shoulders. When you lead the movement with dumbbells, you will not optimally stimulate the desired rear deltoid muscle. Try to make sure to move the whole arm together.

❷ Contract the rear deltoid muscle as hard as you can and hold for one second at the top of the exercise (shoulder level or slightly higher), then slowly lower the dumbbells back to the starting position. Your rear deltoid muscles should still be working while you lower the weight

❸ When you reach the starting position, do not rest. Slowly begin lifting the dumbbells out to each side of your body in a smooth, controlled, fluid motion, without using momentum. Repeat the recommended number of repetitions.

Seated Bent-Over Lateral Raise

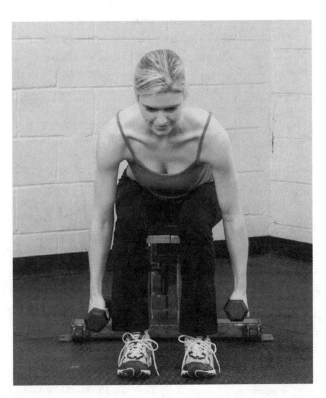

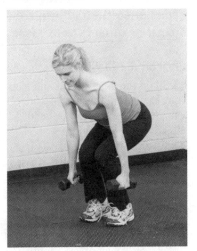

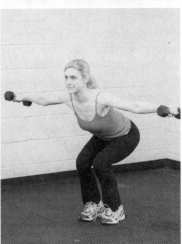

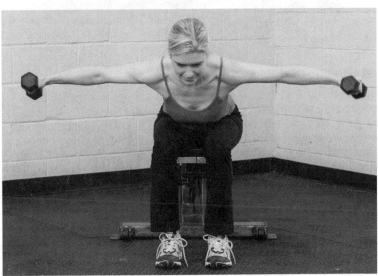

Military Press

Unlike behind-the-neck presses, which risk damaging the rotator cuffs, military presses are a great exercise to develop all three heads of the shoulder or deltoid muscles. You will find that a narrower grip focuses more on the muscles of the medial and rear deltoids with an emphasis on the triceps. The wider you go, the more you'll incorporate the front and medial deltoids. Look at your shoulders in a mirror and decide where you would like to see a little more muscle development or muscle tone. Based on that you can vary your grip for a customized exercise variation.

PROPER ALIGNMENT

❶ Sit on the military seat and place your feet flat on the floor in front of you. Your knees should be facing straight ahead.

❷ Take hold of the barbell with your grip of choice. Remember that grip variation will stimulate certain muscles more than others. The best thing you can do for your body is to assess your shoulder muscles and decide what portion of the three heads are in need of further development for overall muscle balance and symmetry.

❸ Sit all the way back in the seat, making sure that your back is straight and flat against the back pad.

❹ A mistake made when doing either this exercise or the dumbbell shoulder press is to stick the chest way out when pressing up. Do not do this! Remember, when you stick the chest out during the press, you take primary stimulation away from the shoulder muscles and direct it to the chest muscles. You want to relax the chest at all times during this exercise. If you see your chest rise or feel your chest muscles handling the majority of the work, stop and correct yourself. You may either be going too heavy, or you just need to practice your form without weight.

❺ As you hold the bar, make sure that your arms and elbows are as wide as possible (as if you were trying to touch your elbows behind your back).

❻ Keep your upper arm horizontal to the floor and don't let the biceps and triceps region sink below shoulder height as this is the ideal level for a full range of motion for this exercise.

❼ Keep your forearms in a vertical position (they should point directly towards the ceiling at all times).

❽ Make sure that your head and neck are as relaxed as possible throughout the entire exercise. Please note that you must never turn your head while doing any of these exercises. Position your body into the proper alignment, keeping your head straight, and stay that way throughout the exercise! If you don't, you could end up seriously injured.

TECHNIQUE AND FORM

Before you begin the exercise, close your eyes and visualize yourself doing the movement. Focus on the shoulder muscles you are about to stimulate. Remember what we discussed about assessing your shoulder muscles and comparing the balance and symmetry of the muscles. This goes for all muscles. Pay close attention to the muscles that are lagging behind others and concentrate all of your energies to those areas during the exercise. If your muscles are already in balance and symmetric, focus on the muscle as a whole.

❶ You should now be in position to begin. First, pick up the bar and begin the exercise from the top position.

❷ With the arms and elbows wide and head level, slowly bring the bar down to an area slightly below the chin. The upper arm, from the elbow to the shoulder, should end up slightly below parallel to the floor, with your forearms perpendicular to the ceiling.

❸ When you reach the bottom of the movement as your upper arms are lowered slightly below chin level slowly begin pressing upward in a smooth, controlled, fluid motion, without resting. Make sure that you do not use any momentum.

❹ When you reach the top of the movement, do not lock out the elbow joint. When you lock out the elbow joint, you distribute all of the weight from the shoulders to the elbow joint, thus interrupting muscle stimulation. This can hurt the elbow joint and limit shoulder muscle stimulation.

❺ From this point, slowly begin to lower the bar in a smooth, controlled, fluid motion, without resting.

Military Press

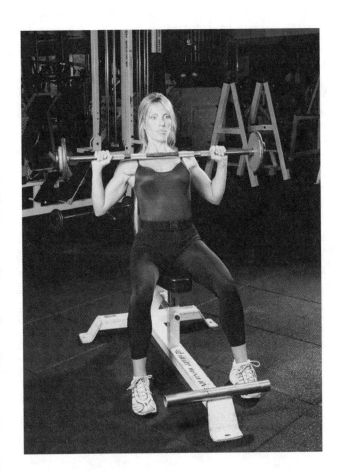
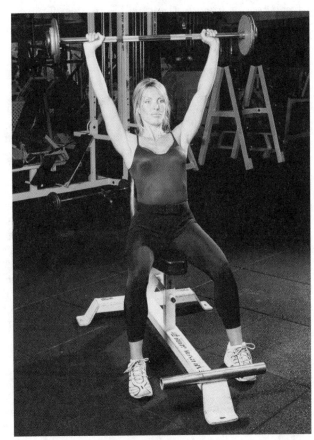

FAQ:

Why do I constantly see so many people leaning back while doing this exercise?

ANSWER:

Leaning back while doing the military press will bring your upper chest muscles into the movement. This stops isolating the shoulder muscles. Many people do this because they are lifting too heavy a weight-or perhaps their shoulders became tired and they leaned back to get the weight up. If you have trouble staying upright during the military press, either go lighter, or plant your feet behind you to help maintain your upright position.

Front Raise

This exercise is great for working the shoulder muscles, as long as you keep yourself in perfect form to not engage the chest muscles. There are several variations to experiment with, including performing with one hand alone, alternating hands, or using a barbell instead of dumbbells.

PROPER ALIGNMENT

1 Stand with a straight torso and the dumbbells resting in front of your thighs with the palms of your hands facing you. Align the body from the bottom up, beginning with the feet. Make sure the feet are pointing straight ahead.

2 Keep knees pointing straight ahead and slightly bent to prevent any unnecessary back strain.

3 Remember that as you lift the dumbbells your palms should be facing downward so that your shoulder muscles do the work, not your biceps muscles.

TECHNIQUE AND FORM

1 While standing still, lift the dumbbells straight to the front, with a slight bend of the elbow and the palms of the hands facing down.

2 While exhaling, continue until your arms are parallel to the floor. Pause for a second at the top of the movement.

3 Inhale and lower the dumbbells slowly in a controlled fashion to the starting position while maintaining your posture and body alignment. Make sure you choose a weight that allows you to practice perfect form. If you use a weight that is too heavy, momentum will force muscles other than the shoulders to do the work.

Front Raise

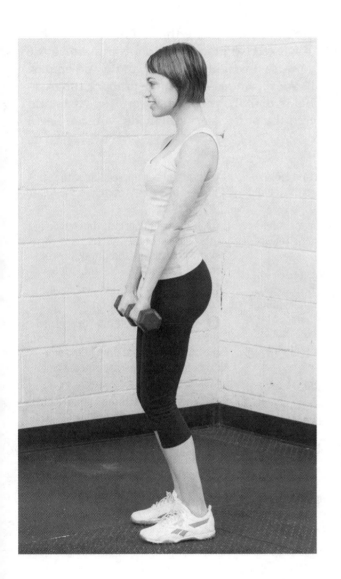 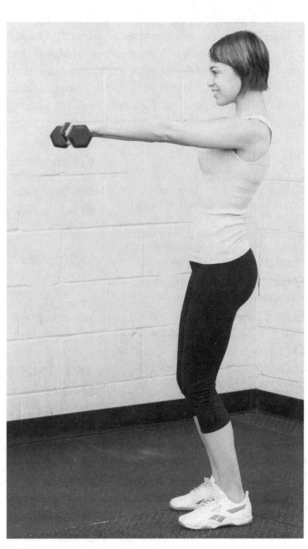

Upright Row

Upright rows are a great exercise to develop the tie-in muscles, aesthetically tying your shoulders and trapezius muscles together for a beautifully fluid look. You must make certain that you use very strict form with this exercise, and avoid using momentum at all times. The rotator cuff muscles of the shoulder are extremely delicate and are prone to injuries that occur as a result of using poor form and excessive weight. The upright row exercise movement alone can stress the rotator cuff muscles. This makes it imperative that you use a weight you can handle and employ perfect form and technique and no momentum at all. We recommend that you practice the exercise using a cambered (E-Z Curl Bar) bar at first. This is usually much easier on the wrists and shoulders than a straight barbell. After you've mastered the perfect form methods, you can begin using two separate dumbbells for variety.

PROPER ALIGNMENT

❶ Choose a weight for the cambered bar that is easy enough so you can focus only on your form. Once you have mastered the correct form, it will become second nature and you will find it easy to move up in weight, thereby stimulating the shoulder muscles.

❷ Grasp the bar using a shoulder-width grip.

❸ Place your feet shoulder-width apart and point them straight ahead.

❹ Keep your knees slightly bent at all times during the movement to take stress off the lower back region. Also, keep the knees pointing straight ahead.

❺ Contract the abdominal muscles slightly to help keep your postural alignment.

❻ Keep your back straight and body still as you do the exercise.

❼ Relax the musculature of your chest and back.

❽ Keep your head level and look straight ahead at all times during the exercise.

❾ Hold the bar across your thighs and keep your palms facing toward your body.

❿ Begin focusing on the muscles of the shoulder including the trapezius muscles. Although you will be pulling the weight up with your hands, you must let the elbows lead the motion, keeping them high as you pull up.

TECHNIQUE AND FORM

❶ Before you begin the exercise, close your eyes and once again visualize yourself actually doing the movement while focusing on the shoulder and trapezius muscles.

❷ With proper form and postural alignment, begin pulling the bar up slowly, concentrating on feeling the stimulation of the focused muscles.

❸ Pull the bar up, leading with your elbows, to a point where it comes close to your chin.

❹ The most important thing to do at this position of the exercise is to consciously focus on and physically contract the muscles of the trapezius.

❺ Hold the contraction here for a count of one to two seconds.

❻ With just enough time to contract the trap muscles, slowly begin lowering the bar while maintaining the same exact form and posture you did when pulling up.

❼ When you reach the bottom (start) position, slowly begin pulling the bar back to the top position of the exercise using a smooth, controlled, fluid motion. Make sure that you do not jerk or use momentum to lift the bar at any time during this exercise.

Upright Row

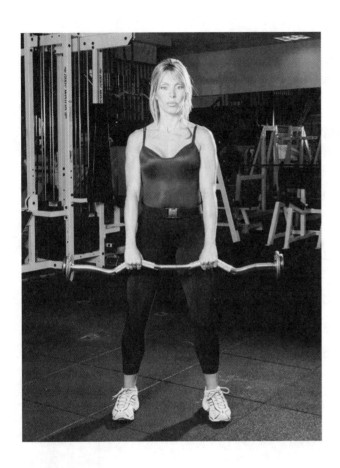

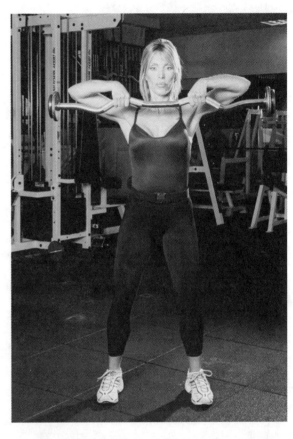

VARIATION

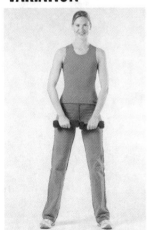

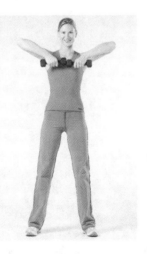

FAQ:

When I do this exercise it sometimes hurts my shoulder joints and rotator cuff muscles. Why?

ANSWER:

To avoid pain, try this: When you begin the movement with the bar lying on your upper thigh, as you pull it up, bring the bar about four to six inches away from your body. This distances will take some pressure off of the joints and the rotator cuff. It will be more challenging, so you may need to go a bit lighter than previously.

Bent-Arm Bent-Over Row

This exercise can also be done standing, but those with lower back problems are better off performing it seated.

PROPER ALIGNMENT

❶ Place a couple of dumbbells parallel to and in front of a flat bench.

❷ Sit on the end of the bench with your legs together and the dumbbells behind your calves.

❸ Bend at the waist while keeping your back straight in order to pick up the dumbbells. As you pick them up, the palms of your hands should be facing behind.

❹ Bend at the elbows until there is a 90-degree angle between the forearm and upper arm.

TECHNIQUE AND FORM

❶ Keep your torso forward and stationary with arms bent at a 90- degree angle at the elbows, and lift the dumbbells straight to the side until both upper arms are parallel to the floor. The forearms should be pointed to the floor in this contracted position. Exhale as you lift the weights. Avoid swinging the torso or bringing the arms back rather than to the side.

❷ After a one second contraction at the top slowly lower the dumbbells back to the starting position.

❸ Repeat for the recommended number of repetitions.

Bent-Arm Bent-Over Row

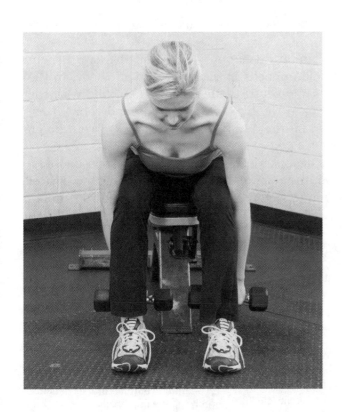 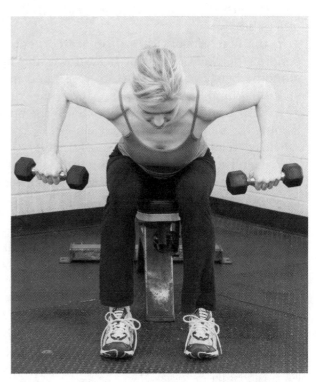

Bent-Over Lateral Raise on Incline Bench

The bent-over lateral raise is a great exercise for developing the rear deltoid muscles of the shoulder, which in our opinion is one of the most poorly trained muscles in the body. By using this exercise to develop these muscles, you will give your shoulders a very sexy, three-dimensional look.

There are three ways that you can do this exercise. We will describe one in depth and the others briefly.

In the first version, called the seated bent-over lateral raise, you sit on the edge of a bench, bend at the waist with your head down and lift the dumbbells to each side of your body. In the standing bent-over lateral raise, you stand in the same postural alignment as you did with the standing dumbbell lateral raise. This time, bend over at the hips. Once again, bend your knees, keep your back straight and parallel to the floor and lift the dumbbells to the sides of your body, leading the movement with your elbows.

The exercise we will discuss now, however, is the best exercise for developing the rear deltoids. This exercise is the bent-over lateral raise done on an incline bench. It will give you the best of both of the exercises we first discussed, allowing you to stay very strict while keeping you almost parallel to the floor.

PROPER ALIGNMENT

❶ Choose two light dumbbells so that you may practice perfect form.

❷ Rest your entire torso, from your pelvic bone to your chest, on the incline bench's angled pad with your head and eyes looking straight ahead.

❸ Position your feet shoulder-width apart, pointing them straight ahead at all times during the exercise.

❹ Make sure that your knees are bent so there is no unnecessary lower back stress.

❺ Bring the dumbbells down to each side of your body with your palms facing each other.

❻ Make sure that you are positioned steadily on the bench incline.

❼ Bring your head up to the level of your torso, which must be close to or parallel to the floor. Look straight ahead.

❽ As you prepare to do the exercise, focus all of your attention and concentration on the rear deltoid muscles of the shoulder. Know where these muscles are located and how they feel when stimulated. This is why we suggest that you go light, so that you may isolate these muscles without incorporating others into the movement.

❾ As you lift the dumbbells to the sides of your body, your elbows will be leading the motion. Many people who do this and similar exercises lead the movement with the dumbbells and take all of the focus off the shoulders. When you lead the exercise movement with the dumbbells, you will not optimally stimulate the desired rear deltoid muscles.

TECHNIQUE AND FORM

❶ Slowly and without momentum, begin lifting the dumbbells out to each side of your body.

❷ Try to move your whole arm together, or at least make sure that the elbows are leading the movement.

❸ Do not lift your torso as you lift. If you find that you are in fact lifting your torso for momentum assistance, stop! Either lighten the weight or rest for one minute and do your next set. Don't just go through the motions just to get the weights up. Focus on isolation of the rear deltoid muscles, and make them work hard.

❹ Make sure that you lift the dumbbells straight out to your sides rather than behind you. This is very important for rear deltoid isolation.

❺ Maintain your postural alignment and bring the dumbbells up to level with your shoulders or slightly higher.

❻ Squeeze the dumbbells back while you contract the rear deltoid muscles as hard as you can. Hold this contraction for one second.

❼ From this point, slowly begin lowering the dumbbells, making sure that you make the rear deltoid muscles continue to work during the lowering portion of the exercise.

❽ As you reach the start position, do not rest. Slowly begin lifting the dumbbells out to each side of your body in a smooth, controlled and fluid motion, without using momentum.

Bent-Over Lateral Raise on Incline Bench

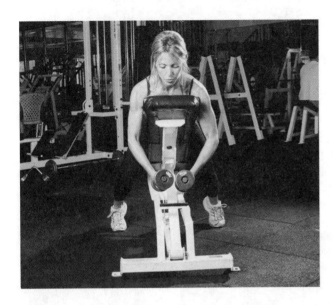 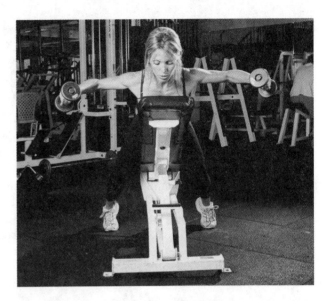

FAQ:

I don't feel the stimulation in my rear deltoids as much as I feel it in my triceps and upper back muscles. Why is this?

ANSWER:

If this is the case, try bringing your arms a little further in front of your body as you lift. This slight variation should redirect the stimulation to the rear deltoids. As far as the triceps are involved, you must work to maintain that slight bend in the elbows throughout the exercise. You will experience the triceps involvement if you can't maintain it. The place where this customarily happens is at the top of the movement, where the elbow is extended.

Two-Arm Cable Lateral Raise

Using cables to perform laterals provides resistance during the positive and negative phases of your repetition. You may need to use lighter weights than usual for this exercise. Any pain in your neck is an indication that the weight you are lifting may be too heavy. Make sure to keep your head in line with your spine throughout this exercise.

PROPER ALIGNMENT

❶ Place the pins at the desired weights in the cable machine.

❷ Stand in the center of the cables, lean slightly forward from your hips while maintaining erect posture.

❸ Keep your knees bent and your abdominals engaged. Hold a handle in each hand.

❹ Pull the handles in until your arms cross under your chest.

TECHNIQUE AND FORM

❶ Extend your arms in an upward arc-like movement, until they are parallel to the floor.

❷ At the top position, hold for a couple of seconds before returning to the crossed position.

❸ Repeat for the desired number of repetitions.

Two-Arm Cable Lateral Raise

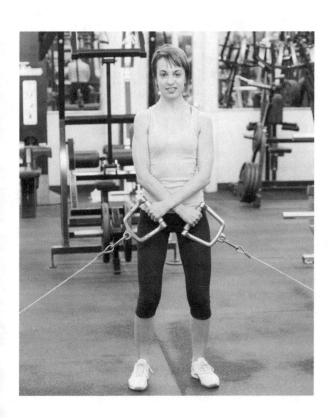
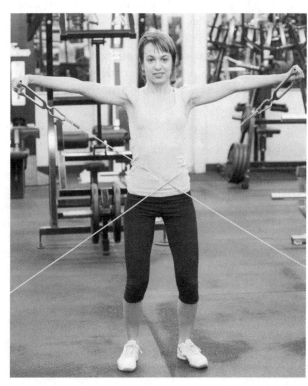

Seated Rear Delt Machine

The seated rear-delt machine is a great exercise to use when you're looking to add variety to your shoulder training. It will give you the ability to really focus on isolating the rear deltoids without the possibility of lower back injury and the burden of having to bend over at the hips. This is a perfect exercise for those who feel dizzy when bent over or feel too much chest compression from having to lean on the incline bench. All you have to do to begin exercising is set the pin to the desired resistance and position the level of the seat.

VARIATION: A variation you can try without a machine sues a bench and one dumbbell. Simply place one knee and one hand on a bench, bend over, keeping the lumbar curve in your lower back, and lift the dumbbell up, bending your elbow so your arm creates a 90-degree angle.

PROPER ALIGNMENT

❶ Sit yourself on the machine and position your body so that you are sitting upright with your chest flush against the vertical pad. There should be a seat adjustment that will allow you to raise and lower the seat. Bring the seat to a height where your chin can rest neutrally on the edge of the pad in front of you. This is a good height to optimize the proper anatomical position for this shoulder exercise.

❷ Keep your feet flat on the floor and pointing straight ahead during the movement. Also, keep your knees pointing straight ahead at all times. On most rear-delt machines, you will find inner thigh pads for added stability. Keep your thighs snug against the pads to give you the added support needed to secure your core musculature.

❸ This machine is often used as a pec deck and gives you the option of adjusting the arm bars to your liking. For this particular exercise, you will want the arm bars brought to the back position so they are just about touching one another. You also might have the option of taking your handgrip in a palms facing position or an over-hand position. Take the overhand position since this will take much stress off the wrists and allow better muscle control and isolation of the rear shoulders, thus negating the triceps muscles as much as possible from the movement.

❹ Make sure that you keep a slight bend in the elbows at all times. This bend of the arms will help maintain focus of resistance on the rear delts and off the triceps. You might reach a level of fatigue where you are forced to use the triceps muscles to move the weight. When you reach this point, either resist the temptation or simply lower the weight.

❺ Keep your chest cavity against the chest pad at all times during the exercise with your torso totally upright.

TECHNIQUE AND FORM

❶ Begin the exercise with your feet flat on the floor, thighs pinned snug against the thigh pads, and body upright with chest against the pad and chin rested on the edge.

❷ With hands holding the grips in an overhand position, make sure that your elbows are pointed directly out to the sides. This is very important for isolation of the rear delt muscles.

❸ Before you begin the movement, make sure you are consciously focused on the rear delt muscles and begin to isometrically contract them before moving the weight. This might take some practice to perfect, but you will soon multiply your muscle isolation abilities ten-fold.

❹ Begin bringing the bars away from each other and maintain your anatomical positioning at all times. Bring the bars as far back as possible without jerking or using momentum to do so.

❺ As you reach the top of the movement, with arms fully extended outward, try to hold this position for one count while feeling the rear shoulder muscles taking the brunt of the resistance. At this point, really squeeze the rear delts.

❻ Slowly allow the arms to return to the start position, resisting the bars on the negative portion of the exercise.

❼ Once you have reached the position where the bars are just about touching each other, do not allow the weight stack to touch the bottom. You want to keep constant tension on the muscles and must stop right before the weights touch bottom. From here immediately begin to bring the bars apart once again with great form.

Seated Rear Delt Machine

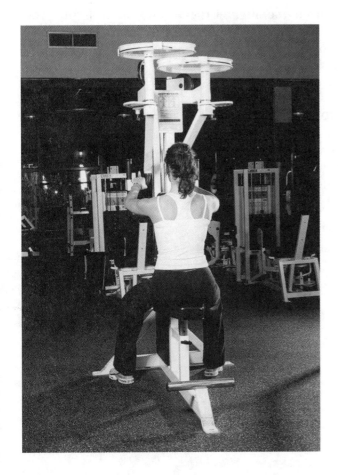

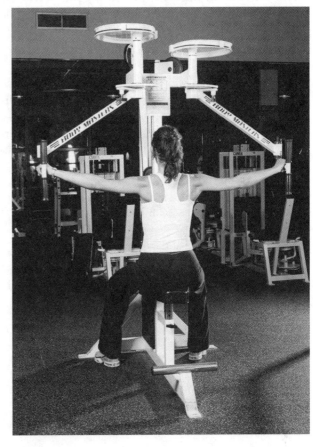

FAQ:

The overhand grip hurts my wrists. Can I use another grip?

ANSWER:

Yes. There are several other grips available on this machine. Try a couple to see which one feels comfortable and helps to elicit the best recruitment of the rear deltoid muscles.

VARIATION

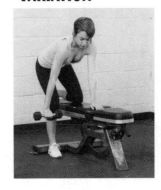

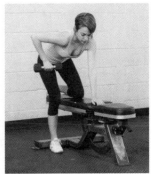

Rotator Cuff

The four small muscles of the rotator cuff need strengthening, as they are prone to injury. You will need to use a noticeably lighter weight for this exercise than for other arm exercises. To make sure that you get the maximum benefit from this exercise, make sure you maintain the 90-degree angle in the arms throughout the range of motion.

PROPER ALIGNMENT

❶ Stand in a neutral position. Your feet should be just under shoulder width apart, your knees slightly bent, your shoulders back and your chest out.

❷ You should be holding a light weight in each hand, your palms facing behind you.

❸ Bend your arms so that the upper and lower arms are at a 90 degree angle, your arms parallel to the floor and extended before you.

TECHNIQUE AND FORM

❶ Exhale and rotate your shoulders so that your hands rise about you elbows and your palms face front.

❷ Slowly return to the start position. At no time should your arms not be in a 90-degree angle, as this could cause stress or injury on your rotator cuff.

❸ Repeat for the desired number of repetitions.

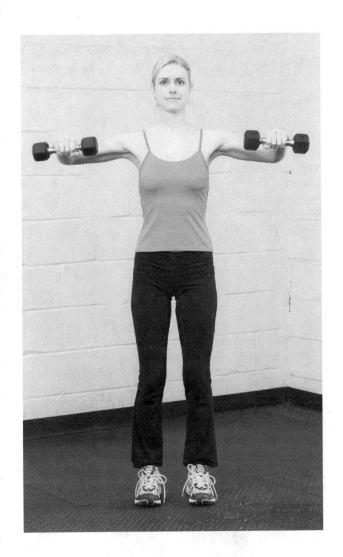

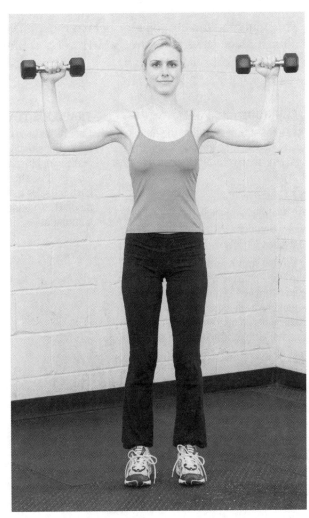

Reverse Fly Machine

This machine targets the rear deltoid most effectively. This is one of the few machines which I feel is almost as effective as its free weight version (the Bent-Over Lateral Raise) due to the degree of isolation that it provides.

TECHNIQUE AND FORM

❶ Adjust the seat so that the handles are at shoulder height and sit on the machine with your torso pressed against the pad.

❷ Grasp the handles.

❸ Slightly bend your elbows and rotate your shoulders so that the elbows are to the sides. This is your starting position.

❹ Using your rear deltoid muscles, pull the levers apart and to the rear until elbows are just behind back. There should be a slight bend at the elbows. Exhale as you perform this movement and hold the contraction for a second.

❺ Slowly return to the starting position as you inhale.

TRAINER'S TIPS

Ensure that the elbows do not drop below the shoulders in order to maximize rear deltoid involvement. If you let the elbows drop, then you start using the back muscles more to perform the movement, thus taking away from deltoid stimulation.

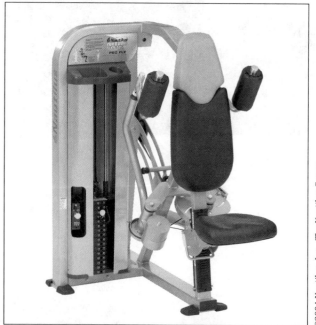

Chapter 10
Triceps

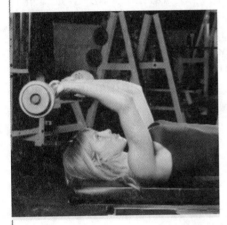

The triceps muscle, located on the back of the upper arm, can be tricky to develop, which is why many women worry about having flabby arms. That's because this three-headed muscle requires different angles of training for full development. A lot of people don't realize that just one exercise for most body parts simply won't cut it, unless you want a simple looking body with simple looking muscles. Specific exercises will stimulate specific muscles to work as primary muscles and incorporate other muscles to work as the secondary muscles. The following exercises incorporate all angles of training, providing total triceps muscle development for flab-free and superbly toned arms. The most important thing to remember with this and all exercises is to concentrate on keeping your form and technique correct during the exercise movement.

For immediate Body Sculpting Bible support & coaching directly from James & Hugo, please visit www.BodySculptingBibles.com

10

THE BODY SCULPTING BIBLE FOR WOMEN

Overhead Dumbbell Extension

The overhead dumbbell extension focuses on the middle and inner heads of the triceps muscle. You can do this exercise either while seated or while standing. We recommend you do the seated version, as you will be less likely to cheat using momentum and injuries will be less likely to occur. One very important thing to remember is to keep the elbows pointed to the ceiling above you at all times during the movement. This will help create a full range of motion for the triceps. You also need to hold the upper arms close to your head as you extend the weight overhead. Finally, and one of the most important things to remember and perfect with this exercise, is your handgrip on the dumbbell. It is not easy to get a perfectly even grip for both hands with this exercise. If you fail to grip the dumbbell evenly, you may end up directing the force of the dumbbell resistance to one arm more than the other. This will create muscle imbalance between the two muscles. To fix this, you must learn to either grip the top, inner portion of the dumbbell with a separate, even grip for both hands or with an overlapping grip having one hand overlap the other. We recommend that you choose, if available, a dumbbell that adequately allows two separate and even hand grips. Unfortunately, most dumbbells will not allow a great deal of space to securely grip in this fashion, but you might luck out considering your hands may be smaller than most men's hands. If this is not the case, you must learn to perfect your overlapping grip for better balance and muscle symmetry.

PROPER ALIGNMENT

❶ Choose a weight that you believe to be light enough to practice perfect form. Place the dumbbell on top of your thigh. You can also have someone hand the dumbbell to you from behind. This is especially useful when using very heavy weight and to avoid injuring the shoulder joints.

❷ Sit on a bench with a 90-degree angled back pad.

❸ Sit all the way back into the seat, making sure that your back is flat against the pad at all times during the movement.

❹ Before lifting the weight into position overhead, make sure that your feet are placed flat on the floor and pointed straight ahead. Make sure that your knees are also pointing straight ahead.

❺ Keep the head level and facing straight ahead at all times during the movement.

❻ Position the dumbbell overhead or have someone hand it to you from behind.

❼ In the above position, choose your grip of choice on the dumbbell.

❽ Point your elbows straight to the ceiling above you while holding your arms and elbows close to your head for triceps isolation.

TECHNIQUE AND FORM

❶ With the dumbbell overhead and in position, begin lowering the dumbbell while keeping the elbows pointed directly to the ceiling. It is important to do this because it will help isolate the triceps muscle and provide a full range of productive motion. It will also help you avoid hitting the dumbbell on the back of your head while extending and lowering the dumbbell.

❷ As you lower the dumbbell, focus on the triceps muscle and feel the stretch.

Always take this negative portion slow and stay in control.

❸ Lower the dumbbell to a point where your forearms are slightly below parallel to the ground. You should feel a big stretch in the triceps.

❹ Without any rest and avoiding the use of momentum, begin pressing the weight back up to the top position. Make sure that you are using perfect form, while maintaining the correct postural alignment.

❺ All of your attention must be on the triceps muscle, focusing on the isolation of the muscles.

❻ As you approach the top of the movement, contract the triceps muscles as hard as you possibly can while avoiding intensely locking out the elbow joints.

❼ Hold this contraction for a one to two second count and begin your descent, lowering the dumbbell in a slow, controlled and fluid manner.

Overhead Dumbbell Extension

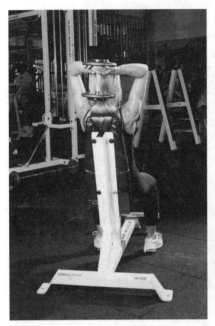

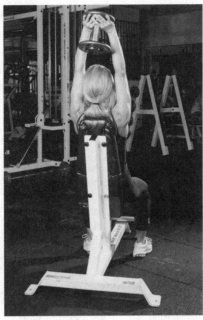

FAQ:

This exercise really hurts my elbows. What can I do to prevent this?

ANSWER:

This can be a very good exercise, but make no mistake; it can also be very tough on those elbow joints. Think about the position you're in: you are holding a moderate to heavy weight over your head, with your elbows flexed. All of the pressure is coming from two different points, compression caused by the dumbbell being overhead, and the force of the dumbbell pulling on your elbow joint. If you have elbow problems or simply feel pressure or pain from this exercise, you should switch it immediately with something less strenuous.

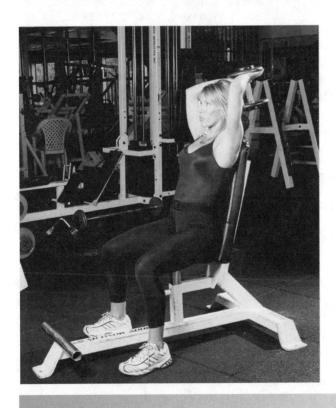

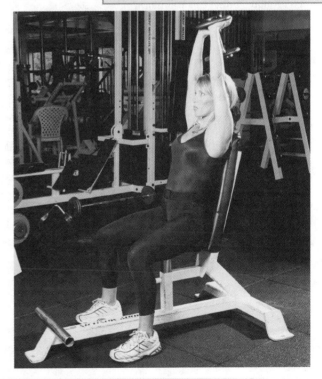

Lying Dumbbell Extension

This exercise is a favorite for both women and men. The lying position provides greater stability to lift more safely, preventing a chance of injury to your lower back. Much like the flat dumbbell press, it also allows greater leverage to occur, allowing better strength output with a smoother exercise movement. Always make sure to move the dumbbells slowly from start to finish and squeeze the triceps muscles at the top of the movement to really feel the triceps working. If you had to choose one exercise for the triceps, this might very well be the one.

PROPER ALIGNMENT

❶ Pick up two dumbbells, making sure that they are light enough for you to practice perfect form or for simply warming up your triceps muscles.

❷ Sit at the end of a flat bench with the weights positioned upright on top of your thighs.

❸ It is very important to grip both dumbbell handles all the way at the end closest to your thighs. Make sure to slide your hands all the way to the bottom of the handle so that the pinky side of your hand is up against the weight plate. Doing this will help you control the weight better while also allowing you to contract the triceps muscles harder at the top of the movement.

❹ Thrust each dumbbell up just as you would when doing a dumbbell bench press.

❺ Lay back on the bench and place your feet flat onto the floor.

❻ As you are lying down, keeping the long side of the dumbbells and the palms of your hands facing each other at all times, press the weights up using your chest muscles (chest press). You will begin the exercise in this position to avoid stressing the elbow joint. If you start at the bottom position of this exercise, you can easily create too much pressure on the elbow joint capsule, risking long-term injury. Remember, throughout the movement, the palms of your hands and your inner elbows must always face each other. You want to make sure that your whole arm is in a direct line with your front shoulder (anterior deltoid).

❼ You must also make sure that your elbows are pointing directly at the ceiling at all times during the exercise.

❽ Begin the exercise with the arms fully extended overhead, holding the dumbbells high to the ceiling.

TECHNIQUE AND FORM

❶ Once you are in the proper body alignment with the dumbbells overhead, slowly lower the dumbbells down toward your shoulders. While doing this, your elbows will remain pointing directly at the ceiling; and your entire arm from the elbows to the shoulders will be frozen at all times. These steps are necessary for proper triceps stimulation during this exercise. Remember to consciously focus all of your attention on proper form and stimulation of the triceps muscles.

❷ As you lower the dumbbells, stop just before the dumbbells reach your shoulders and begin to slowly and smoothly extend your arms from the elbows to the hands back up to the starting position of the exercise. Remember to keep your upper arm frozen in place.

❸ As you reach the top of the exercise, contract the triceps muscles as hard as you possibly can for complete muscle stimulation. Make sure that you avoid excessively locking the elbow joint. Once you reach the position of full elbow extension, do not thrust the elbow joint into a locked position. Instead, contract the triceps muscles as hard as you possibly can. Practice using light weights with this technique as practice will make for perfect execution of the exercise and better results. Also, make sure that there is a smooth transition when switching from lowering the dumbbells to raising the dumbbells. Do not rest between lowering and raising the dumbbells.

Lying Dumbbell Extension

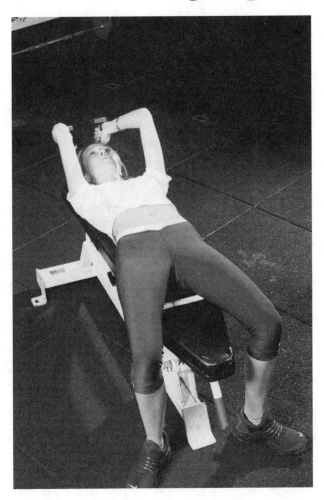 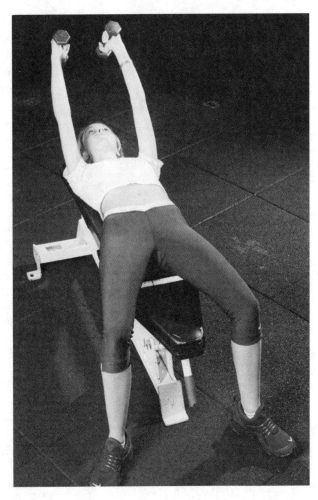

FAQ:

I feel the same pain and pressure as I did with the overhead dumbbell extension.

ANSWER:

Your elbows are under the same pressure here. However, you can take a bit of the shearing force off of the elbow joints by making sure to keep your arms angled back throughout the exercise. If you still feel discomfort, switch this exercise with another.

Lying E-Z Bar Extension

This triceps exercise is one that will fully stimulate all three muscles of the triceps. It is performed with an E-Z Bar curl bar, a curved looking bar usually found in the free weight section of your gym or health club. You might want to start with this exercise, considering it can help build your strength and coordination, preparing you for the Lying Dumbbell Triceps Extensions. If you don't have access to this type of bar, just stick with the lying dumbbell triceps extension, as these exercises are very similar.

PROPER ALIGNMENT

1 Set up a cambered bar (E-Z curl bar) with some light weight on each side or get one that is already pre-weighted. You can rest the curl bar on your thighs and lay back, set it in place so that it is at the base of your head while you lie down, or simply have someone hand it to you when you are already lying down.

2 Before lifting the bar or having it handed to you, lay back on the bench and place your feet flat onto the floor, pointing straight ahead.

3 As you are lying down, lift the bar into place by pressing it up using your chest muscles (like the chest press). Hold it up above your head and stay there. You will begin the exercise in this position to avoid stressing the elbow joint. If you start at the bottom position of this exercise, you can easily create too much pressure on the elbow joint capsule, risking long-term injury. Once you begin the movement from the top, the pressure in the elbow joints will be reduced as you reach the bottom position.

4 Remember, your inner elbows must always face each other during the exercise.

5 Make sure that your whole arm is in a direct line with your front shoulder (anterior deltoid).

6 This exercise will be done slightly differently from the lying two-dumbbell extension. Take a grip on the bar and position your hands about 8 to 10 inches apart; bring the E-Z bar overhead and position your elbows so that they are pointing directly to the ceiling above you but now, you will point your elbows slightly behind you and toward the ceiling on an angle. Doing this with the E-Z curl bar in your hands will automatically distribute the resistance from resting on the elbow joints to the triceps muscles. We don't recommend that you do this with the lying dumbbell extension because the two movements will stimulate different areas of the triceps muscles.

Begin the exercise just as we described it to you and maintain that technique, form and postural alignment throughout the exercise.

TECHNIQUE AND FORM

1 Once you are in the proper body alignment with the E-Z curl bar overhead, slowly begin to lower the bar down toward your forehead. While doing this, your elbows will remain pointing slightly behind you on an angle toward the ceiling.

2 Make sure that your entire arm from the elbow to the shoulder is frozen in place at all times during the exercise. These steps are necessary for proper triceps stimulation during this exercise.

3 Remember to consciously focus all of your attention on proper form and stimulation of the triceps muscles.

4 As you lower the bar, stop just before it reaches your forehead and begin to slowly and smoothly extend your arms back up to the starting position of the exercise.

5 As you reach the top of the exercise, make sure you are consciously contracting the triceps muscles as hard as you possibly can for complete muscle stimulation.

6 Hold this contraction for one second.

7 Make sure there is a smooth transition when switching directions. There should be no rest at all when switching from the bottom position to the upward extension of the bar.

Lying E-Z Bar Extension

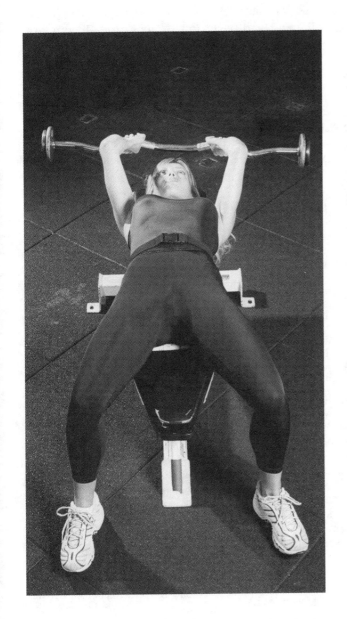
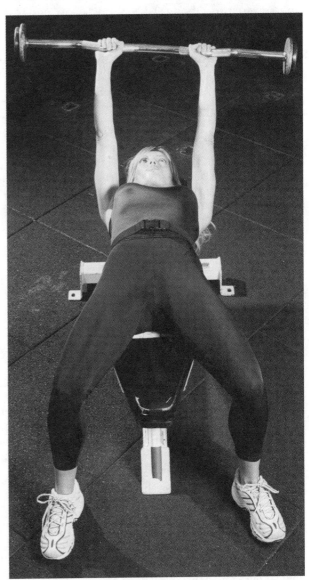

Triceps Dip

The triceps dip is a great muscle-enhancing exercise focusing on the lower triceps, which are closer to the elbow. To isolate the triceps, you will need a dip station or machine. If you are working out in your home, you can purchase an inexpensive dip unit from one of the sports-related retail chains or a wholesale fitness supply store. Just remember that the dips are not an easy exercise. Do not get discouraged if you can't yet do this exercise, because you soon will be able to, GUARANTEED!

PROPER ALIGNMENT

❶ First, place your hands on the parallel bars as you position yourself for postural alignment. The best way to do this is to raise yourself up onto the dip bars by locking out your arms. Align your body starting with your head and moving down to your feet. We have found a fantastic way of doing triceps dips that makes it very easy to isolate the triceps muscles. To make it as easily understood as possible, your entire body from head to toes should be as straight as possible throughout the exercise.

❷ As you lower yourself from the lockout position, keep your head in a neutral or level position.

❸ Your chest and shoulders must be completely upright and as straight as possible.

❹ Your arms and elbows will ride close to your body as you lower yourself and when pushing to triceps lockout.

❺ Your abdominal muscles should be contracted slightly to hold you in position.

❻ Your legs must be completely straight, and your feet flat as if you were standing up. Now, don't think that because the setup is easy, the exercise will be easily executed. Yes, the set-up for the exercise is easier than most; but this easy set-up makes the triceps isolation and stimulation incredibly powerful.

TECHNIQUE AND FORM

❶ As you lower yourself down, lean back to help hold your body in the upright position.

❷ Lower yourself slowly while resisting your body weight all the way to the bottom position.

❸ Keep the elbows close to your body, helping to better isolate the triceps muscles.

❹ Keeping your legs straight and feet flat to the floor, lower yourself to the floor. You can do two things here: You can either stop lowering your body right before your feet touch, or you can lower yourself to the point where you tap your feet flat on the ground and immediately begin your return upward. We prefer the latter since we know that when we tap bottom, we have completed the full range of motion for complete muscle stimulation and should explode into the upward press. Some people will not be tall enough to touch their feet at the bottom of the training apparatus being used. Also, you would never want to lower yourself to a point where you could injure yourself just to touch your feet flat on the floor. There is such a point! In any of these cases, just lower your body until your upper arms (from your elbows to your shoulders) are parallel to the floor. Then, immediately begin your return upward.

❺ No matter what technique you use at the bottom position, after you've reached that point, slowly and with a smooth transition begin to press your body upward, maintaining your upright posture.

❻ As you begin pressing upward, make sure that all of your focus is directed to your triceps muscles. This alone will help stimulate the triceps by increased muscle control and as a reminder to maintain proper alignment.

❼ As you near the top of the motion, your goal is not to lock the joint but instead to contract and squeeze the triceps muscles as hard as you possibly can for a one to two second count. It is important to let the triceps muscles hold you in this position rather than lock the elbow joints. Otherwise, you can injure the joint. In addition, you take all of the resistance off the triceps muscles and put it onto the joints and bones. Remember that there should be no rest at the top of the exercise after the contraction period. From that lockout position, once again slowly lower yourself back to the bottom position as you resist the weight of your body. If you get to a point where your body weight is too light for the exercise, you may use a dip belt to hook some additional weight to your body, thus increasing the resistance. Please make sure that if you do use additional weight, you do so in incremental stages.

Triceps Dip

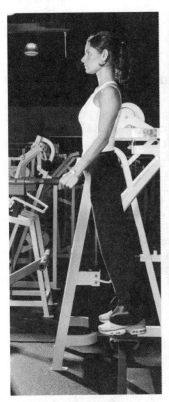
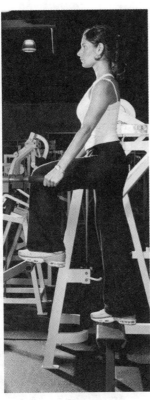
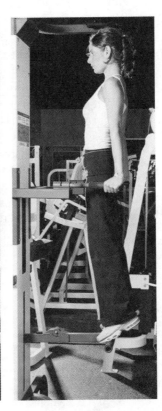
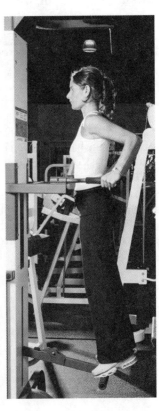

FAQ:
When I do triceps dips, I feel a lot of pressure and pain in my shoulders. Why?

ANSWER:
The triceps dip can be a very powerful and productive exercise. You do, however, need to make sure that you protect yourself from injury, keep a few things in mind when doing the triceps dip. Don't go too heavy unless you know your muscles, joints, and connective tissue can handle it. Although you may be very strong and feel that your flexibility is great, you still may not be as strong as necessary to do this exercise at its full capacity.

Bench Dip

Triceps dips can also be performed between benches if you are unable to perform them on the parallel bars for whatever reason. Just like parallel bar triceps dips, this exercise will primarily focus on the three heads of the triceps, located on the back of the arms, helping you achieve fat free and toned looking arms. This is a great exercise for developing the strength necessary to do the Triceps Dips exercise on the parallel dip bar unit.

PROPER ALIGNMENT

❶ Place two benches parallel to each other (side by side) with sufficient space in between them to allow for the palms of the hands to be on one bench and the back of your feet on top of the other bench.

❷ Sit between the two benches with your palms on the bench behind you and with your legs on top of the other bench. If you are aligned correctly, your body should resemble an L.

TECHNIQUE AND FORM

❶ Use the strength of your triceps to lower you towards the ground in a gradual and controlled movement.

❷ Continue to lower yourself until the upper arm and the forearms create a 90 degree angle.

❸ Use your triceps to push yourself back up to the starting position.

Important Notes

❶ Do not move up and down in a jerky or uncontrolled manner, as this exercise can place extreme stress on the shoulder girdle.

❷ If unable to perform this exercise, you may use the assistance of a partner who should support part of your weight.

❸ If you would like to add weight to the exercise, ask a partner to gently place a weight on your thighs, as illustrated at right.

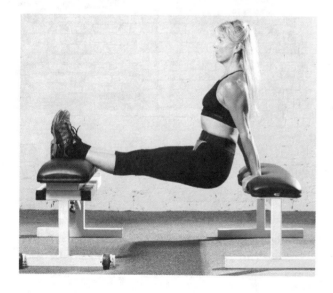

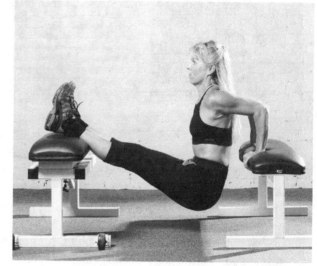

Bench Dip

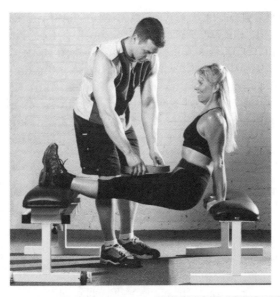

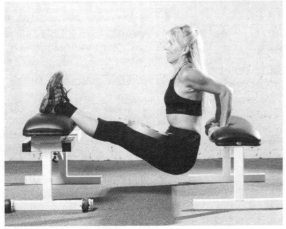
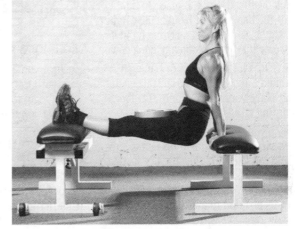

FAQ:

I saw someone perform this with five 45-pound plates on his lap. Is this safe?

ANSWER:

It may be safe for him, but if you're not used to this exercise, you should start with your body-weight first. This can be a very effective triceps exercise, but you'll want to perfect your form before progressing too quickly. Just be careful not to strain your shoulders with this exercise. just like the chest and triceps dip, going too low can seriously damage your shoulders.

E-Z Curl Bar Close-Grip Press

This exercise can be done one of two ways. It can be done alone as a triceps and inner chest exercise or as a secondary superset exercise with the E-Z Bar Triceps Extension exercise. How you incorporate it will depend on the phase of training you have reached. The conventional way to do the close-grip bench press is with a barbell. It also calls for the arms to widen at the bottom, putting more emphasis on the inner chest muscles than the triceps. Our version of this exercise will be done with the E-Z curl bar and with a different arm position than the conventional version. This puts emphasis on the triceps with a secondary workload to the inner chest muscles, two of the areas women are most concerned with targeting.

PROPER ALIGNMENT

This exercise will incorporate many of the same alignment positions as the lying E-Z bar triceps extension exercise.

❶ Set up the E-Z bar with some weight or get one that is pre-weighted. You can rest the bar on your thighs and bring it back overhead, set it in place so that it is at the base of your head while you lie down, or simply have someone hand it to you when you are already lying down.

❷ Before lifting the bar or having it handed to you, lay back on the bench and place your feet flat onto the floor, pointing straight ahead.

❸ As you are lying down lift the bar into place by pressing it up using your chest muscles (just like the chest press). Hold it above your head and stay there. You will begin the exercise in this position to avoid stressing the elbow joint.

❹ Remember to make sure that your whole arm is in direct line with your front shoulder (anterior deltoid). Your arms must stay close to your body and follow in a straight line from shoulder, to elbow, to arm. This is what will create primary isolation on the triceps muscles and allow better control of the bar.

❺ Take a position on the bar so that your hands are in the outer curved position of the bar. The inner curved position will create too much wrist strain. The proper width will be about 8-10 inches apart.

TECHNIQUE AND FORM

❶ Once you are in the proper alignment with the E-Z curl bar overhead, slowly begin to lower the bar down as if you were lowering the bar during a bench press. But remember, your arms will now stay close to your body with your front shoulders and arms in a straight line.

❷ As you lower the bar, keep your arms riding closely to the sides of your body. This technique is essential for proper triceps stimulation.

❸ Remember to consciously focus all of your attention on proper form and intense stimulation of the triceps during the movement.

❹ As you continue to lower the bar, do so in a controlled manner and bring the bar down to around mid-chest. Without resting, and without momentum, use your triceps muscles to push the bar off your chest and back to the start position. Remember to maintain your proper form with the arms riding close to the sides of your body.

❺ As you reach the top of the movement, squeeze the triceps muscles as hard as you can without locking out your elbow joints.

❻ Hold this contraction for one second.

❼ Make sure that there is a smooth transition when switching directions from the top position going into the lowering of the bar, and also from the bottom position going into the extension or raising of the bar. There should be no rest at all when switching from the bottom position into the upward extension of the bar.

E-Z Curl Bar Close-Grip Press

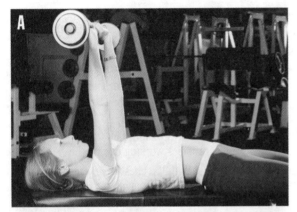

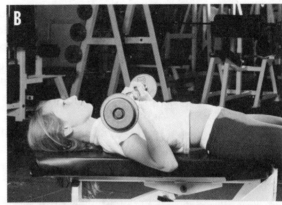

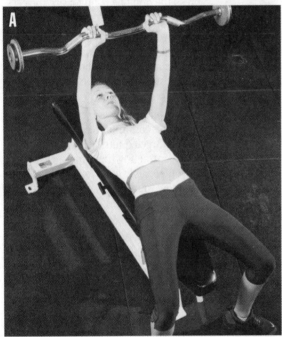

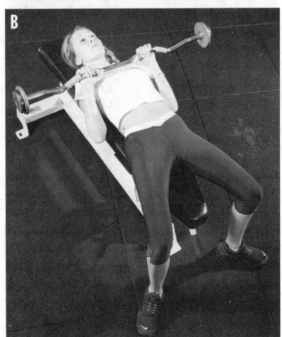

FAQ:
I thought that it was necessary and much more effective to keep the hands close together in order to work the triceps.

ANSWER:
Not at all. keeping your hands too close together can seriously damage your wrists and shoulders. You will get more than enough triceps stimulation by keeping your hands 8 to 10 inches apart.

Close-Grip Dumbbell Press

The close-grip dumbbell press is an excellent compound movement that not only targets the triceps muscles, but also, as a bonus, targets the middle of your chest. The alignment used for this exercise is the same as the alignment used for chest exercises with the exception that you will need to retract the scapula (bring the shoulder blades towards one another) in order to bring the chest above the shoulders. The reason for this technique is to make sure that the chest muscles receive the secondary emphasis over the shoulders.

PROPER ALIGNMENT

This exercise will incorporate virtually the same alignment positions as the E-Z curl bar close-grip press.

❶ Choose your dumbbells and, from a seated position, place them on your lap.

❷ Bring the dumbbells back into position as you learned earlier in the proper lifting and dumbbell positioning techniques.

❸ Before lifting the dumbbells, lay back on the bench and place your feet flat onto the floor, pointing straight ahead.

❹ Remember to make sure that your whole arm is in direct line with your front shoulder (anterior deltoid). Your arms must stay close to your body and follow in a straight line from shoulder, to elbow, to arm. This is what will create primary isolation on the triceps muscles and allow better control of the bar.

❺ Take a position on the dumbbells so that your hands are positioned directly in the middle of the dumbbell handles.

TECHNIQUE AND FORM

❶ With the dumbbells on your thighs, thrust one leg up, leveraging one dumbbell up to around your chest level.

❷ Immediately thrust the second dumbbell upward while simultaneously allowing momentum and the dumbbells to guide you back into the lying position; use your abdominal muscles to help safely ease you into position.

❸ Lay back and align your body using the alignment instructions presented for chest exercises but retracting the scapula to bring the chest above the shoulders.

❹ Once you are in position, instead of bringing the dumbbells to the outside of the chest, hold them close to your chest. The handles of the dumbbells and palms of your hands must face each other with the elbows riding close to your body during movement. Your forearms must be perpendicular to the ceiling during the entire exercise. This close-grip movement will stimulate the inner chest muscles while a primary emphasis will be delivered to the triceps muscles as well.

❺ Because your shoulder muscles are more likely to move the weight than your chest muscles, you must retract the shoulder blades back or together against the flat bench. This slight variation will take the shoulders out of the chest movement, allowing the chest and triceps muscles to be the primary muscles working during the exercise.

❻ With the chest in its elevated position, the elbows out and wide and the forearms perpendicular to the floor, press the dumbbells up toward the ceiling.

❼ As you press the weight up, put your mind into the chest and triceps muscles by concentrating on and feeling the muscles contract as you push upward.

❽ As you reach the top of the exercise, you must continue to consciously focus on the targeted muscles while physically contracting these muscles as hard as you possibly can. Your goal is to get the most intense contraction possible in the top position!

❾ In this position, squeeze and hold for a count of one to two seconds.

❿ Slowly begin lowering the weight while holding proper postural alignment throughout the exercise.

⓫ As the dumbbells are lowered to the start position, they should touch your chest. This allows for a full stretch of the chest and triceps muscles.

⓬ Without rest, slowly begin to press the dumbbells up again in a controlled, smooth, fluid motion, without using any momentum.

Close-Grip Dumbbell Press

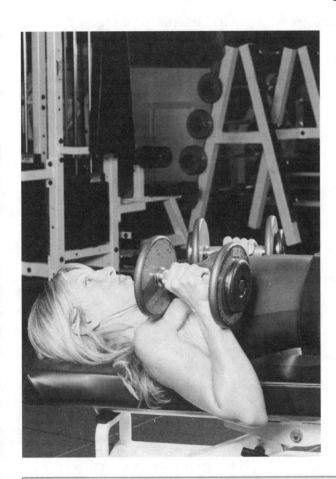
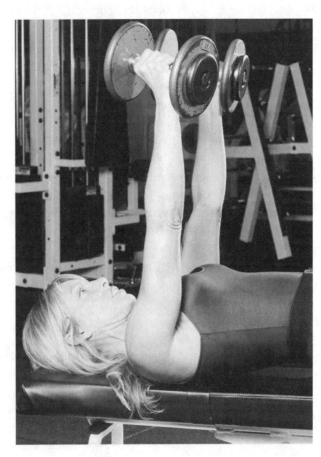

FAQ:
When I do this exercise, I feel all the stimulation in my chest muscles instead of my triceps.

ANSWER:
Because this exercise uses dumbbells, your range of motion is more open to improper form than with the E-Z bar. Focus on keeping your arms pulled in close to your sides. This will put the emphasis of the resistance on your triceps.

Triceps Pushdown

This exercise often is performed incorrectly. Some common mistakes include the following:

A) Too much bending at the hips, thus incorporating chest muscle activity. Using proper form for this exercise means staying as straight as possible with a very slight bend at the hips, to prevent lower back injury.

B) Bending over with the cable set on one side of the trainee's head. This causes the crucial balance of the resistance to be thrown off because force is greater at one side of the body than the other. Many professional trainers and athletes do this all the time. For proper form keep the cable right at the center of your body.

C) Allowing the arms to come up during the negative portion of the exercise. Proper form calls for the upper arms (from the elbows to the shoulder) to stay locked at the sides of the body and remain there until the end of the exercise, when you have to return to the start position. Only the forearms should move.

This is a great exercise if done correctly. Follow the proper form and techniques and you will soon have the fat free and firm triceps you desire.

PROPER ALIGNMENT

You have the option of using a v-bar, a short cambered bar attachment, a rope, or a straight bar attachment for this exercise. Choose the bar that gives you the most comfortable grip. You can also change bars over time in order to add variety to your program.

❶ Stand in front of the cable and take hold of the bar. Bring the bar down by bringing your arms (from the elbow to your shoulder) to the sides of your body and lock them there.

❷ Position your feet shoulder width apart with your feet pointing straight ahead.

❸ Slightly bend your knees and keep your torso upright throughout the movement.

❹ Keep your head pointing straight ahead and avoid looking down; otherwise you will tend to bend over.

TECHNIQUE AND FORM

❶ Holding the bar with your arms positioned in place at your sides, begin by isometrically contracting the triceps muscles before moving the bar down.

❷ Begin pushing the bar down while keeping your elbows pinned to your sides.

❸ Push down until you have reached full extension. Avoid locking the elbow joint out hard. Make sure you squeeze the triceps muscles as hard as you possibly can at lockout. You are to focus on squeezing the triceps muscles hard, not the elbow joint. There is a major difference that practice will perfect.

❹ When you've reached the bottom position, squeeze the triceps muscles and hold for a count of one second.

❺ Begin to allow the bar to rise while maintaining your posture and arms at the sides.

❻ Let the bar come up to the point where your forearms are slightly higher than parallel to the floor. At this point, without resting, begin once again pushing down to the bottom position.

❼ Follow this form throughout this exercise and your triceps will burn with delight. If you continue with this proper alignment, technique and form, your triceps will very soon develop into arms of beauty!

Triceps Pushdown

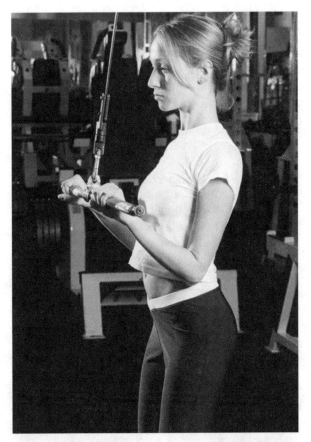

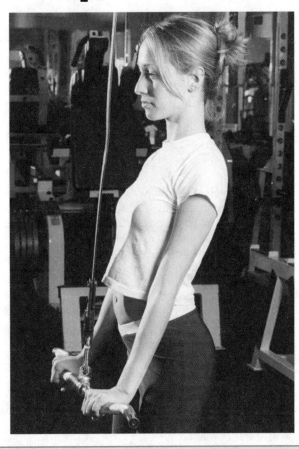

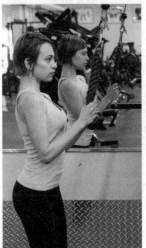

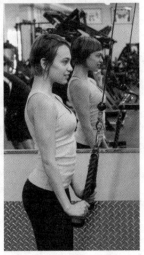

FAQ:

I always see people doing this exercise with their body in line with the cable, but with their head to one side.

ANSWER:

Pulling your head to one side of the cable will create an imbalance in the distribution of weight. One side will be working much more than the other, and there are risks to your spine, as it is enduring the lateral pull to your core.

To avoid this, keep your head directly in the middle of the cable, stand up straight to avoid the chest's muscles involvement, keep your elbows pointed to the round, and lock those shoulders in place. Don't let them flex upward.

Triceps Kickback

We see so many people doing this exercise the wrong way. It is vital that you do it with proper form and technique, or you will be wasting your time.

Notice the model demonstrating the exercise. Do you see how her upper arm remains stationary from the start to finish? This is vital to the development of your triceps. Too many people use momentum to bring the dumbbell to the extended top position of the movement. They don't realize that this does absolutely nothing productive in developing the triceps muscles. Lighten the weight if necessary and be conscious of your form and technique.

PROPER ALIGNMENT

❶ With this exercise, you will be training one arm at a time. Starting with the right triceps, lean down on a flat bench and place your left knee and your left hand on the bench for support. Your right leg will remain in a semi-straight position, with the foot flat on the floor. Maintain a flat back throughout the exercise.

❷ Pick up a dumbbell with the right hand using an overhand grip, making sure that the weight is light enough to maintain proper form throughout the exercise.

❸ In the bent-over position, place the upper arm (right humerus) flush against the right side of your body.

Make sure to allow your lower arm to remain loose.

❹ Take note that when you are ready to begin this exercise the upper and lower arm form a 90-degree angle.

❺ Follow the same protocol when training the left triceps.

TECHNIQUE AND FORM

❶ Once again, make sure that the lower and upper arm are at a 90-degree angle, and the dumbbell is held with an overhand grip.

❷ Begin the exercise by extending the lower arm back until it is at full extension.

❸ Make sure that you keep the upper arm pressed against the right side of the body during the exercise.

❹ Once the elbow reaches the point of full extension, contract the triceps as hard as possible. Make sure to avoid hyperextension of the elbow.

❺ Slowly lower the dumbbell back to the 90-degree angle.

FAQ:

I'm not sure if I'm getting the dumbbell up high enough for a full range of motion.

ANSWER:

There's nothing wrong with looking in the mirror every so often to check if your form and technique are good. If you see that you aren't bringing the dumbbell up high enough, maybe you need to go lighter with the weights. Make sure to avoid momentum.

Triceps Kickback

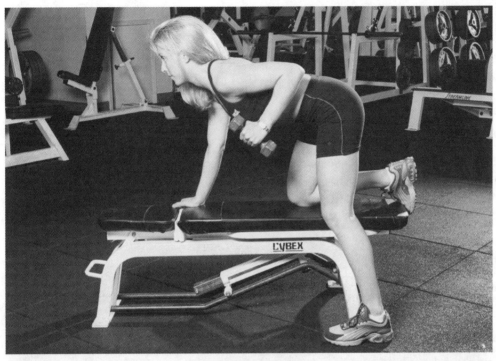

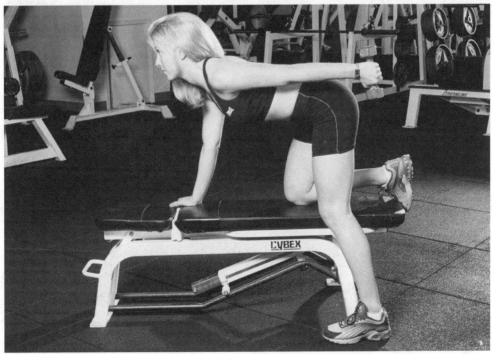

Fixed Bar Bodyweight Triceps Extension

This is a very advanced exercise that should only be performed by people with strength and gym experience.

PROPER ALIGNMENT

❶ Fix a horizontal bar in front of you at waist height. Do this by using the bar of a Smith machine or a regular Olympic bar placed at the end of a squat rack with adjustable pins.

❷ Grasp the bar at shoulder width with an overhand (pronated) grip. Your arms should extend forward at an angle of 50 degrees from the head to the arms.

❸ Keep the rest of the torso straight but slanted forward so your arms are holding your weight and your legs are behind you like a modified push-up position.

❹ Keep your arms stationary and your elbows in.

TECHNIQUE AND FORM

❶ Inhale, bend at the elbows, and lower your body until your forehead lightly touches the bar.

❷ Use your triceps to press against the bar, and then exhale while bringing you torso back to the starting position.

Fixed Bar Bodyweight Triceps Extension

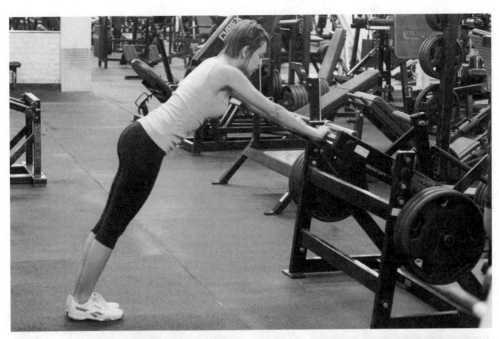

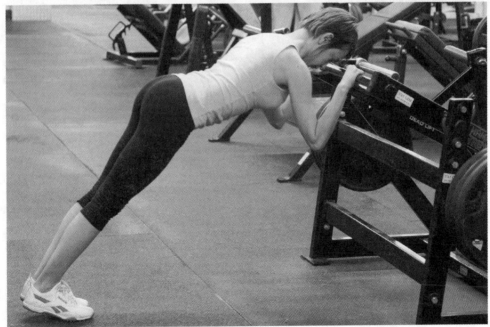

Triceps Extension Machine

This movement targets the triceps brachii. For an equivalent dumbbell exercise, try the Lying Dumbbell Triceps Extension.

TECHNIQUE AND FORM

1 Sit on the machine and adjust the seat of the machine so that your upper chest is placed just above the arm pad provided by the machine.

2 Grasp the handles with a neutral grip (palms facing each other) and position the elbows on top of the arm pad at shoulder width distance. This will be your starting position.

3 Push the lever down until the arm is fully extended. Breathe out as you perform this movement.

4 Go back to the starting position as you breathe in.

TRAINER'S TIPS

1 Keep the elbows always in contact with the pad. This will ensure full triceps stimulation.

2 The upper body should remain stationary as well.

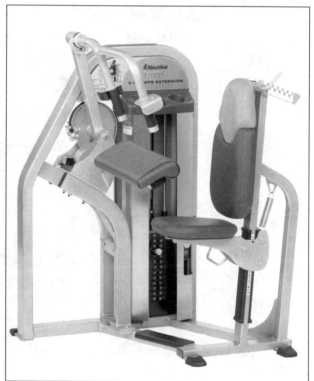

©2004 Nautilus Inc., The Nautilus Group

Chapter 11
Biceps

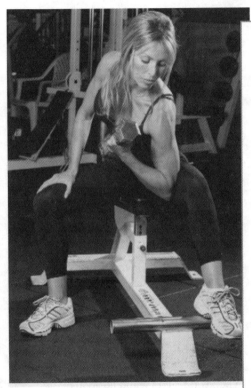

The biceps muscles are located on the front of the upper arms. This two-headed muscle helps to lift the forearms upward. Biceps are probably one of the more simple muscles to train. However, just like chest muscles, if you go to any gym in the country you will see 90 percent of the people training them using incorrect form. Look at our model to the left and notice how beautifully her biceps, triceps and shoulders tie into one another. This not only comes from working hard, but also from working smarter!

For immediate Body Sculpting Bible support & coaching directly from James & Hugo, please visit www.BodySculptingBibles.com

11

THE BODY SCULPTING BIBLE FOR WOMEN

Dumbbell Curl

(Using two dumbbells simultaneously)

The dumbbell curl is a more traditional exercise, focusing on the two heads of the biceps muscles. We believe that using two dumbbells simultaneously, while standing, is the best way to perform this exercise. There are many who believe that training one arm at a time is better; however, by training both arms at the same time you have a few advantages.

1. First, working the arms simultaneously keeps the biceps working without rest through the exercise. You'll have time to rest when the set is over.

2. Second, you train the arms with equal strength output. When you train one at a time you can very likely put much more effort into one arm than the other.

3. Third, you stay balanced. When you train one arm at a time, you will have a tendency to lean to the side of the arm you are lifting with. No Good!

PROPER ALIGNMENT

We suggest that you do this exercise standing up and supporting yourself against a wall for good body mechanics and strict form.

❶ Choose two light dumbbells so that you can practice perfect form.

❷ With the dumbbells in hand, begin the alignment of your body by placing your feet about shoulder width apart and pointing straight ahead of you.

❸ Slightly bend at the knees.

❹ Allow the dumbbells to hang down at your sides with your palms and dumbbells facing forward, as shown in the picture.

❺ Make sure that your elbows stay pointed to the ground at all times during the biceps curl exercise. Do not allow them to move from that position.

❻ Keep your upper body straight by sticking out your chest and keeping your shoulder blades squared off.

❼ Keep your head level, and your eyes pointing straight ahead of you.

TECHNIQUE AND FORM

❶ Once you are in proper postural alignment against the wall, focus all of your attention on the biceps muscles and the exercise you are about to do.

❷ With the dumbbells at your sides, begin curling them up, making sure to keep your elbows pointed toward the ground.

❸ Once you've reached the top position of the exercise, contract the biceps muscles as hard as you possibly can and hold that contraction for a count of two seconds.

❹ From the top position, slowly and smoothly begin to lower the dumbbells back to the starting position.

❺ As you reach the bottom of the exercise, immediately begin curling the weights up toward your shoulders again. Make sure that there is a smooth transition when switching directions from both the top position and also from the bottom position. Both scenarios must be done with no rest in between either of the direction changes, unless you are so fatigued by the end of the set that you need a few seconds of rest in order to get a couple more repetitions.

VARIATION: SUPINATION

For added stimulation of the biceps muscles, you can try a technique called supination. Instead of beginning the exercise with your palms facing forward, begin with your palms facing in toward the sides of the body. As you lift the weights, rotate your wrists until the palms of your hands are facing back toward you by the time you reach the top of the movement. Supination or rotation of your wrists should last the entire distance from the sides of your body up to your shoulders. In other words, don't just rotate your hands completely at the bottom position; allow them to gradually rotate during the entire distance. When you reach the top position of the exercise, your pinkies should be above your thumbs. Make sure your elbows remain pointed to the ground. Then, as you lower the weight, reverse the supination by rotating the wrists in the opposite direction, again prolonging the rotation throughout the entire distance. When you finish, the palms of your hands should once again be facing the sides of your body.

Dumbbell Curl

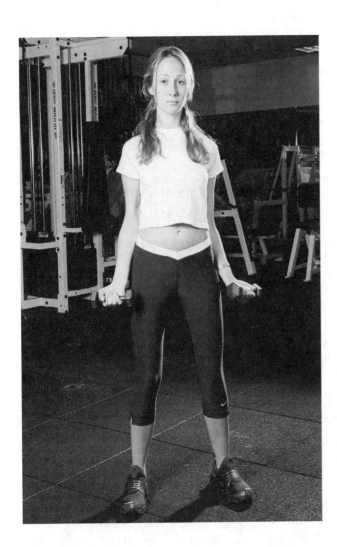 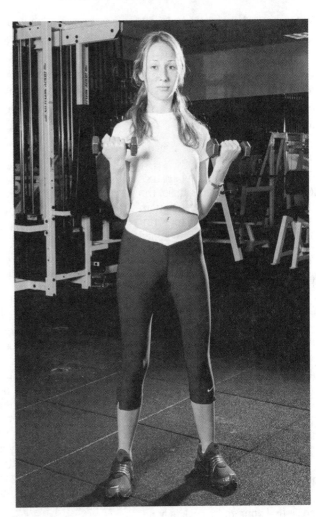

FAQ:

Why don't my biceps get larger?

ANSWER:

Your biceps are really not a very big muscle. Beginners might see some dramatic difference, but the more advanced you are, the less likely you will see larger biceps. If you want to get the most out of your biceps training, make sure that you avoid momentum, keep those elbows pointed to the ground, and stop allowing those shoulders to flex upward. Remember to squeeze and contract fully at the top of each repetition!

Incline Dumbbell Curl

(Using two dumbbells simultaneously)

The incline dumbbell curl is a great exercise for developing great looking biceps muscles. Because the exercise requires strict form and isolation, you should start doing the exercise with a weight lighter than what you'd usually use for a regular dumbbell curl. Remember, form is everything. In the start position of the exercise you will notice a nice stretch in the biceps region. Because of this, you must make sure to take it slowly. Make sure to avoid momentum and keep the form strict.

PROPER ALIGNMENT

❶ Go to an incline bench and set the bench incline to a 45-degree angle. Due to the full stretch and range of motion of this exercise, it is designed to work the full length of the biceps with added emphasis on the outer head of the biceps muscle.

❷ Pick two dumbbells with a weight that you can handle using perfect form. This exercise must be done very strictly in order to receive the desired effects.

❸ Decide if you'd rather start the exercise holding the dumbbells at the sides of your body or with them resting on top of your thighs, which we prefer. Starting with the dumbbells on your thighs will give you some quality time to visualize and focus on the exercise you are about to do. This preparation can set up the proper mindset for even greater lifting performance.

❹ Lean all the way back into the bench so that your entire back is lying flat against the back pad. Stay that way for the entire exercise and do not take your back off the bench until the exercise is complete. Once you are properly positioned and ready to begin, firmly grip on the dumbbells and allow them to hang at your sides.

❺ Make sure that the palms of your hands are facing the wall in front of you for the entire exercise. No supination or hand twisting with this exercise.

❻ Make sure to keep your elbows pointed directly at the floor during the entire exercise. When people usually do any type of biceps curl, they allow their elbows to drift up with the curling movement, allowing the shoulders to flex forward. When this happens, you can forget about fully stimulating the biceps muscles since the anterior shoulders become the prime movers of the weight being curled. There is only one instance in which you may lift the shoulders while doing a biceps curl. That is when you have come to a point in your training where you add repetitions (forced reps) with the help of a spotter. Before you reach this point in your training, you must keep the elbows to the ground for full and proper stimulation of the biceps muscles.

TECHNIQUE AND FORM

❶ Once you are in position, focus all of your attention on the exercise you are about to do and on the biceps muscle itself.

❷ Begin curling the dumbbells at the same time, making sure that the elbows stay positioned towards the ground without moving upward as you curl.

❸ Curl the weights up until you can no longer curl, while simultaneously contracting the biceps muscles as hard as you can. Hold that position for a second or two.

❹ Slowly and smoothly begin to lower the dumbbells until your arms are fully elongated and back at your sides.

❺ Without rest and without using any momentum, slowly and steadily begin curling the dumbbells back up toward your shoulders. If you jerk or in any way use momentum to begin curling the dumbbells, you risk serious injury to the biceps muscles. Once again, make sure that the changes of direction from the top position going into the lowering phase, and from the bottom position going into the curling phase, are always smooth and controlled.

Incline Dumbbell Curl

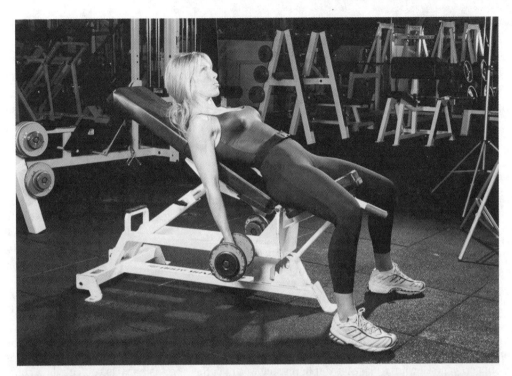

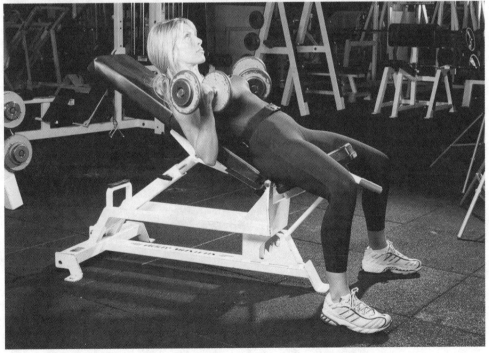

One-Arm Preacher Curl

(Using a preacher machine or inclined bench)

The preacher curl is yet another of the great biceps exercises. It develops the lower portion of the biceps muscle, helping to build balance in the biceps muscles. For this exercise, you may use two dumbbells together or one at a time, as it will help to create concentration and balance. This exercise will also cause a greater contraction at the top of the movement because of the independent range of motion involved. It can be done on a preacher bench or simply on the back support of an incline bench. Because the exercise is very strict, it is important that you choose a dumbbell weight you can handle while practicing perfect form.

PROPER ALIGNMENT

❶ If using a preacher machine, sit on the machine's seat and bring your chest against the pad in front of you. If using an incline bench, stand at the end of the bench so the incline portion is touching your stomach.

❷ Position your feet flat on the floor and keep them there for the entire exercise.

❸ Allow one arm to hang over the angled support of the preacher bench or incline bench. Support yourself with your other arm. Make sure that the back of your arm is positioned flat against the angled support and lying in a straight line. In order to comfortably keep the arm in this position, you may have to angle your body to one side, making sure you are not using leveraging techniques to assist you in the curl.

❹ It is important to focus all of your attention on the biceps muscles while doing the exercise instead of calling upon the assistance of other muscles to help curl the weight. Also, as you curl the weight up, make sure that you lean into the front chest support rather than lean back for cheating leverage. Make sure that the majority of the resistance is being focused on the biceps muscles throughout the exercise. When you reach the top position of the exercise, you must contract the biceps muscle as hard as you possibly can. Because you are on an angled support, the upper position of this exercise makes it very easy for you to rest the weight of the dumbbell on the bones rather than the biceps muscle sustaining the weight. You must overcome this bone support with a very hard contraction of the biceps muscle.

TECHNIQUE AND FORM

❶ Once you are in position with one arm lying flat against the angled support, hold the body steady and begin curling the weight up toward your shoulder.

❷ Focus all of your attention on the arm you are exercising, making sure to squeeze hard on the curling phase and resisting the weight as you come back down.

❸ As you begin curling, relax the shoulder on the arm you are training as it can assist in the lift.

❹ As you reach the top of this exercise, again contract the biceps muscle as hard as you can for a count of two seconds.

❺ Slowly return to the starting position of the exercise.

❻ As you reach the bottom position, immediately once again begin curling the weight up toward your shoulder. Once you are done with the desired amount of repetitions with that arm, switch arms and do the same amount of repetitions.

One-Arm Preacher Curl

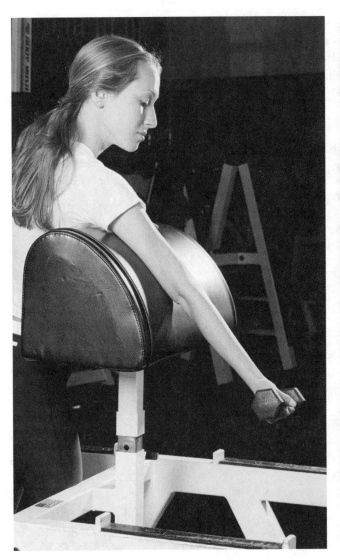
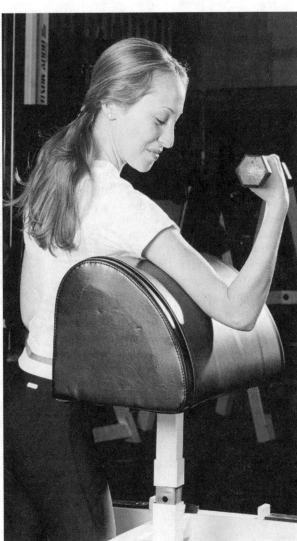

E-Z Reverse Preacher Curl

This exercise targets the brachialis, also known as the outer biceps, and forearm muscles. Remember to keep your head level, looking straight ahead, and to engage your abdominals to avoid using your lower back.

There are a couple variations, including the regular preacher curl, which requires grasping the E-Z bar with your palms facing you. You can also use a low pulley with an E-Z bar attachment instead of an E-Z bar. You will need to position the bench in front of the pulley, and may also use a closer grip. You can use a straight bar as well: just remember that straight bars place more stress on the wrist joint.

PROPER ALIGNMENT

❶ This exercise requires a preacher bench and an E-Z bar. Have your spotter hand you the bar or use the front bar rest. Grasp the E-Z curl bar at the wide outer handle with the palms of your hands facing downward due to the shape of the bar, arms fully extended. Your thumb should be higher than your little finger.

❷ Position your chest and upper arms against the preacher bench pad and hold the E-Z curl bar at shoulder length.

❸ Keep your head and eyes facing straight ahead throughout the movement.

TECHNIQUE AND FORM

❶ As you inhale, slowly lower the bar until your upper arm is extended and the biceps are fully stretched.

❷ Exhale and use the biceps to curl the weight up until your biceps is fully contracted and the bar is at shoulder height.

E-Z Reverse Preacher Curl

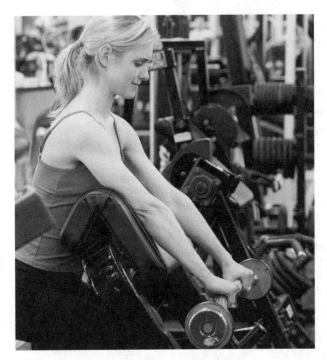

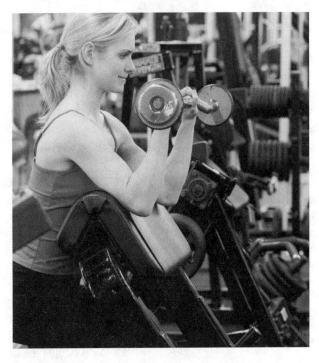

VARIATION

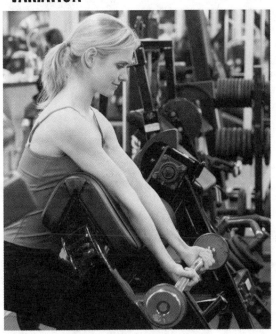

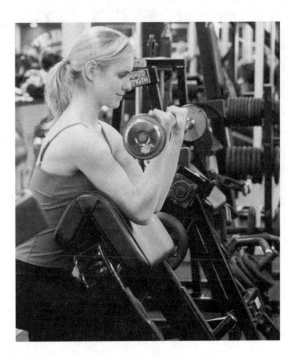

Concentration Curl

(One arm at a time)

The name concentration curl should not just be applied to this version of the biceps curl. It should be applied to every exercise we've discussed or will discuss in the book. Putting your mind into the muscle and focusing every bit of your attention on the exercise you are about to do is the surest way to reach your fitness goals in the quickest amount of time possible. In the picture of our model demonstrating the concentration curl, look at how her eyes are focused on the exercise movement. Her results and the results you will soon achieve are a direct result of the focus and intensity you put into every set and rep of an exercise.

PROPER ALIGNMENT

❶ You can do the concentration curl in a seated position or while standing.

❷ Whatever position you choose, bend over at the hips and take a dumbbell in one hand. The dumbbell weight should at first be light so that you can practice perfect form.

❸ Sit at the edge of a bench and support your arm by resting your elbow on your thigh.

TECHNIQUE AND FORM

❶ Do not curl the weight straight up to your chest. You must curl the weight with your arm angled in toward your body. This will help make certain that the exercise motion is correct, following the direction towards your shoulders rather than your chest. To start, bend over at the hips and fully extend the arm that you will be exercising while the other arm is resting on your thigh.

❷ Begin curling the weight while you also begin rotating your wrist.

❸ Curl the weight towards your shoulder and contract the biceps muscle as hard as you possibly can, while keeping your arm pointing at the ground.

❹ Once you reach the top of the movement, hold for a two-second count.

❺ Slowly lower the dumbbell back to the starting position, resisting the weight the entire way down.

❻ Without rest or momentum, once again start curling the weight towards the shoulder with great focus and concentration. Once you have completed the desired amount of repetitions, switch arms and do the same amount of repetitions.

Concentration Curl

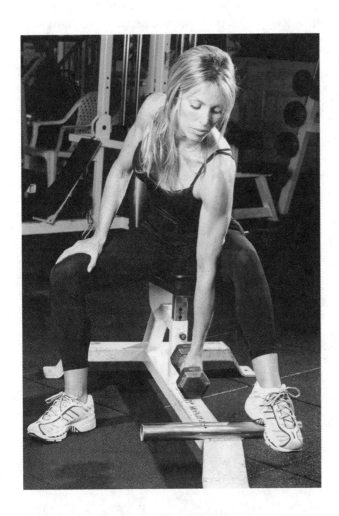
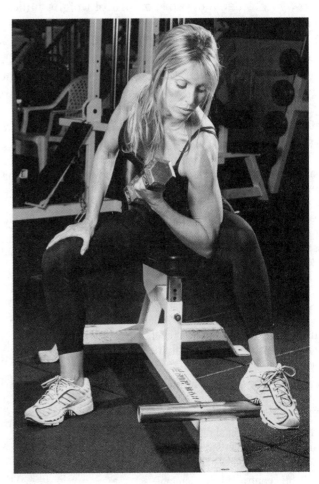

FAQ:

Why do I feel this exercise more than any other biceps exercise?

ANSWER:

You can bet that it's because you're focused on truly squeezing and contracting the biceps at the top of the movement. Most people just go through the motions of exercises and pay little attention to making sure that they are consciously squeezing and contracting. This additional bit of mental focus really works your muscles. This applies to all exercises!

Standing E-Z Bar Curl

Do not underestimate this exercise because of its name. E-Z bar curls are versatile exercises that allow you to use a decent amount of weight while being much easier on your wrists than straight bar curls. If you have a pending strain such as tennis elbow or tendinitis, we would recommend this exercise over straight bar curls. The two-curved hand positions on the bar allow you to do both close- and wide-grip curls. The inner grips will enable you to develop the outer biceps, and the outer grip will enable you to develop the inner biceps. You can truly develop the sculpted arms you desire with the help of this great exercise.

PROPER ALIGNMENT

❶ First, decide what hand position you will take on the bar. Remember what we discussed earlier about assessing your body and focusing on the unbalanced or weak body parts to create muscle balance and symmetry. Look at your biceps muscles and assess the inner and outer muscle heads. Decide if one head needs more work then the other. If you find a weakness or imbalance in one of the two muscle heads, then address that problem by simply using the hand position that will bring the smaller portion of the biceps muscle up to par with the others.

❷ Hold the bar across your thighs with your palms facing away from your body.

❸ Position your feet shoulder width apart and point them straight ahead. Next, bend your knees slightly.

❹ Slightly contract the abdominal muscles.

❺ Stand straight up and stay that way throughout the movement.

❻ Stick your chest out and keep your shoulders back, which will help you maintain a straight back.

❼ Keep your head level and do not move it from that position for the rest of the exercise.

TECHNIQUE AND FORM

❶ With the bar across your thighs, lock your elbows to the sides of your body and begin curling the bar up towards your shoulders in an arc-like motion.

❷ Keep the elbows pointing directly to the ground as you curl upward to avoid using the shoulders in the curling motion.

❸ As you curl upward to the shoulders with an arc-like movement, concentrate and focus all of your attention on the biceps muscles. Feel the muscles contracting as you curl the bar upward.

❹ As you reach the top of the movement with the bar close to your shoulders, contract the biceps muscles as hard as you possibly can.

❺ Hold this position for a count of one to two seconds.

❻ Slowly begin lowering the bar while making sure that the biceps endure the negative resistance on the way down to the bottom position.

❼ As you reach the start position with the arms fully straightened, do not rest. Begin curling the bar once again in a smooth controlled and fluid motion without using momentum.

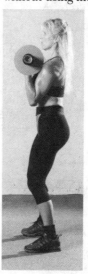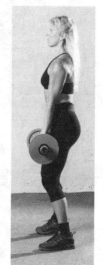

FAQ:

Why do my wrists and forearms hurt when I do this exercise?

ANSWER:

This exercise can definitely stress those areas. If you feel discomfort, we recommend warming up a bit more or simply switching the exercise for something more effective.

Standing E-Z Bar Curl

WIDE GRIP

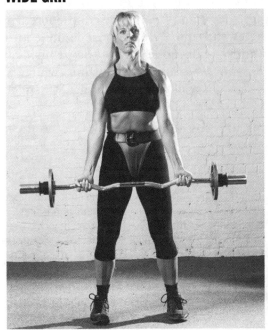 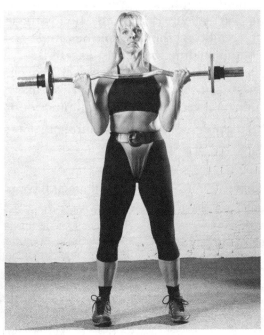

NARROW GRIP

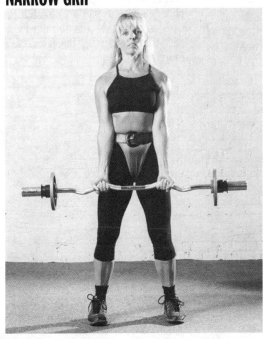 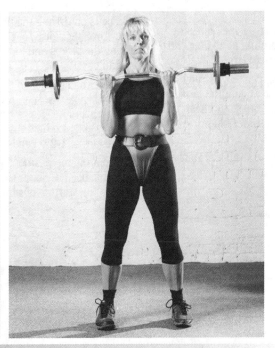

Hammer Curl

(Outer biceps and forearms)

The dumbbell hammer curl is a great exercise for building the outer area of the biceps muscles also known as brachialis muscle. It also builds those very sexy extensor muscles of the forearms, located on the area below the back of the hands on the lower arms. This exercise is done in the same way as standing dumbbell curls, except that you hold the dumbbells with the palms facing each other throughout the entire exercise. You can do this exercise either sitting, which will make it much stricter, or standing which will allow you to get a bit more leverage. We suggest that you include both versions in your training routine.

VARIATION: To get an additional burn in your forearms, try this same movement on an incline bench.

PROPER ALIGNMENT

❶ Choose two light dumbbells so that you can practice perfect form.

❷ With the dumbbells in hand, begin the alignment of your body by placing your feet about shoulder width apart and pointing straight ahead of you.

❸ Slightly bend the knees.

❹ Allow the dumbbells to hang down at your sides with your palms and dumbbells facing the sides of your body.

❺ Make sure that your elbows stay pointed at the ground at all times during the biceps curl exercise.

❻ Keep your upper body straight by contracting your abdominal muscles slightly, sticking out your chest and keeping your shoulder blades squared off.

❼ Keep your head level, and your eyes pointing straight ahead.

TECHNIQUE AND FORM

❶ Once you are in proper postural alignment stand against a wall. Make sure to focus all of your attention on the biceps and forearm muscles. It is very easy to get distracted during exercise, but the rewards of staying focused throughout your training sessions will be well worth your efforts.

❷ Begin curling the dumbbells up with palms and dumbbells facing each other.

❸ Focus on driving the thumbs to your front shoulders, concentrating on feeling the biceps and forearm muscles working.

❹ Once you've reached the top position of the exercise, contract the biceps and forearm muscles as hard as you possibly can and hold that contraction for a count of 1-2 seconds.

❺ From the top position, slowly and smoothly begin to lower the dumbbells back to the starting position.

❻ As you reach the bottom of the exercise, the palms of your hands and dumbbells should remain facing each other and held to the sides of your body.

❼ Make sure that there is a smooth transition when switching directions from both the top position going into the lowering of the dumbbells, and also from the bottom position going into the curling or raising of the dumbbells. Both scenarios must be done with no rest in between either of the direction changes, unless you are so fatigued by the end of the set that you need a few seconds rest in order to get a couple more repetitions.

Hammer Curl

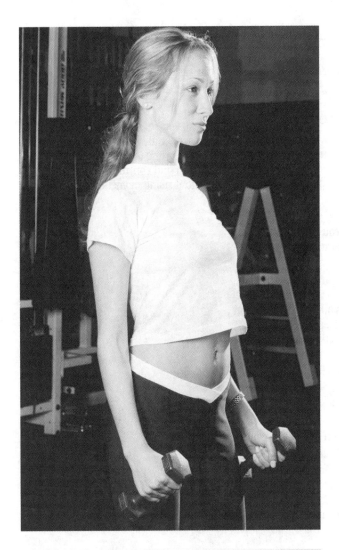

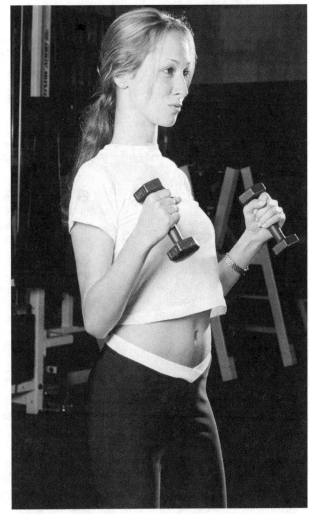

FAQ:
I don't feel this in my biceps.

ANSWER:
That's fine. You should instead feel it in your forearm extensor muscles (the backs of your forearms). The secondary muscles here are the brachiallis muscles of the upper arm (the outer biceps).

VARIATION

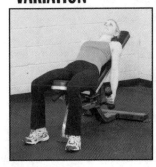

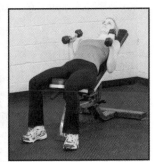

Reverse Curl

This exercise is best performed with an E-Z bar and it targets the outer area of the biceps muscles known as the brachialis, along with the upper forearm muscles. The exercise alignment and execution is much the same as that of the E-Z curls except that the hands are holding the bar with the palms facing the thighs and positioned on the inner handles of the bar.

PROPER ALIGNMENT

To prepare for the exercise, you will align your body similar to the way you did with the standing dumbbell biceps curl.

1 Place your hands with an overhand grip on the outer handles of the bar.

2 Hold the bar across your thighs with your palms facing towards your body.

3 Position your feet shoulder width apart and point them straight ahead. Next, bend your knees slightly.

4 Slightly contract the abdominal muscles.

5 Stand straight up and stay that way throughout the movement.

6 Stick your chest out and keep your shoulders back, which will help you maintain a straight back.

7 Keep your head level and do not move it from that position for the rest of the exercise.

TECHNIQUE AND FORM

1 Now in position with the bar across your thighs, lock your elbows to the sides of your body and begin curling the bar up towards your shoulders in an arc-like motion.

2 Keep the elbows pointing directly to the ground as you curl upward to avoid using the shoulders in the curling motion.

3 As you curl upward to the shoulders with an arc-like movement, concentrate and focus all of your attention on forearms and biceps muscles. Feel the muscles contracting as you curl the bar upward.

4 As you reach the top of the movement with the bar close to your shoulders, contract the biceps muscles as hard as you possibly can.

5 Hold this position for a count of one to two seconds.

6 Slowly begin lowering the bar while making sure that the forearms and biceps endure the negative resistance on the way back down to the bottom position.

7 As you reach the start position with the arms fully straightened, do not rest. Begin curling the bar once again in a smooth and controlled, fluid motion without using momentum.

Reverse Curl

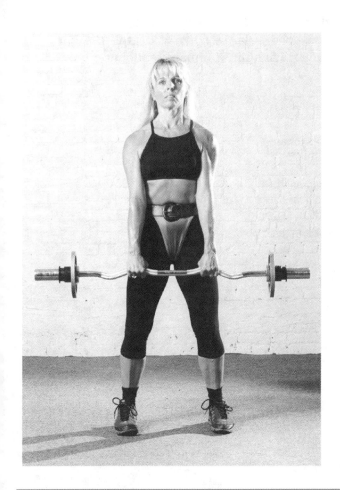
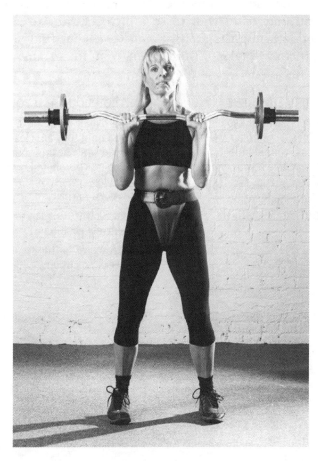

FAQ:
I feel like I tend to rest at the top of the exercise when the bar is just under my chin.

ANSWER:
If this is happening to you, try using an E-Z bar cable attachment, and stand in front of that cable machine. Because of the line of pull, it keeps tension on the muscles, even at the top of the movement.

High Cable Curl

This movement targets the biceps brachii with a secondary emphasis on the brachialis.

You may slant your torso a bit backward to maintain good balance when you grab the bar before starting the exercise, but remember that your upper arms must remain stationary: moving them will take off stimulation from the biceps.

PROPER ALIGNMENT

❶ Stand between two high cable machines. Your abdomen should be pulled in, your shoulders back, and your head in line with your spine.

❷ Grasp the handles with a palms-up grip, positioning your upper arms as close to parallel to the floor as possible.

TECHNIQUE AND FORM

❶ Exhale and curl the handles toward you until they are close to your forehead while flexing your biceps. The upper arms should remain still- only the forearms should move. Hold for one second in the contracted position.

❷ Slowly bring your arms back to the starting position as you inhale.

❸ Repeat for the recommended number of repetitions.

High Cable Curl

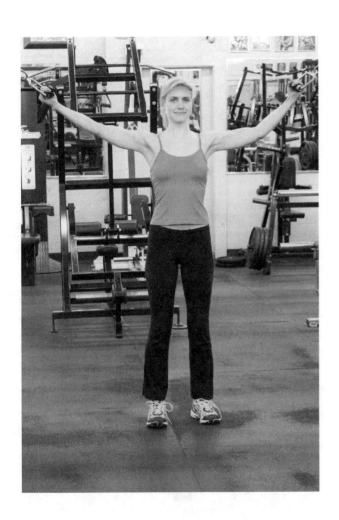
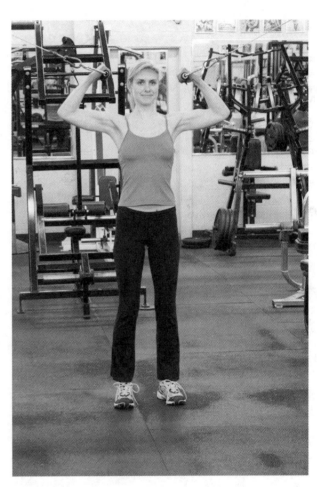

Biceps Curl Machine

This movement targets the biceps brachii with secondary emphasis on the brachialis. For a similar dumbbell exercise, try the Dumbbell Curls.

TECHNIQUE AND FORM

1 Sit on the machine and adjust the seat of the machine so that your upper chest is placed just above the arm pad provided by the machine.

2 Grasp the handles with an underhand grip and position the elbows on top of the arm pad at shoulder width distance. This will be your starting position.

3 Raise the handle bars as you breathe out until the biceps are fully flexed with the back of the upper arm remaining on the pad.

4 Go back to the starting position as you breathe in.

TRAINER'S TIPS

Keep the elbows always in contact with the pad. This will ensure full biceps stimulation.

The upper body should remain stationary as well.

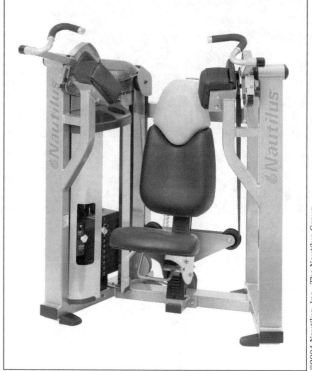

©2004 Nautilus, Inc., The Nautilus Group

Chapter 12
Abdominals

In this section we will talk about how to exercise the most visually stunning and most sought-after muscles: the abdominals. Let us recall that these exercises only firm and build these muscles. We are constantly being asked to recommend the "best" exercises responsible for creating flat and toned tummies. As we tell everyone, you can create the most beautifully toned tummy muscles in the world, but unless you remove the overlying fat covering them, you will be the only one who knows what is underneath! In order to increase the visibility of the abdominal muscles, both the diet and the aerobic training have to be in order, as these are the components that burn body fat.

For immediate Body Sculpting Bible support & coaching directly from James & Hugo, please visit www.BodySculptingBibles.com

12

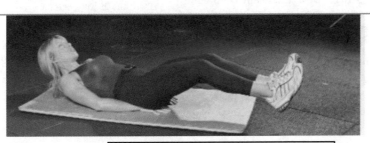

Crunch

Crunches are a great exercise for the abdominal muscles. They are easier to do than the traditional sit-up but do not mistake their being easy for easy looking results. By far, crunches are one of the best abdominal exercises for creating great looking abs.

VARIATION: A variation of this exercise is a crunch on the ball. For this, you use a fitness ball which allows for greater range of motion and increased recruitment of core stabilizers. Simply sit on a fitness ball, then slide down until your lower back is on the ball. Elevate your shoulders and upper back, keep your feet flat on the floor, focus your eyes on the ceiling, and crunch slightly to your feet. You'll be keeping your head in line with your spine.

PROPER ALIGNMENT

❶ Lay down with your back flat on a carpet or mat.

❷ Bend your knees and lay your feet flat on the floor.

❸ Cross your hands at the chest and put a thumb on each side of your chin. This will help keep your head in a neutral position throughout the movement.

TECHNIQUE AND FORM

❶ To really optimize this exercise you'll want to focus on the motion of bringing your chest plate to your pelvic area. Our focus is to squish the stomach area between the chest and pelvis. The abdominal muscles are what will actually move your chest towards your pelvic region, so what better than to crunch them in-between the two. The reason we say this is because many trainers simply teach their clients to "crunch." Many times, instead of flexing their spines with their abdominal muscles, these clients often end up using their hip flexors as the primary muscles to "crunch."

❷ Begin by isometrically contracting the abdominal muscles before moving.

❸ As you begin the crunch, focus on moving your chest (not your head) toward your pelvis.

❹ Exhale as you move up toward your knees. This will allow you to get a more forceful contraction of the abs.

❺ Remember that the distance from start position to end position is not very far at all. It is not like a sit-up. Once again, your focus is not just to move but also to crunch your abs in between your chest and pelvis.

❻ As you reach the top (end) position, make sure that you are contracting the abdominal muscles as hard as you possibly can. This is the most important position of the exercise.

❼ Hold the contraction for a one to two second count.

❽ Return to the bottom position and, without rest or momentum, return to the upward movement.

FAQ:
My neck hurts when I keep my thumbs under my chin.

ANSWER:
You can put your hands behind your head, but make sure not to pull on your head to assist in the exercise. You can also stretch your hands out to the sides of your body. Imagine trying to touch an object a bit far in front of you. This will both help to take your mind off the ab muscle burn, while making sure that you are really squeezing and contracting those ab muscles. This also applies to the trunk curl and crunch.

Crunch

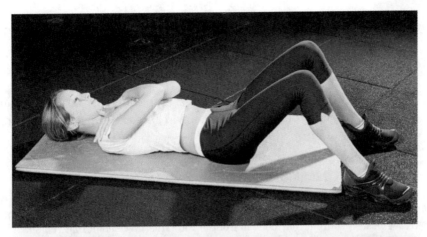

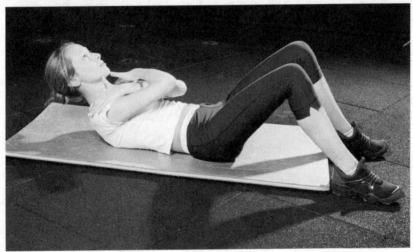

VARIATION

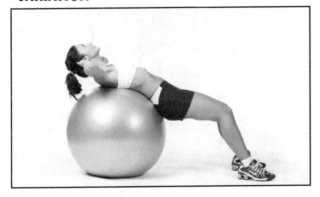

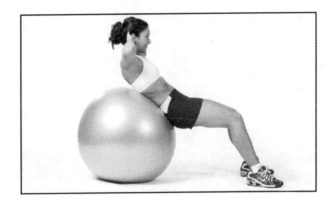

Trunk Curl and Crunch

This is yet another great abdominal exercise that works to incorporate and simultaneously involve the upper and lower abs. You should find this easier than the V-Ups but just as effective. The object is to bring the knees to the chest and chest to the knees at the same time. Once you master these movements, you will become a master of abdominal training.

VARIATION: A difficult variation to this exercise is the jackknife on the ball. From a push-up position, bend your knees, bringing your lower body towards your chest in a reverse trunk curl and crunch.

PROPER ALIGNMENT

❶ Lay flat on your back with knees bent, but lower legs and feet suspended (The correct thigh and lower leg position should look like the number 7).

❷ As you did with the crunch curl, cross your hands across your chest with your thumbs touching each side of your chin.

❸ Once again, the object will be to simultaneously crunch your chest to your knees and your knees to your chest. The elbows will meet with the knees as an indicator of one full rep.

TECHNIQUE AND FORM

❶ Cross your hands over your chest and bring the thighs and feet away from your body in front of you. This will provide a full range of motion for this exercise.

❷ Isometrically contract the abdominal muscles before moving.

❸ At the same time, crunch your chest to your knees and bring your knees to your chest. Your back should come off the ground while your buttocks should also slightly lift off the ground.

❹ By touching your elbows to the knees and vice-versa you will know you have done one full rep. It is at this point that you should squeeze the abdominal muscles as hard as you possibly can. Do not cheat by failing to bring your thighs away from your body in front of you. With each rep, reach out with your feet and allow the lower abs to bring them back in for the knee-elbow touch. At the same time, do not fail to effectively crunch your upper body from the bottom of the floor up to the elbow-knee touch.

Trunk Curl and Crunch

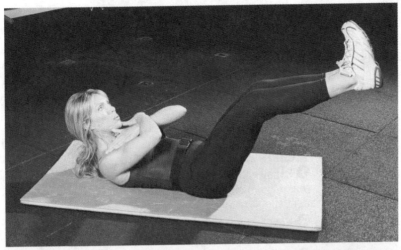

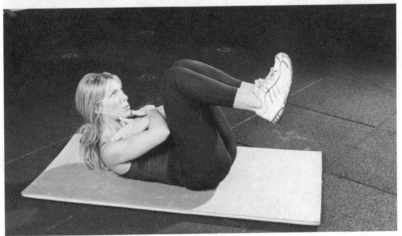

VARIATION

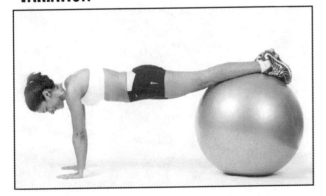

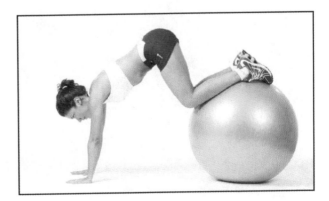

Twist on the Ball

This exercise maximizes recruitment of the obliques while working the entire core. If you do not have a fitness ball, perform this exercise on a mat, keeping your shoulders elevated throughout the exercise as you twist from side to side. make sure you are leading with your shoulder and not pulling on your neck.

To increase the challenge of this exercise, life your opposite leg off the ball as you perform the twist.

PROPER ALIGNMENT

❶ Position yourself on the ball so your lower back is supported.

❷ Your arms should be bent at the elbows and your head should be relaxed into the palms of your hands.

❸ Your chest should be open.

❹ Keep your feet flat on the floor and facing forward for balance.

TECHNIQUE AND FORM

❶ Exhale, lift your chest, and twist over to your left knee, leading with your right shoulder.

❷ Hold for one second and return to the starting position.

❸ Lift and twist, leading with your left shoulder, to your right knee.

❹ Return to start position.

❺ Repeat for the desired number of repetitions, alternating the leading shoulder on each repetition.

Twist on the Ball

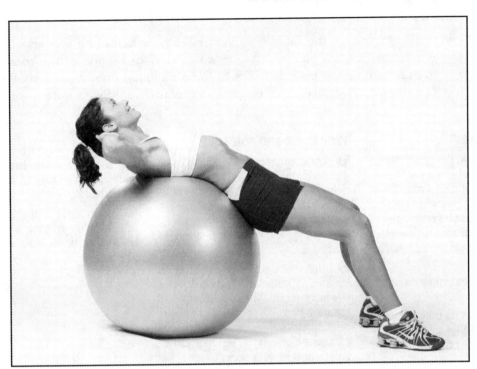

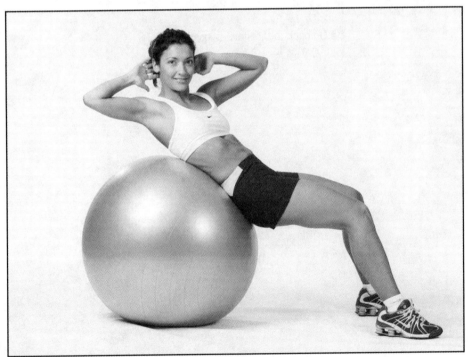

Bicycle Crunch

This exercise, commonly known as the bicycle, is very effective when done properly. In a study conducted by the American Council on Exercise, it was found to be one of the most effective exercises you can do to stimulate the muscle fibers in the abdominal area. You cannot add resistance to this exercise but you can concentrate on perfect execution and slow speed.

PROPER ALIGNMENT

❶ Lay on your back, flat on the floor, keeping your hands behind your head and your knees bent. Press your lower back to the ground. Be careful not to strain your neck as you perform this exercise. Try to keep your back pressed against the floor; avoid having it arch up.

❷ Lift your shoulders into the crunch position.

❸ Bring your knees up until they are perpendicular to the floor, with your lower legs parallel to the floor.

TECHNIQUE AND FORM

❶ Now simultaneously go through a pedal motion, kicking forward with the right leg and bringing in the knee of the left leg. The extended leg should be a few inches off the floor--if you place it too close to the floor you can strain your back.

❷ Bring your right elbow close to your left knee by crunching to the side as you breathe out. When you twist toward your knee, actively think about twisting with your waist, rather than with your elbow. If you feel that you are pulling against your neck, you may be using your arms rather than your waist to twist.

❸ Go back to the starting position as you breathe in.

❹ Immediately crunch to the opposite side as you cycle your legs and bring your left elbow closer to your right knee and exhale.

❺ Continue alternating in this manner until all of the recommended repetitions for each side have been completed.

Bicycle Crunch

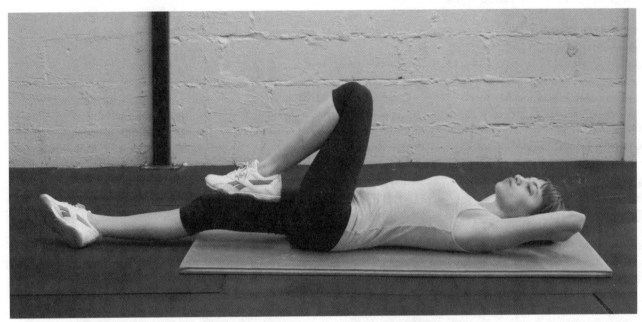

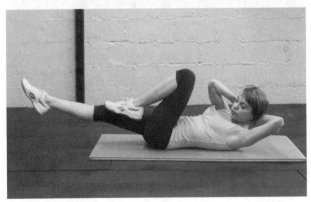

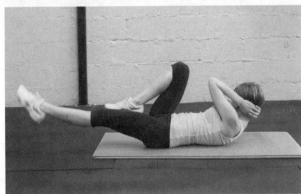

V-Up

This is a very good exercise for simultaneously incorporating the upper and lower abdominal muscles. It is a variation of the crunch, but much more intense. You will simultaneously exercise the upper and lower abs. Start out easy, but try! You will soon breeze through these as if you had been doing them for years.

PROPER ALIGNMENT

❶ Sit on a carpet or mat.

❷ Put your arms by your side for support, slightly behind your torso. Your torso should be at an incline of 45 degrees between your lower back and the floor.

❸ Keep the legs straight and flat on the ground.

❹ Focus on keeping the head and neck in line with your chest.

❺ The object is to simultaneously lift your legs and torso, thus crunching your mid-section.

TECHNIQUE AND FORM

❶ Begin by isometrically contracting the abdominal muscles before moving.

❷ At the same time, crunch forward by moving your torso toward your feet (as if trying to make your chest touch your legs), while you lift your legs and reverse crunch.

❸ You must truly focus on the contraction of your abdominal muscles here. If you do, the contraction will be very intense; a sure sign of amazing abs soon to come!

❹ Hold the crunched position for a count of one second.

❺ Slowly return to the start position, but do not allow your legs to touch the ground. This is a true measure of "time under muscular tension" and is very important if you want to obtain great results from your efforts.

❻ Without rest or momentum, slowly begin once again to lift your chest and legs to the middle meeting point.

FAQ:
I don't feel this one very much in my lower abs.

ANSWER:
You may be sitting too far upright. This can engage the hip flexors to a higher degree. Try leaning back a bit more and concentrate on those lower abdominals. This also applies to the knee-in.

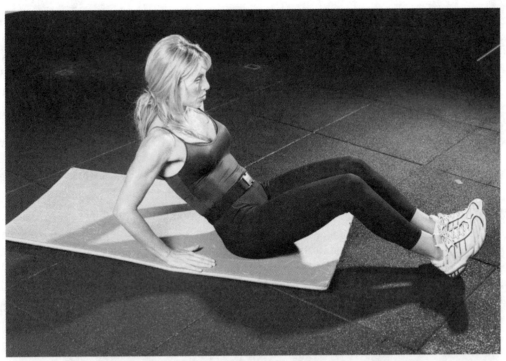

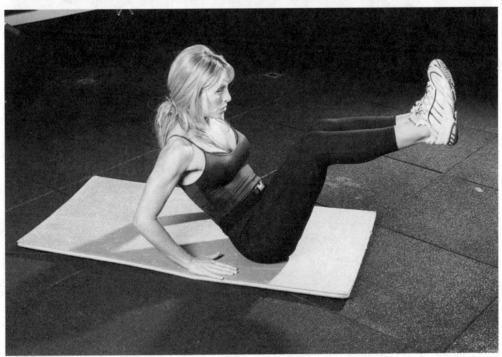

Knee-In

This is another great variation exercise for developing the lower abdominal muscles. It is more convenient than some of the other lower abdominal exercises and just as effective. This exercise also gives you the ability to really squeeze the lower abs when the knees are brought in towards your chest. For a change of pace, why not vary your speed from one workout to the next? The next time you do this or any of the exercises we recommend, move slowly while exercising. Deliberately squeeze the abdominal muscles at the peak contraction position. Then the next time you train your abdominal muscles again, go a little quicker. This variation in the speed of your movements will yet again help to keep your body from hitting a plateau, while keeping you motivated by changing the pace of your movements.

PROPER ALIGNMENT

❶ Sit on the floor (or on the edge of a chair or exercise bench) with your legs extended in front of you.

❷ Your hands should be holding on to the sides of the bench or to the floor for support.

TECHNIQUE AND FORM

❶ Keeping your knees together, pull them in towards your chest until you can go no farther.

❷ Keeping the tension on your lower abdominal muscles, return to the start position.

❸ Repeat the movement until you have completed your set.

Knee-In

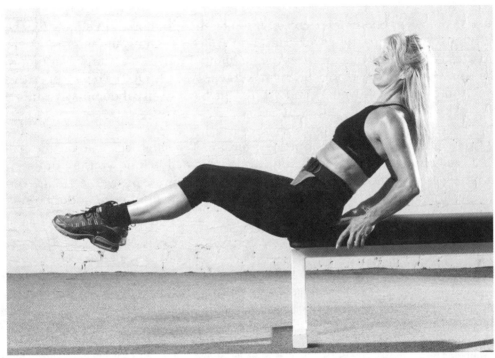

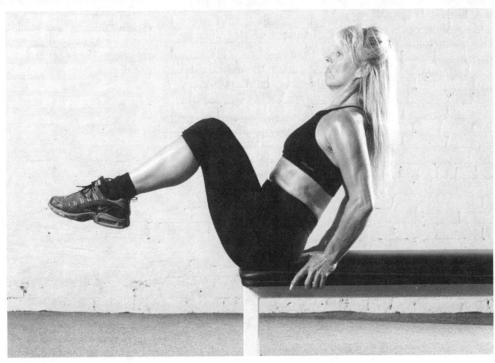

Lying Leg Raise

Leg raises are a great lower abdominal exercise. It is not enough though to simply lift the legs off of the floor. Doing so can hurt the lower back and will do nothing for improving your lower abdominal muscles. You must focus and feel the abdominal muscles actually working while you raise your legs up. When you are ready for the next step, WATCH OUT! The advanced version of the leg raise will not only blow your minds, but will blast your abdominal results into the stratosphere!

VARIATION: There are a few variations on this exercise. Try lying leg raise on the ball, where you lie on a ball, holding onto a rack with your arms extended behind you, and raise your legs up and down. There is also the hanging leg raise, which requires an overhead bar. You will be hanging with your arms fully extended, using either wide or medium grip, and then raising and lowering your legs.

PROPER ALIGNMENT

❶ Lay flat on the floor with your legs straight and flat on the floor as well.

❷ Put your hands face down underneath your buttocks, with fingertips facing each other. Your ring finger and pinky finger will most likely sit between the insertion point of your buttocks and hamstrings. This is a preventative measure against lower back injury.

❸ You will also put a very slight bend in the knees for the same reason.

TECHNIQUE AND FORM

❶ Begin by lifting your legs about five inches off the ground and holding. This is for preparation.

❷ Lift your legs straight up until they are perpendicular to the ground.

❸ Make sure you are focused on the abdominal muscles working while you move the legs up.

❹ When you reach the vertical point, squeeze the abs as hard as you can and hold momentarily.

❺ Slowly return the legs to the bottom position but remember to stop five inches from the floor. From here you will once again lift the legs up.

ADVANCED VERSION

This time, when your legs reach the perpendicular position, holding the vertical position, lift your buttocks off of your hands and reach your feet into the air as if you are trying to put footprints on the ceiling. This little movement will greatly enhance the stimulation of the lower abdominal section. It is like doing an instant super-set and is sure to be one of your favorites.

FAQ:
This exercise hurts my lower back.

ANSWER:
Try bending your knees a bit more for additional support, or switching to another exercise.

Lying Leg Raise

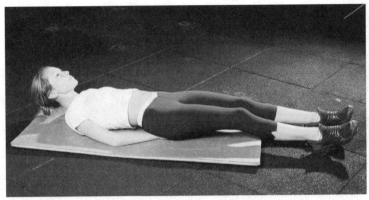

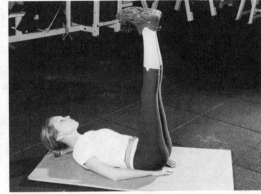

ADVANCED

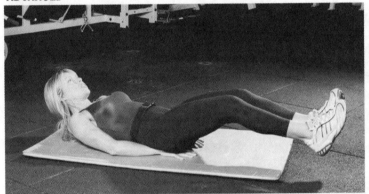

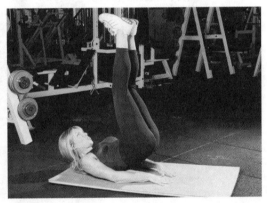

VARIATION

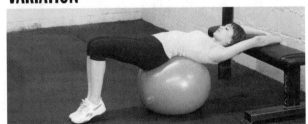

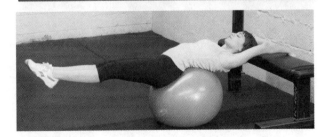

VARIATION

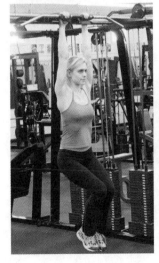

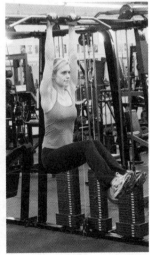

Crunch/Pelvic Lift Combination

This exercise targets both the inner and outer abdominals. Try not to bring your shoulders down to the floor for the entire set. By keeping them slightly elevated, you maintain tension and work in the muscles throughout the range of motion. A great variation is the reverse crunch with ball. In this exercise, you lay on a mat, your arms extended to your sides, and hold a ball between your legs, lifting and raising for a predetermined number of repetitions.

PROPER ALIGNMENT

❶ Lay on your back with your legs extended so that the soles of your feet face the ceiling. Your legs should make a 90-degree angle with your body.

❷ Bend your arms behind your head.

❸ Make sure you keep your head back and that your neck is relaxed.

TECHNIQUE AND FORM

❶ Exhale and slowly lift your torso, keeping your head in line with your spine.

❷ At the same time, press your heels up to the ceiling by pressing your abs deep down through your spine. For the pelvic lift segment of the exercise is it important that you mentally focus on the lower part of your abdominals. Try to minimize action in the hips. The movement is very small-your buttocks should rise just an inch or two from the floor.

❸ Hold at the top position for a second or two before returning to a point where your shoulders do not quite touch the floor.

❹ Repeat for the desired number of repetitions.

Crunch/Pelvic Lift Combination

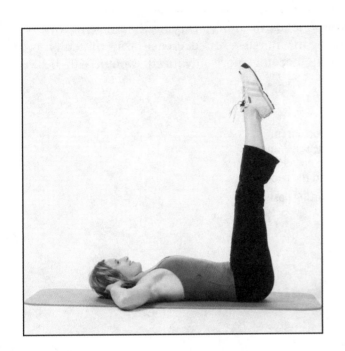
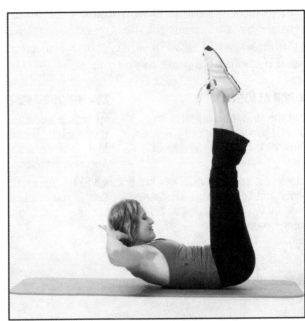

VARIATION

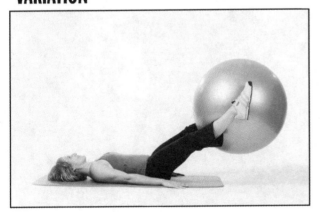
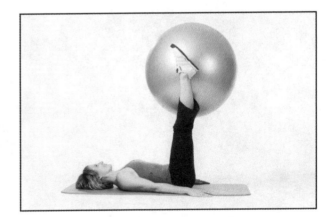

Incline Board Partial Sit-Up

This exercise can be hard on the lower back, so avoid it if you have an unhealthy back. Avoid performing this exercise by swinging your torso as this leads to injury. Varying the angle of this exercise by choosing smaller or steeper inclines can increase or decrease the difficulty. Beginners should always start with no angle. As you become more advanced, weight can be added by holding a plate to your chest.

PROPER ALIGNMENT

1 Set the abdominal board to an incline. The more advanced you are, the steeper the incline you should choose.

2 Hook your feet under the foot brace provided and lie on it with your hands crossed on top of your chest or kept alongside your body.

3 Keep your head straight and your eyes looking ahead.

TECHNIQUE AND FORM

1 Exhale and raise your torso from the bench by bending at the waist and hips until you achieve a 30-degree angle between the torso and the bench.

2 Slowly return to the starting position as you inhale.

Incline Board Partial Sit-Up

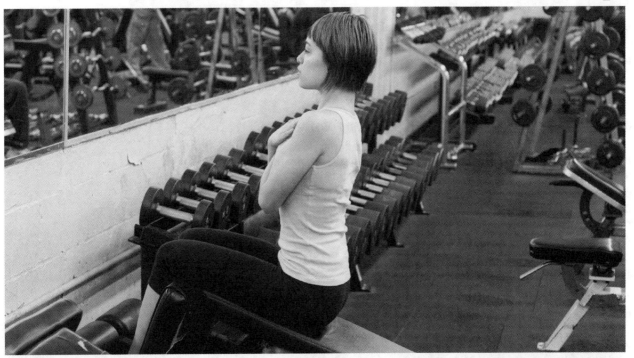

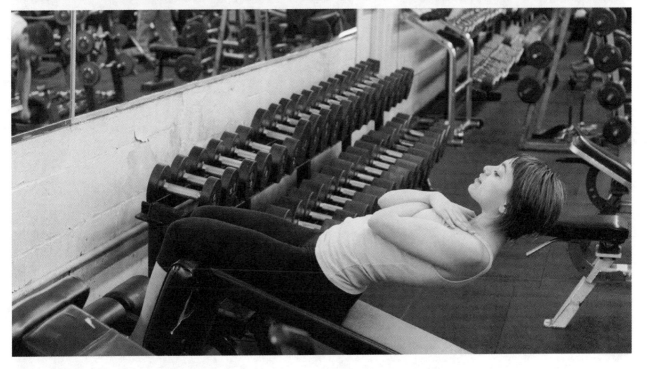

Ab Bench Crunch

For this exercise you will need a bench created by Ironman called the Ab Bench. it has a rounded back that allows for a full stretch of abdominals. As always, be very careful when adding weight to this exercise: if you add too much too quickly you could injure yourself.

PROPER ALIGNMENT

❶ Sit on the Ab Bench with your back on the rounded pad and hold onto the handlebars.

❷ Your feet should be firm on the ground and your torso should be tilted back to stretch the abdominals.

❸ Keep your head steady and your eyes looking straight ahead for the duration of the exercise.

TECHNIQUE AND FORM

❶ Exhale and pull your torso forward and maintain full contact with the back pad. Hold this contraction for a second.

❷ Inhale and slowly return to the starting position.

Ab Bench Crunch

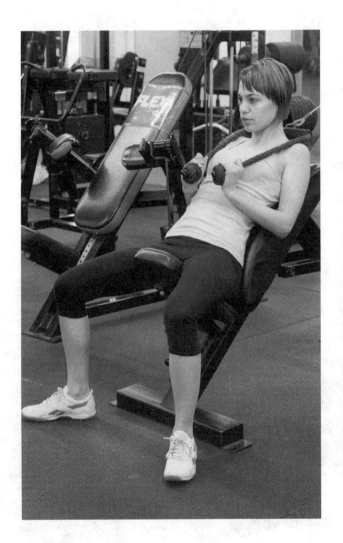
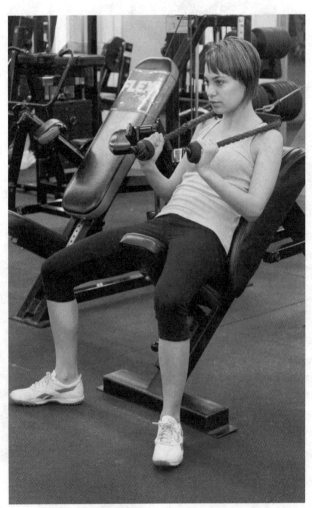

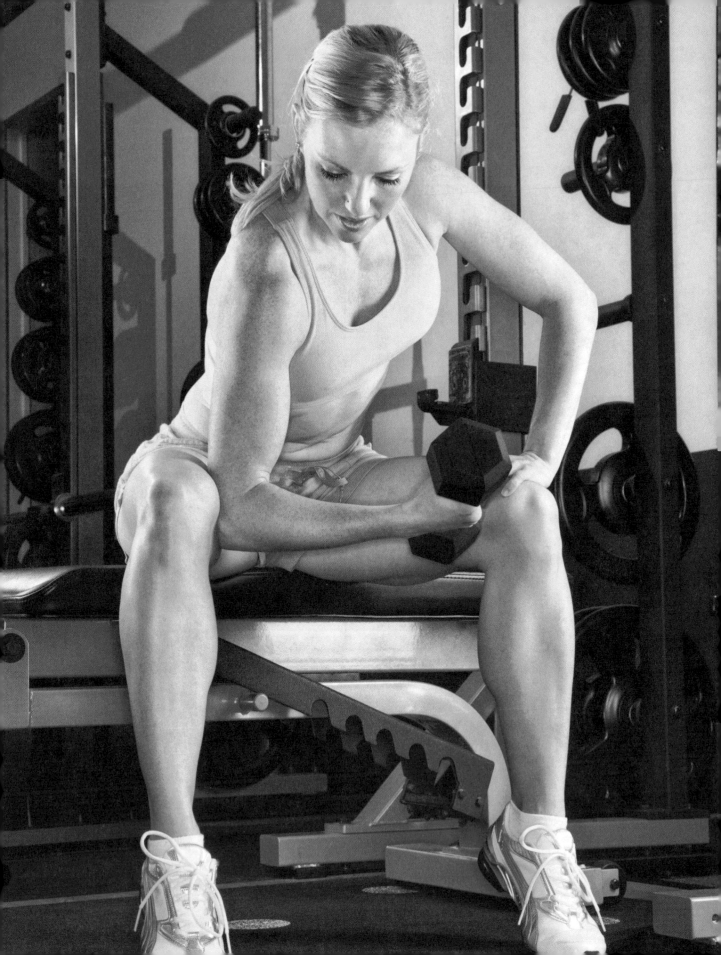

Chapter 13

Combination Exercises

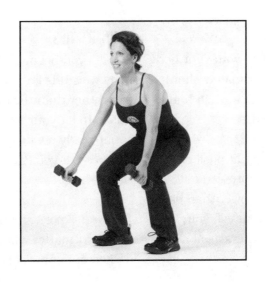

13

THE **BODY SCULPTING BIBLE** FOR **WOMEN**

SQUATS WITH DUMBBELL ROWS

This exercise pairs the squat for your hamstrings, quadriceps, and gluteals with the row for your back.

TECHNIQUE AND FORM

1 Begin in a standing position, with your body in neutral form, your feet approximately shoulder width apart. Hold a dumbbell in each hand, your arms are down by your sides.

2 Inhale and lower into the squat position with your knees bent, your hips pressed out behind you, and your thighs no lower than parallel to the floor. As you lower yourself, your arms slowly extend in front of your legs at an angle.

3 Exhale and pull your abdominals in toward your spine as you straighten your legs. At the same time as you straighten, bend your arms to bring the weights in toward your waist, pulling your elbows behind you.

4 Extend your arms and lower your body back down into the starting position.

TRAINER'S TIPS

As you begin to lift, make sure that your body weight is balanced over the heels of your feet rather than the toes. A good way to check this is to lift your toes while you are in the squat-ready position to see if you remain balanced. If you can't balance, try shifting your weight back toward your heels.

Your knees should be in line with your toes. It doesn't matter whether your legs are slightly turned out or straight ahead.

Keep your head in line with your spine and look straight ahead as you lift and perform the row.

Squats with Dumbbell Rows

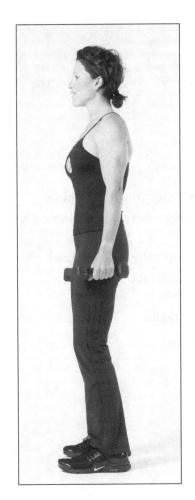
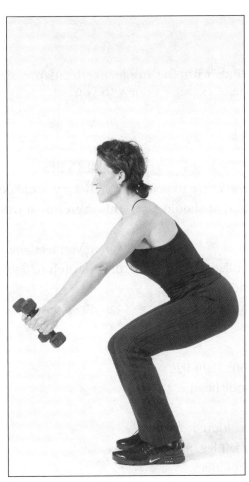
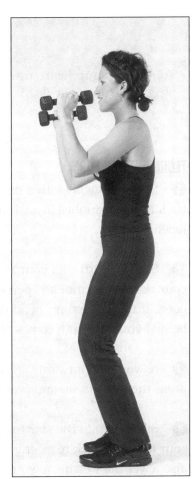

LUNGES WITH OVERHEAD PRESS

You'll feel your heart rate climb with the lunge/overhead press combo, so go easy on the weights—especially if this type of exercise is new to you.

TECHNIQUE AND FORM

1 Stand straight, with a natural curve to your back and a dumbbell in each hand at shoulder height.

2 Step forward with your right leg, bending your right knee until it is perpendicular to the floor. At the same time, bend your left knee behind you, so that it comes close to the floor.

3 As you step forward with your right leg, press the weights up and over your head.

4 Straighten to the starting position, bringing your right leg back to meet your left leg, as you also lower the weights to your shoulders.

5 Repeat beginning with the left leg.

6 Alternate right/left lunges.

TRAINER'S TIPS

✪ Keep your abdominals pulled in tight for this exercise—it will help you remain balanced.

✪ If you feel any sharp pain in your shoulders, switch to lighter weights.

✪ Keep your head straight.

Lunges with Overhead Press

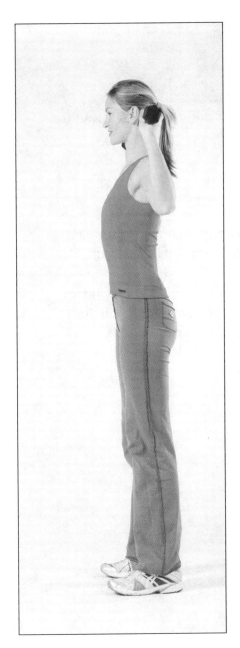
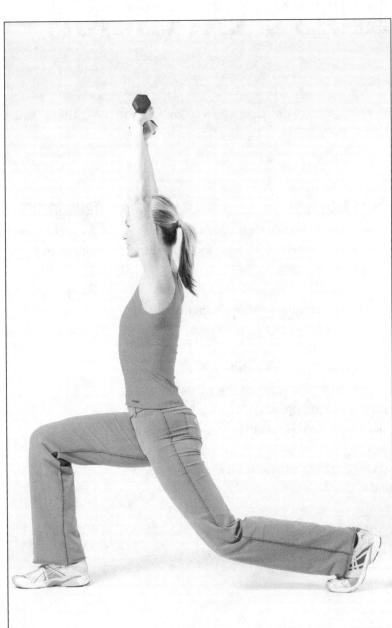

PLIÉ SQUATS WITH TRICEPS EXTENSION

The plié squats with triceps extension works your glutes, your inner and outer thighs, and the backs of your arms.

TECHNIQUE AND FORM

1 Take a wide stance with your legs more than a few feet apart. Bend your legs, pressing your knees to the side.

2 With both hands, hold one weight behind your head, arms bent at your elbows.

3 Exhale and pull your abdominals in toward your spine as you straighten your legs and extend your arms up over your head, pressing the weight toward the ceiling.

4 Hold the top position for a couple of seconds.

5 Lower to start position.

TRAINER'S TIPS

When extending your arms, keep your elbows in by your heard and facing front.

Keep a slight bend in your knees and in your arms, even as you straighten. You don't want to lock out your joints.

Plié Squats with Triceps Extension

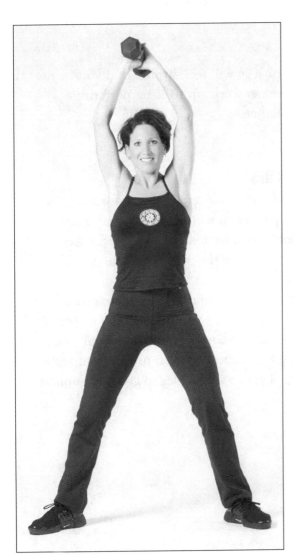
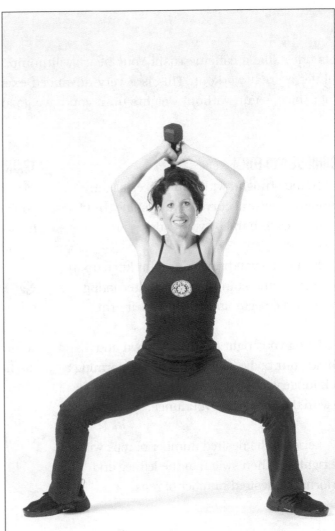

KNEE-UP INTO BACK LUNGE WITH BICEPS CURL

This one's like a caffeine rush! Your heart will pump, your legs will feel strong, and your arms will get a great workout. This is a very advanced exercise, so work up to it by performing the lunge/biceps curl without weights until you have good balance.

TECHNIQUE AND FORM

1 Stand straight, with your knees slightly bent and a natural curve to your spine. Hold a weight in each hand by your sides.

2 Exhale as you bring your right knee up in front of you and start to perform alternating biceps curls, beginning with your left arm.

3 Bring your right knee back down and behind your body, so that you are performing a back lunge with your right leg. Bring the knee close to the floor when you lunge.

4 Perform the desired number of reps with the right leg, then switch to the left leg and perform the desired number of reps.

TRAINER'S TIPS

To modify this exercise if you are a beginner you can perform it without weights or alternate from right to left leg instead of performing consecutive reps with the same leg leading.

Balance is so important in this exercise. Use your core to pull your abs in tight as you lift your knee up. Ground yourself with your standing leg—concentrate on pressing through the heel of your standing leg to give you support.

Knee-Up Into Back Lunge with Biceps Curls

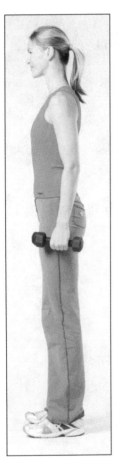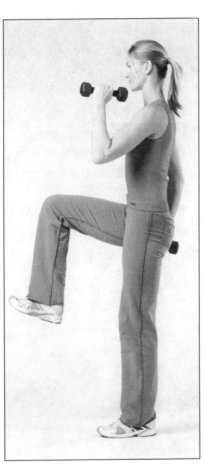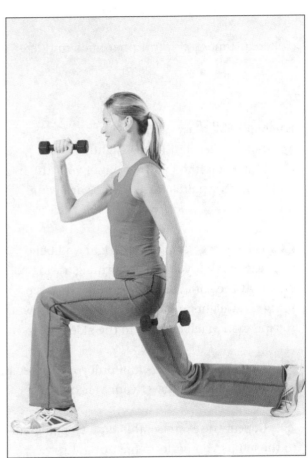

UPRIGHT ROW WITH SIDE-TO-SIDE PLIÉ SQUATS

A great toner for your upper back and legs, this fast moving exercise has cardio benefits too!

TECHNIQUE AND FORM

1 Stand with your knees slightly bent, a weight in each hand at the front of your thighs, and with your palms turned in toward your body.

2 Take a large step to your right and bend your legs so that you are performing a wide plié squat. At the same time as you take the step, bring the weights up to your chest in an upward rowing motion (elbows out to the side).

3 Straighten your legs and pull your left leg in to your body as you lower your weights.

4 Repeat the exercise, this time stepping out to the left as you perform the upright row.

TRAINER'S TIPS

⚓ Keep your elbows slightly above the weights as you perform the row.

⚓ Lift the weights only as high as your chest or you could injure your shoulders.

Upright Row with Side-To-Side Plié Squats

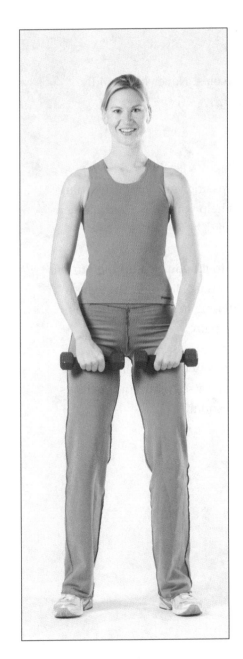

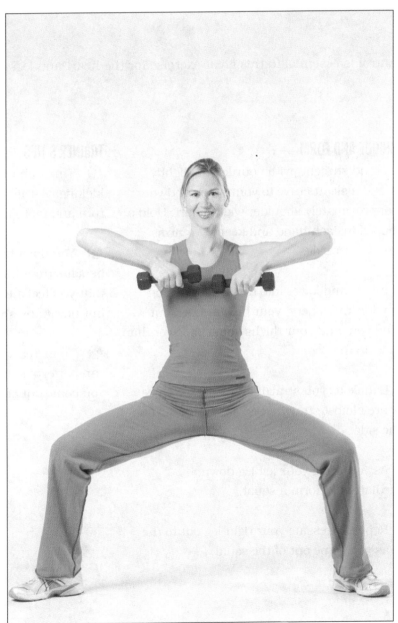

SQUAT WITH ALTERNATING LEG KICK

Control is essential in this great exercise for the heart and legs muscles. Never kick wildly.

TECHNIQUE AND FORM

1 Stand straight, with your knees slightly bent and a slight curve to your spine and your feet approximately shoulder width apart. Hold a dumbbell in each hand and keep your arms down by your sides.

2 Inhale and lower into the squat position with your knees bent, your hips pressed out behind you, and your thighs going no lower than parallel to the floor.

3 Exhale as you straighten your legs. Once they are almost straight, press your left leg out to the side.

4 As you bring your left leg down, immediately perform a squat.

5 Repeat, pressing your right leg out to the side as you come out of the squat.

TRAINER'S TIPS

Think about pressing your leg rather than kicking it—this will help you to use less momentum and more muscle.

You don't have to lift your leg up high to get benefits from this exercise, lift high enough so that you feel a tightening in your outer thighs, but never any sharp pain.

To increase intensity of this exercise you can perform side arm raises with dumbbells as you come out of the squat.

Squat with Alternating Leg Kick

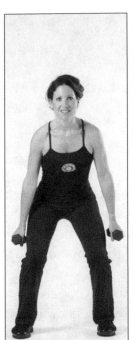 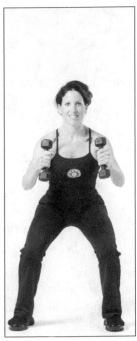 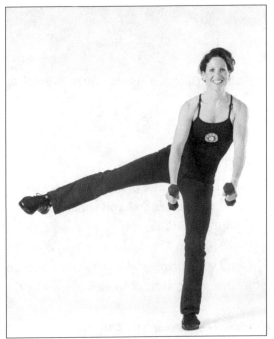

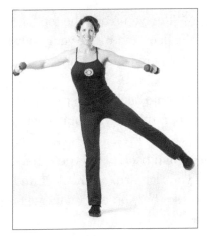

VARIATION

PUSH-UP WITH SIDE ROTATION

A toughie, this exercise requires significant core (ab/back) strength. Work up to it.

TECHNIQUE AND FORM

1 Face the floor in a push-up-ready position with your arms extended and wider than your chest, your back flat.

2 Bend your arms and lower your chest so that it hovers a couple of inches above the floor.

3 Push back up as you exhale.

4 When you reach the top, lift your right arm off the floor and rotate your body so that you are balancing on your left arm and left foot.

5 Rotate back and return your right hand to the floor, then lower your chest again.

6 Push back up as you exhale, this time lifting your left arm off the floor and rotating your body so that you are balancing on your right side.

TRAINER'S TIPS

To work up to this exercise, begin by performing regular push-ups on bent knees. Progress to performing push-ups with straight legs before adding the rotation.

Think about using your abs and lower back muscles to stabilize your body as you lift. Also think about grounding your body with the opposite arm and leg.

Push-Up with Side Rotation

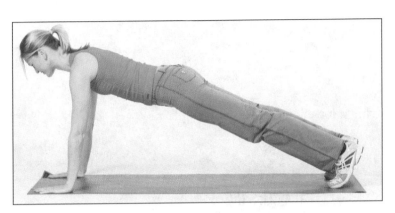

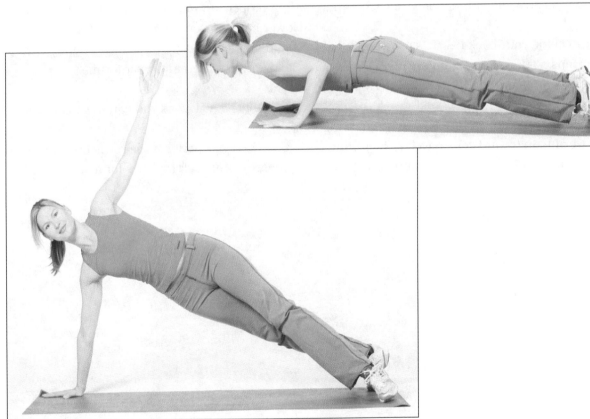

DEADLIFT/ ROW COMBO

Perform this exercise for your hamstrings, lower back, and mid-back.

TECHNIQUE AND FORM

1 Stand straight with a weight in each hand.

2 Keeping your back nearly straight, bend at your hips so that the weights are just below your knees. Your palms should face your legs.

3 Exhale and straighten. As you do so, bring the weights in toward your navel, pulling your elbows behind your back to perform a row.

TRAINER'S TIPS

⊗ Proper form is vital to avoid injury to the lower back. Never curve your back when you bend forward. Pulling in your abs tightly can help you to maintain proper form.

⊗ Only go as low as you can in good form.

⊗ When you perform the row, concentrate on squeezing the back muscles for a second or two.

Deadlift/Row Combo

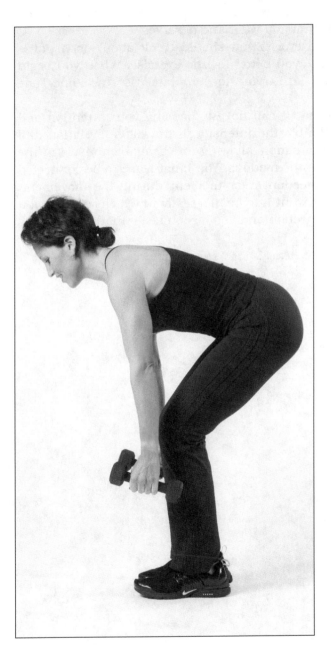

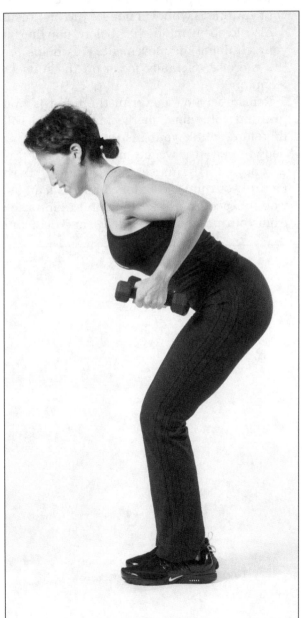

FINAL POINTERS ON EXERCISE FORM

Remember that without knowing how to perform an exercise correctly, no matter how good your routine is, you will not get the fast results that you want and deserve.

Also keep in mind that before starting any exercise, you should think about or visualize yourself doing the movement. This helps prepare you better for the exercise. When you begin the exercise, mentally focus on the muscle you are trying to stimulate. Use the Zone-Tone technique.

Remember how powerful the mind is and what it can do! By focusing your attention and "putting your mind in the muscle" you will double the intensity of muscle stimulation and therefore double your results. This is opposed to simply allowing any available muscle in the body to move the weight merely by going through the motions. You must learn to be connected as one with the muscle, observant of the connection every moment during the movement. Picture your muscle as toned and as lean as you want it to be. It's really much easier than you would expect to master the mind-to-muscle connection and you'll soon see remarkable results from your newfound knowledge and dedication.

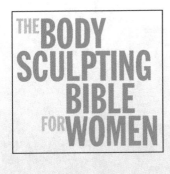

Part 4
Workout Charts

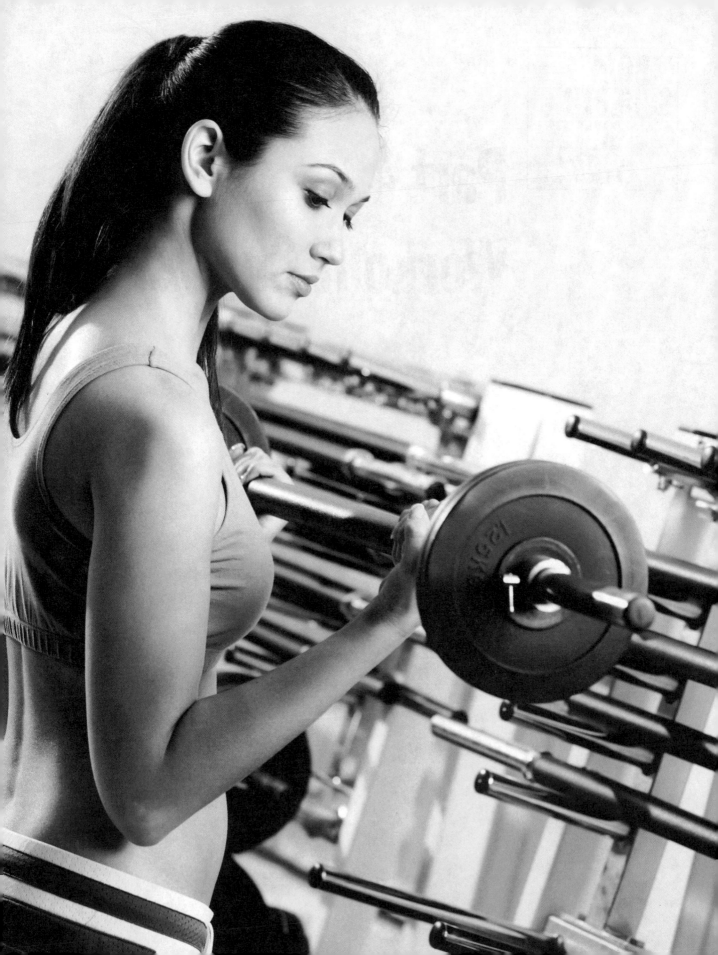

Chapter 14
Workout Charts

14

THE BREAK-IN PROGRAM

In this program you will train with weights 3 days a week and perform aerobic activity 3 days a week. Sundays are your days off. You may do Day 1 on Mondays, Day 2 on Wednesdays, Day 3 on Fridays, and Cardio with Abs on Tuesdays, Thursdays, and Saturdays. Any other combination like Day 1 on Tuesdays, Day 2 on Thursdays, Day 3 on Saturdays, and Cardio with Abs on Wednesdays, Fridays, and Sundays is also valid.

This program is designed to be performed in the comfort of your home with minimum equipment, namely a pair of dumbbells or a pair of dumbbells with an adjustable bench. As you get stronger you may wish to purchase a pair of secure adjustable dumbbells such as Powerblocks (visit our websites www.custom-physiques.com and www.fitnessingear.com for information on these).

You will notice that we present two Break-In Routines. The first assumes that the only equipment available is a pair of dumbbells. The second routine assumes that you also have access to an adjustable exercise bench with a leg curl/leg extension attachment. Choose the routine that you can do with the equipment that you have available.

HOW TO PROGRESS WITH BREAK-IN ROUTINES 1 AND 2

For the first 6 weeks, follow the routine exactly as it is laid out. If you have never worked out before, it will take your body approximately 6 weeks to get used to the movements and to be recruiting muscle fibers. It will also give your cardiovascular system a chance to get used to this type of training. By the end of the 6 weeks, you should have lost a significant amount of weight, and will begin seeing more

muscle tone and definition in your body. You should also be able to reach your target heart rate by the end of this period.

After week 6, add one more set to all of the exercises. You will now be performing 3 sets instead of 2. Increase the weights and perform fewer repetitions (13-15, except for Abs and Calves where the repetition range stays the same). Also, increase your aerobic activity to 20 minutes. Follow this workout for the next 4 weeks.

After week 10, you are ready to go up to 4 sets per exercise and 30 minutes of cardio. Increase the weights and perform fewer repetitions (10-12, except for Abs and Calves where the repetition range stays the same). Also, reduce the rest in between sets to 60 seconds. Follow this workout for 3 more weeks; you should not only look dramatically different, but now you will also be in shape to start the 14-Day Body Sculpting Program.

THE 14-DAY BODY SCULPTING WORKOUT

In this workout you will train with weights three days a week and perform aerobic activity three days a week. Sundays are your days off. You may choose to do Day 1 on Mondays, Day 2 on Wednesdays, and Day 3 on Fridays with Cardio and Abs on Tuesdays, Thursdays and Saturdays. Any other combination like Day 1 on Tuesdays, Day 2 on Thursdays, Day 3 on Saturdays, and Cardio with Abs on Wednesdays, Fridays and Sundays is also valid.

This workout is designed to be performed in the comfort of your home with minimum equipment, namely a pair of dumbbells or a pair of dumbbells with an adjustable bench. As you get stronger you may wish to purchase a pair of secure adjustable dumbbells such as Powerblocks.

You will notice that we present two 14-Day Body Sculpting Workouts. The first routine assumes that the only equipment available to you is a pair of dumbbells. The second two routines assume that you also have access to an adjustable exercise bench with a leg curl/leg extension attachment. Choose the routine you can do with the equipment you have available.

THE EXPRESS WORKOUTS

The Body Sculpting Bible Express program offers two workouts. One is the all dumbbell workout that can be performed either in the comfort of your home, or at a gym, with an adjustable bench and a set of dumbbells. The second workout is one that makes use of selectorized weight machine equipment (or weight stack machines). This is a good workout to use while on vacation at a hotel gym that does not offer dumbbells.

These workouts are designed to be done three days each week within a 21-minute limit. They are fast-paced, providing good cardiovascular conditioning as well as toning and strengthening. On the days off you can perform some abdominal work in the comfort of your home along with some optional cardiovascular exercise. For the fastest results, you are encouraged to use the dumbbell workout in addition to adding the optional cardiovascular exercise component on your days off.

THE 14-DAY RAPID BODY SCULPTING WORKOUT

This program was created especially for women who do not have a lot of time to work out. The program is very fast paced and will get you the most effective and efficient workout possible in 30 minutes or less!

Use this program either as a means to introduce variety into your workouts after you have gone through the 14-Day Body Sculpting Workouts #1 and #2 or use the 14-Day Rapid

Body Sculpting Workout right after the Break-In Routines if 30 minutes is all the time that you can devote to exercise.

The 14-Day Rapid Body Sculpting Workout comes in two workouts. Workout #1 only requires a pair of dumbbells, while workout #2 also requires a weight bench.

THE ADVANCED 14-DAY BODY SCULPTING WORKOUT

In this workout you will train with weights six days a week and perform aerobic activity six days a week. Sundays are your off days. You may do Day 1 on Mondays and Thursdays, Day 2 on Tuesdays and Fridays and Day 3 on Wednesdays and Saturdays.

This workout is designed to be performed at either a commercial gym or a very well equipped home gym. The reason for this is that we will be using a variety of exercises and training different angles and areas of the muscles in order to stimulate all muscle fibers.

Note that these routines provide alternate exercises. Alternate exercises are to be performed the next time that you perform the workout for that specific body part in order to provide varied stimulation. For example, if on Monday of week one you perform reverse curls as your first biceps exercise, on Friday you will perform preacher curls instead. This variation will help to avoid a plateau, keeping your muscle building capabilities in paramount shape.

Cardio and abs are to be performed on a daily basis preferably first thing in the morning on an empty stomach. The weight training workouts are to be performed in the afternoon or at any other convenient time. If your schedule does not allow for two separate sessions, then you may merge both sessions by performing the abs first, and then the weight training followed by the cardiovascular exercise.

THE 14-DAY BODY SCULPTING DEFINITION WORKOUT

This program was created for those people with faster metabolisms—and consequently, low body fat—who are interested only in gaining muscle and building definition. We created the program with the assumption that you will be working out at a well-equipped gym. If you are working out at home, just substitute exercises that you can do with your equipment for those designed for the gym. However, be aware that to add serious muscle you will have to lift some heavy weights, which means that you need sturdy, high-quality equipment. At this point, you should have already completed the Break-In Routines described earlier. If you are a complete beginner, start with the Break-In Routines. Once you have completed them, you can graduate to this level.

You will notice that every two weeks the exercises change along with the set, rep and rest schemes to provide a fresh shock to the body. If you work out at a gym, once you have completed this routine, feel free to add other exercises, such leg press hack squats for the leg routines. As long as the exercises are basic (using mostly free weights), there is no problem with substituting them for other exercises.

THE 14-DAY BODYWEIGHT BODY SCULPTING WORKOUT

This program was created for people who, for one reason or another, do not have access to any weight-bearing equipment. This is also a great workout to do if you are traveling. All you need is a portable pull-up bar, which you can find at any sporting goods store. This is also a great functional program for soldiers who may be overseas and have limited access to weights.

While you won't be able to manipulate the amount of repetitions in the same manner that you would with the other Body Sculpting Workouts, you can certainly manipulate the number of sets and rest time in between sets in order to get the results you want. You will notice that there is no direct shoulder work, but due to the compound nature of the exercises used, you will be giving your shoulders plenty of stimulation.

You will be training with bodyweight exercises four days a week while you perform aerobic activity twice a week. This is how your schedule will look:

Monday (Day 1): Chest/Back/Abs/Calves/Thighs/Biceps/Triceps/Hamstrings

Wednesday (Day 2): Thighs/Hamstrings/Calves/Abs

Friday (Day 3): Chest/Back/Abs/Calves/Thighs/Biceps/ Triceps/Hamstrings

Tuesday, Thursday, Saturday: Cardio

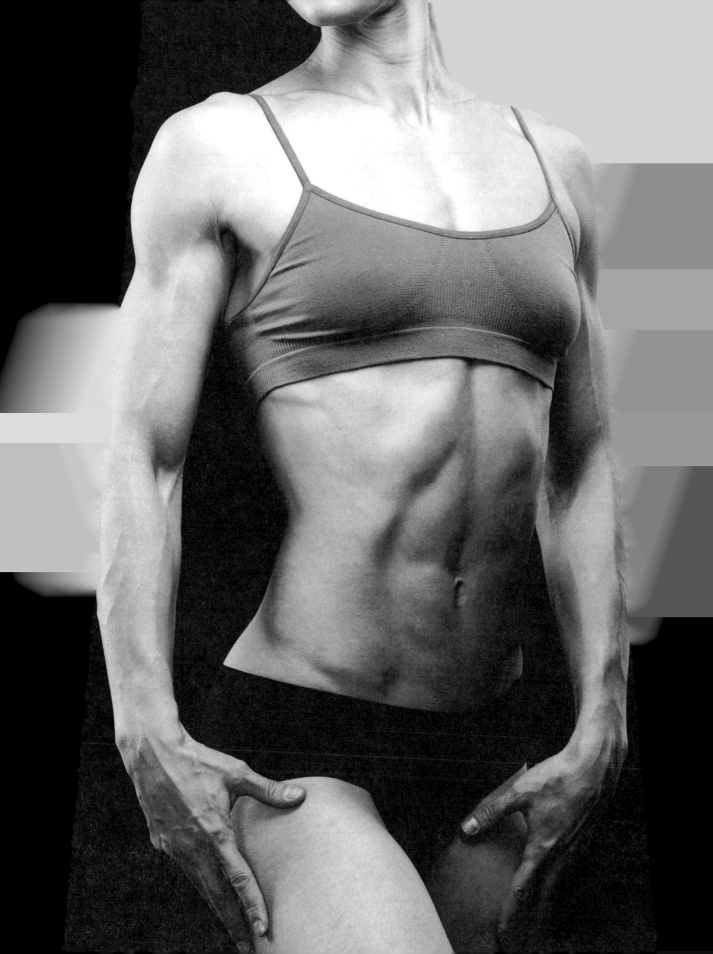

Break-In Routine #1

SPECIAL INSTRUCTIONS FOR WEEKS 1 & 2

Use Modified Compound Supersets. Perform Modified Compound Supersets by performing the first exercise, resting for the prescribed rest period, performing the second exercise, resting the prescribed rest period and going back to the first one. Continue in this manner until you have performed all of the prescribed number of sets, and then continue with the next modified compound superset.

DAY 1 — MONDAY

		EXERCISE	PAGE NO.	REPS	SETS	REST (seconds)
MODIFIED COMPOUND SUPERSET # 1	back	Dumbbell One-Arm Row	162	15-20	2	90
	chest	Push-Up (against wall if unable to perform on floor)	198	15-20	2	90
MODIFIED COMPOUND SUPERSET # 2	shoulders	Dumbbell Shoulder Press	204	15-20	2	90
	calves	Dumbbell Calf Raise (one leg)	144	15-20	2	90
MODIFIED COMPOUND SUPERSET # 3	biceps	Dumbbell Curl	250	15-20	2	90
	triceps	Overhead Dumbbell Extension	228	15-20	2	90
MODIFIED COMPOUND SUPERSET # 4	thighs	Dumbbell Squat	112	15-20	2	90
	hamstrings	Stiff-Legged Deadlift	142	15-20	2	90

NOTES ON PUSH-UPS

Depending on your body weight, you may find this exercise difficult to do in the traditional way. If this is the case, then start by performing them standing against the wall (stand 1.5-2 ft. in front of the wall, extend your arms and perform the exercise). In this position you will not be lifting your full bodyweight. As you become stronger, you may perform push-ups against the floor "from your knees." Once you master that position, you will be able to perform the traditional push-up.

DAY 2 — WEDNESDAY

		EXERCISE	PAGE NO.	REPS	SETS	REST (seconds)
MODIFIED COMPOUND SUPERSET # 1	thighs	Dumbbell Squat	112	15-20	2	90
	hamstrings	Dumbbell Lunge	122	15-20	2	90
MODIFIED COMPOUND SUPERSET # 2	thighs	Ballet Squat	114	15-20	2	90
	hamstrings	Stiff-Legged Deadlift	142	15-20	2	90
MODIFIED COMPOUND SUPERSET # 3	calves	Dumbbell Calf Raises (one leg)	144	15-25	2	90
	shoulders	Dumbbell Upright Rows	214	15-20	2	90
MODIFIED COMPOUND SUPERSET # 4	calves	Dumbbell Calf Raise (two legs)	144	15-25	2	90
	triceps	Triceps Kickback	244	15-20	2	90

DAY 3					FRIDAY
EXERCISE	**PAGE NO.**	**REPS**	**SETS**	**REST (seconds)**
MODIFIED COMPOUND SUPERSET # 1 — back — Two-Arm Row	164	15-20	2	90
chest — Flat Dumbbell Fly (lying on the floor)	190	15-20	2	90
MODIFIED COMPOUND SUPERSET # 2 — shoulders — Bent-Over Lateral Raise	218	15-20	2	90
calves — Dumbbell Calf Raise (two legs)	144	15-20	2	90
MODIFIED COMPOUND SUPERSET # 3 — biceps — Hammer Curl	262	15-20	2	90
triceps — Lying Dumbbell Extension	230	15-20	2	90
MODIFIED COMPOUND SUPERSET # 4 — thighs — Ballet Squat	112	15-20	2	90
hamstrings — Dumbbell Lunge	142	15-20	2	90

Cardio and Abs

				TUESDAY/THURSDAY/SATURDAY	
EXERCISE	**PAGE NO.**	**REPS**	**SETS**	**REST (seconds)**
MODIFIED COMPOUND SUPERSET # 1 — Abs — Lying Leg Raise	282	as many as possible	2	90
Abs — Crunch	270	as many as possible	2	90

AEROBIC ACTIVITY

10 minutes of fast walking, stationary bike, or any other type of aerobic activity that you like. Don't be concerned at this stage with reaching the target heart rate; just concentrate on performing the activity at a comfortable but steady pace.

REPETITIONS

You will note that the repetition ranges are higher than what we normally recommend. The reasons for this are the following:
- To start getting the joints and the muscles accustomed to weight training exercise while preventing injuries.
- To start creating neural pathways (links) between the brain and the muscles so that you start gaining better control and feel of the muscles in your body.

PUSH UPS

Depending on your body weight, you may find this exercise difficult to do in the traditional way. If this is the case, then start by performing them standing against the wall (stand 1.5-2 feet in front of the wall, extend your arms and perform the exercise). In this position you will not be lifting your full bodyweight. As you become stronger, you may perform push-ups against the floor "from your knees". Once you master that position, you will be able to perform the traditional push-up.

Break-In Routine #2

<table>
<tr><td colspan="2" align="center">**SPECIAL INSTRUCTIONS FOR WEEKS 1 & 2**</td></tr>
<tr><td colspan="2">Use Modified Compound Supersets. Perform Modified Compound Supersets by performing the first exercise, resting for the prescribed rest period, performing the second exercise, resting the prescribed rest period and going back to the first one. Continue in this manner until you have performed all of the prescribed number of sets and then continue with the next modified compound superset.</td></tr>
</table>

DAY 1 — MONDAY

	EXERCISE	PAGE NO.	REPS	SETS	REST (seconds)
MODIFIED COMPOUND SUPERSET # 1 — back	Dumbbell One-Arm Row	162	15-20	2	90
MODIFIED COMPOUND SUPERSET # 1 — chest	Incline Dumbbell Press	186	15-20	2	90
MODIFIED COMPOUND SUPERSET # 2 — shoulders	Dumbbell Shoulder Press	204	15-20	2	90
MODIFIED COMPOUND SUPERSET # 2 — calves	Dumbbell Calf Raise (one leg)	144	15-20	2	90
MODIFIED COMPOUND SUPERSET # 3 — biceps	Dumbbell Curl	250	15-20	2	90
MODIFIED COMPOUND SUPERSET # 3 — triceps	Overhead Dumbbell Extension	228	15-20	2	90
MODIFIED COMPOUND SUPERSET # 4 — thighs	Dumbbell Squat	112	15-20	2	90
MODIFIED COMPOUND SUPERSET # 4 — hamstrings	Stiff-Legged Deadlift	142	15-20	2	90

DAY 2 — WEDNESDAY

	EXERCISE	PAGE NO.	REPS	SETS	REST (seconds)
MODIFIED COMPOUND SUPERSET # 1 — thighs	Dumbbell Squat	112	15-20	2	90
MODIFIED COMPOUND SUPERSET # 1 — hamstrings	Dumbbell Lunge	122	15-20	2	90
MODIFIED COMPOUND SUPERSET # 2 — thighs	Leg Extension	126	15-20	2	90
MODIFIED COMPOUND SUPERSET # 2 — hamstrings	Lying Leg Curl	134	15-20	2	90
MODIFIED COMPOUND SUPERSET # 3 — calves	Dumbbell Calf Raise (one leg)	144	15-25	2	90
MODIFIED COMPOUND SUPERSET # 3 — shoulders	Dumbbell Upright Row	214	15-20	2	90
MODIFIED COMPOUND SUPERSET # 4 — calves	Dumbbell Calf Raise (two legs)	144	15-25	2	90
MODIFIED COMPOUND SUPERSET # 4 — triceps	Triceps Kickback	244	15-20	2	90

DAY 3					FRIDAY
EXERCISE		PAGE NO.	REPS	SETS	REST (seconds)
MODIFIED COMPOUND SUPERSET #1	back · Two-Arm Row	164	15-20	2	90
	chest · Incline Dumbbell Fly	192	15-20	2	90
MODIFIED COMPOUND SUPERSET #2	shoulders · Bent-Over Lateral Raise	218	15-20	2	90
	calves · Dumbbell Calf Raise (two legs)	144	15-20	2	90
MODIFIED COMPOUND SUPERSET #3	biceps · Hammer Curl	262	15-20	2	90
	triceps · Lying Dumbbell Extension	230	15-20	2	90
MODIFIED COMPOUND SUPERSET #4	thighs · Ballet Squat	114	15-20	2	90
	hamstrings · Dumbbell Lunge	122	15-20	2	90

Cardio and Abs

DAY 1, 2, AND 3					TUESDAY/THURSDAY/SATURDAY
EXERCISE		PAGE NO.	REPS	SETS	REST (seconds)
MODIFIED COMPOUND SUPERSET #1	Abs · Lying Leg Raise	282	as many as possible	2	90
	Abs · Crunch	270	as many as possible	2	90

AEROBIC ACTIVITY

10 minutes of fast walking, stationary bike, or any other type of aerobic activity that you like. Don't be concerned at this stage with reaching the target heart rate; just concentrate on performing the activity at a comfortable but steady pace.

REPETITIONS

You will note that the repetition ranges are higher than what we normally recommend. The reasons for this are the following:
- To start getting the joints and the muscles accustomed to weight training exercise while preventing injuries.
- To start creating neural pathways (links) between the brain and the muscles so that you start gaining better control and feel of the muscles in your body.

14-Day Body Sculpting Workout #1

SPECIAL INSTRUCTIONS FOR WEEKS 1 & 2

Use modified compound supersets. Perform modified compound supersets by performing the first exercise, resting for the prescribed rest period, performing the second exercise, resting the prescribed rest period and going back to the first exercise. Continue in this manner until you have performed all of the prescribed number of sets, and then continue with the next modified compound superset. You will repeat Day 1 on Monday, Day 2 on Wednesday, and Day 3 on Friday.

DAY 1 — MONDAY

		EXERCISE	PAGE NO.	REPS	SETS	REST (seconds)
MODIFIED COMPOUND SUPERSET # 1	back	Dumbbell One-Arm Row	162	12-15	2	90
	chest	Push-Up (against wall if unable to perform on floor)	198	12-15	2	90
MODIFIED COMPOUND SUPERSET # 2	shoulders	Dumbbell Shoulder Press	204	12-15	2	90
	calves	Standing Calf Raise (one leg)	144	15-25	2	90
MODIFIED COMPOUND SUPERSET # 3	biceps	Dumbbell Curl	250	12-15	2	90
	triceps	Overhead Dumbbell Extension	228	12-15	2	90
MODIFIED COMPOUND SUPERSET # 4	thighs	Dumbbell Squat	112	12-15	2	90
	hamstrings	Stiff-Legged Deadlift	142	12-15	2	90

NOTES ON PUSH-UPS

Depending on your body weight, you may find this exercise difficult to do in the traditional way. If this is the case, then start by performing them standing against the wall (stand 1.5-2 ft. in front of the wall, extend your arms and perform the exercise). In this position you will not be lifting your full bodyweight. As you become stronger, you may perform push-ups against the floor "from your knees." Once you master that position, you will be able to perform the traditional push-up.

DAY 2 — WEDNESDAY

		EXERCISE	PAGE NO.	REPS	SETS	REST (seconds)
MODIFIED COMPOUND SUPERSET # 1	thighs	Dumbbell Squat	112	12-15	2	90
	hamstrings	Dumbbell Lunge	122	12-15	2	90
MODIFIED COMPOUND SUPERSET # 2	thighs	Ballet Squat	114	12-15	2	90
	hamstrings	Stiff-Legged Deadlift	142	12-15	2	90
MODIFIED COMPOUND SUPERSET # 3	calves	Standing Calf Raise (one leg)	144	15-25	2	90
	shoulders	Upright Row	214	12-15	2	90
MODIFIED COMPOUND SUPERSET # 4	calves	Standing Calf Raise (two legs)	144	15-25	2	90
	triceps	Triceps Kickback	244	12-15	2	90

Weeks 1 & 2

DAY 3					FRIDAY
EXERCISE		**PAGE NO.**	**REPS**	**SETS**	**REST (seconds)**
MODIFIED COMPOUND SUPERSET # 1 — back	Two-Arm Row	164	12-15	2	90
MODIFIED COMPOUND SUPERSET # 1 — chest	Flat Dumbbell Fly (lying on the floor)	190	12-15	2	90
MODIFIED COMPOUND SUPERSET # 2 — shoulders	Bent-Over Lateral Raise on Incline Bench	218	12-15	2	90
MODIFIED COMPOUND SUPERSET # 2 — calves	Standing Calf Raise (two legs)	144	15-25	2	90
MODIFIED COMPOUND SUPERSET # 3 — biceps	Hammer Curl	262	12-15	2	90
MODIFIED COMPOUND SUPERSET # 3 — triceps	Lying Dumbbell Extension	230	12-15	2	90
MODIFIED COMPOUND SUPERSET # 4 — thighs	Ballet Squat	114	12-15	2	90
MODIFIED COMPOUND SUPERSET # 4 — hamstrings	Dumbbell Lunge	122	12-15	2	90

Cardio and Abs

					TUESDAY/THURSDAY/SATURDAY
EXERCISE		**PAGE NO.**	**REPS**	**SETS**	**REST (seconds)**
MODIFIED COMPOUND SUPERSET # 1 — Abs	Lying Leg Raise	282	as many as possible	2	90
MODIFIED COMPOUND SUPERSET # 1 — Abs	Crunch	270	as many as possible	2	90

AEROBIC ACTIVITY
20 minutes of fast walking, stationary biking, or any other type of aerobic activity you enjoy while bringing you to your target heart rate.

14-Day Body Sculpting Workout #1

SPECIAL INSTRUCTIONS FOR WEEKS 3 & 4

Use supersets. Perform supersets by pairing exercises with no rest period in between. Only rest after the two exercises have been performed consecutively. Repeat for the prescribed number of sets and then move on to the next pair of exercises. You will repeat Day 1 on Monday, Day 2 on Wednesday, and Day 3 on Friday.

DAY 1 — MONDAY

	EXERCISE	PAGE NO.	REPS	SETS	REST (seconds)
SUPERSET #1	back — Dumbbell One-Arm Row	162	10-12	3	No Rest
	chest — Push-Up (against wall if unable to perform on floor)	198	10-12	3	60
SUPERSET #2	shoulders — Dumbbell Shoulder Press	204	10-12	3	No Rest
	calves — Standing Calf Raise (one leg)	144	15-25	3	60
SUPERSET #3	biceps — Dumbbell Curl	250	10-12	3	No Rest
	triceps — Overhead Dumbbell Extension	228	10-12	3	60
SUPERSET #4	thighs — Dumbbell Squat	112	10-12	3	No Rest
	hamstrings — Stiff-Legged Deadlift	142	10-12	3	60

NOTES ON PUSH-UPS

Depending on your body weight, you may find this exercise difficult to do in the traditional way. If this is the case, then start by performing them standing against the wall (stand 1.5-2 ft. in front of the wall, extend your arms and perform the exercise). In this position you will not be lifting your full bodyweight. As you become stronger, you may perform push-ups against the floor "from your knees." Once you master that position, you will be able to perform the traditional push-up.

DAY 2 — WEDNESDAY

	EXERCISE	PAGE NO.	REPS	SETS	REST (seconds)
SUPERSET #1	thighs — Dumbbell Squat	112	10-12	3	No Rest
	hamstrings — Dumbbell Lunge	122	10-12	3	60
SUPERSET #2	thighs — Ballet Squat	114	10-12	3	No Rest
	hamstrings — Stiff-Legged Deadlift	142	10-12	3	60
SUPERSET #3	calves — Standing Calf Raise (one leg)	144	15-25	3	No Rest
	shoulders — Upright Row	214	10-12	3	60
SUPERSET #4	calves — Standing Calf Raise (two legs)	144	15-25	3	No Rest
	triceps — Triceps Kickback	244	10-12	3	60

Weeks 3 & 4

DAY 3 FRIDAY

		EXERCISE	PAGE NO.	REPS	SETS	REST (seconds)
SUPERSET # 1	back	Two-Arm Row	164	10-12	3	No Rest
	chest	Flat Dumbbell Fly (lying on the floor) (against wall if unable to perform on floor)	190	10-12	3	60
SUPERSET # 2	shoulders	Bent-Over Lateral Raise on Incline Bench	218	10-12	3	No Rest
	calves	Standing Calf Raise (two legs)	144	15-25	3	60
SUPERSET # 3	biceps	Hammer Curl	262	10-12	3	No Rest
	triceps	Lying Dumbbell Extension	230	10-12	3	60
SUPERSET # 4	thighs	Ballet Squat	114	10-12	3	No Rest
	hamstrings	Dumbbell Lunge	122	10-12	3	60

Cardio and Abs

TUESDAY/THURSDAY/SATURDAY

		EXERCISE	PAGE NO.	REPS	SETS	REST (seconds)
SUPERSET # 1	Abs	Lying Leg Raise	282	as many as possible	3	No Rest
	Abs	Crunch	270	as many as possible	3	60

AEROBIC ACTIVITY

30 minutes of fast walking, stationary biking, or any other type of aerobic activity you enjoy while bringing you to your target heart rate.

14-Day Body Sculpting Workout #1

DAY 1 — MONDAY

	EXERCISE	PAGE NO.	REPS	SETS	REST (seconds)
GIANT SET # 1	thighs Dumbbell Squat	112	8-10	4	No Rest
	hamstrings Stiff-Legged Deadlift	142	8-10	4	No Rest
	back Dumbbell One-Arm Row	162	8-10	4	No Rest
	chest Push-Up (against wall if unable to perform on floor)	198	8-10	4	60
GIANT SET # 2	shoulders Dumbbell Shoulder Press	204	8-10	4	No Rest
	calves Standing Calf Raise (one leg)	144	15-25	4	No Rest
	biceps Dumbbell Curl	250	8-10	4	No Rest
	triceps Overhead Dumbbell Extension	228	8-10	4	60

NOTES ON PUSH-UPS

Depending on your body weight, you may find this exercise difficult to do in the traditional way. If this is the case, then start by performing them standing against the wall (stand 1.5-2 ft. in front of the wall, extend your arms and perform the exercise). In this position you will not be lifting your full bodyweight. As you become stronger, you may perform push-ups against the floor "from your knees." Once you master that position, you will be able to perform the traditional push-up.

DAY 2 — WEDNESDAY

	EXERCISE	PAGE NO.	REPS	SETS	REST (seconds)
GIANT SET # 1	thighs Dumbbell Squat	112	8-10	4	No Rest
	hamstrings Dumbbell Lunge	122	8-10	4	No Rest
	calves Standing Calf Raise (one leg)	144	15-25	4	No Rest
	hamstrings Upright Row	214	8-10	4	60
GIANT SET # 2	calves Ballet Squat	114	8-10	4	No Rest
	thighs Stiff-Legged Deadlift	142	8-10	4	No Rest
	calves Standing Calf Raise (two legs)	144	15-25	4	No Rest
	triceps Triceps Kickback	244	8-10	4	60

Weeks 5 & 6

DAY 3				FRIDAY
EXERCISE	PAGE NO.	REPS	SETS	REST (seconds)
Ballet Squat	114	8-10	4	No Rest
Dumbbell Lunge	122	8-10	4	No Rest
Two-Arm Row	164	8-10	4	No Rest
Flat Dumbbell Fly (lying on the floor)	190	8-10	4	60
Bent-Over Lateral Raise on Incline Bench	218	8-10	4	No Rest
Standing Calf Raise (two legs)	144	15-25	4	No Rest
Hammer Curl	262	8-10	4	No Rest
Lying Dumbbell Extension	230	8-10	4	60

GIANT SET # 1: thighs, hamstrings, back, chest
GIANT SET # 2: shoulders, calves, biceps, triceps

Cardio and Abs

EXERCISE		PAGE NO.	REPS	SETS	REST (seconds)
			TUESDAY/THURSDAY/SATURDAY		
GIANT SET # 1	Lying Leg Raise (abs)	282	as many as possible	4	No Rest
	Crunch (abs)	270	as many as possible	4	No Rest

AEROBIC ACTIVITY

40 minutes of fast walking, stationary biking, or any other type of aerobic activity that you enjoy while bringing you to your target heart rate.

14-Day Body Sculpting Workout #2

> **SPECIAL INSTRUCTIONS FOR WEEKS 1 & 2**
>
> Use modified compound supersets. Perform the first exercise, resting for the prescribed rest period, perform the second exercise, rest the prescribed rest period and then go back to the first exercise. Continue in this manner until you have performed all of the prescribed number of sets, and then continue with the next modified compound superset. You will repeat Day 1 on Monday, Day 2 on Wednesday, and Day 3 on Friday.

DAY 1
MONDAY

	EXERCISE	PAGE NO.	REPS	SETS	REST (seconds)
MODIFIED COMPOUND SUPERSET #1 — back	Dumbbell One-Arm Row	162	12-15	2	90
— chest	Incline Dumbbell Press	186	12-15	2	90
MODIFIED COMPOUND SUPERSET #2 — shoulders	Dumbbell Shoulder Press	204	12-15	2	90
— calves	Standing Calf Raise (one leg)	144	15-25	2	90
MODIFIED COMPOUND SUPERSET #3 — biceps	Dumbbell Curl	250	12-15	2	90
— triceps	Overhead Dumbbell Extension	228	12-15	2	90
MODIFIED COMPOUND SUPERSET #4 — thighs	Dumbbell Squat	112	12-15	2	90
— hamstrings	Stiff-Legged Deadlift	142	12-15	2	90

DAY 2
WEDNESDAY

	EXERCISE	PAGE NO.	REPS	SETS	REST (seconds)
MODIFIED COMPOUND SUPERSET #1 — thighs	Dumbbell Squat	112	12-15	2	90
— hamstrings	Dumbbell Lunge	122	12-15	2	90
MODIFIED COMPOUND SUPERSET #2 — thighs	Leg Extension	126	12-15	2	90
— hamstrings	Lying Leg Curl	134	12-15	2	90
MODIFIED COMPOUND SUPERSET #3 — calves	Standing Calf Raise (one leg)	144	15-25	2	90
— shoulders	Upright Row	214	12-15	2	90
MODIFIED COMPOUND SUPERSET #4 — calves	Standing Calf Raise (two legs)	144	15-25	2	90
— triceps	Triceps Kickback	244	12-15	2	90

Weeks 1 & 2

DAY 3				FRIDAY
EXERCISE	**PAGE NO.**	**REPS**	**SETS**	**REST (seconds)**
MODIFIED COMPOUND SUPERSET # 1 — back — Two-Arm Row	164	12-15	2	90
chest — Incline Dumbbell Fly	192	12-15	2	90
MODIFIED COMPOUND SUPERSET # 2 — shoulders — Bent-Over Lateral Raise on Incline Bench	218	12-15	2	90
calves — Standing Calf Raise (two legs)	144	15-25	2	90
MODIFIED COMPOUND SUPERSET # 3 — biceps — Hammer Curl	262	12-15	2	90
triceps — Lying Dumbbell Extension	230	12-15	2	90
MODIFIED COMPOUND SUPERSET # 4 — thighs — Ballet Squat	114	12-15	2	90
hamstrings — Dumbbell Lunge	122	12-15	2	90

Cardio and Abs

		TUESDAY/THURSDAY/SATURDAY		
EXERCISE	**PAGE NO.**	**REPS**	**SETS**	**REST (seconds)**
MODIFIED COMPOUND SUPERSET # 1 — abs — Lying Leg Raise	282	as many as possible	2	90
abs — Crunch	270	as many as possible	2	90

AEROBIC ACTIVITY
20 minutes of fast walking, stationary biking, or any other type of aerobic activity you enjoy while bringing you to your target heart rate.

14-Day Body Sculpting Workout #2

SPECIAL INSTRUCTIONS FOR WEEKS 3 & 4

Use supersets. Perform supersets by pairing exercises with no rest period in between. Only rest after the two exercises have been performed consecutively. Repeat for the prescribed number of sets and then move on to the next pair of exercises. You will repeat Day 1 on Monday, Day 2 on Wednesday, and Day 3 on Friday.

DAY 1   MONDAY

		EXERCISE	PAGE NO.	REPS	SETS	REST (seconds)
SUPERSET #1	back	Dumbbell One-Arm Row	162	10-12	3	No Rest
	chest	Incline Dumbbell Press	186	10-12	3	60
SUPERSET #2	shoulders	Dumbbell Shoulder Press	204	10-12	3	No Rest
	calves	Standing Calf Raise (one leg)	144	15-25	3	60
SUPERSET #3	biceps	Dumbbell Curl	250	10-12	3	No Rest
	triceps	Overhead Dumbbell Extension	228	10-12	3	60
SUPERSET #4	thighs	Dumbbell Squat	112	10-12	3	No Rest
	hamstrings	Stiff-Legged Deadlift	142	10-12	3	60

DAY 2   WEDNESDAY

		EXERCISE	PAGE NO.	REPS	SETS	REST (seconds)
SUPERSET #1	thighs	Dumbbell Squat	112	10-12	3	No Rest
	hamstrings	Dumbbell Lunge	122	10-12	3	60
SUPERSET #2	thighs	Leg Extension	126	10-12	3	No Rest
	hamstrings	Lying Leg Curl	134	10-12	3	60
SUPERSET #3	calves	Standing Calf Raise (one leg)	144	15-25	3	No Rest
	shoulders	Upright Row	214	10-12	3	60
SUPERSET #4	calves	Standing Calf Raise (two legs)	144	15-25	3	No Rest
	triceps	Triceps Kickback	244	10-12	3	60

Weeks 3 & 4

DAY 3					FRIDAY
EXERCISE	**PAGE NO.**	**REPS**	**SETS**	**REST (seconds)**	
back Two-Arm Row	164	10-12	3	No Rest	
chest Incline Dumbbell Fly	192	10-12	3	60	
shoulders Bent-Over Lateral Raise on Incline Bench	218	10-12	3	No Rest	
calves Standing Calf Raise (two legs)	144	15-25	3	60	
biceps Hammer Curl	262	10-12	3	No Rest	
triceps Lying Dumbbell Extension	230	10-12	3	60	
thighs Ballet Squat	114	10-12	3	No Rest	
hamstrings Dumbbell Lunge	122	10-12	3	60	

SUPERSET #1, SUPERSET #2, SUPERSET #3, SUPERSET #4

Cardio and Abs

				TUESDAY/THURSDAY/SATURDAY	
EXERCISE	**PAGE NO.**	**REPS**	**SETS**	**REST (seconds)**	
abs Lying Leg Raise	282	as many as possible	3	No Rest	
abs Crunch	270	as many as possible	3	60	

SUPERSET #1

AEROBIC ACTIVITY
30 minutes of fast walking, stationary biking, or any other type of aerobic activity you enjoy while bringing you to your target heart rate.

14-Day Body Sculpting Workout #2

SPECIAL INSTRUCTIONS FOR WEEKS 5 & 6

Use giant sets. Perform four exercises with no rest period in between. Only rest after the four exercises have been performed consecutively. Repeat for the prescribed number of sets and then move on to the second group of exercises. You will repeat Day 1 on Monday, Day 2 on Wednesday, and Day 3 on Friday.

DAY 1 — MONDAY

	EXERCISE	PAGE NO.	REPS	SETS	REST (seconds)
GIANT SET #1	thighs — Dumbbell Squat	112	8-10	4	No Rest
	hamstrings — Stiff-Legged Deadlift	142	8-10	4	No Rest
	back — Dumbbell One-Arm Row	162	8-10	4	No Rest
	chest — Incline Dumbbell Press	186	8-10	4	60
GIANT SET #2	shoulders — Dumbbell Shoulder Press	204	8-10	4	No Rest
	calves — Standing Calf Raise (one leg)	144	15-25	4	No Rest
	biceps — Dumbbell Curl	250	8-10	4	No Rest
	triceps — Overhead Dumbbell Extension	228	8-10	4	60

DAY 2 — WEDNESDAY

	EXERCISE	PAGE NO.	REPS	SETS	REST (seconds)
GIANT SET #1	thighs — Dumbbell Squat	112	8-10	4	No Rest
	hamstrings — Dumbbell Lunge	122	8-10	4	No Rest
	calves — Standing Calf Raise (one leg)	144	15-25	4	No Rest
	shoulders — Upright Row	214	8-10	4	60
GIANT SET #2	thighs — Leg Extension	126	18-10	4	No Rest
	hamstrings — Lying Leg Curl	134	8-10	4	No Rest
	calves — Standing Calf Raise (two legs)	144	15-25	4	No Rest
	triceps — Triceps Kickback	244	8-10	4	60

Weeks 5 & 6

DAY 3					FRIDAY
EXERCISE		**PAGE NO.**	**REPS**	**SETS**	**REST (seconds)**
GIANT SET #1	thighs — Ballet Squat	114	8-10	4	No Rest
	hamstrings — Dumbbell Lunge	122	8-10	4	No Rest
	back — Two-Arm Row	164	8-10	4	No Rest
	chest — Incline Dumbbell Fly	192	18-10	4	60
GIANT SET #2	shoulders — Bent-Over Lateral Raise on Incline Bench	218	8-10	4	No Rest
	calves — Standing Calf Raise (two legs)	144	15-25	4	No Rest
	biceps — Hammer Curl	262	8-10	4	No Rest
	triceps — Lying Dumbbell Extension	230	8-10	4	60

Cardio and Abs

					TUESDAY/THURSDAY/SATURDAY
EXERCISE		**PAGE NO.**	**REPS**	**SETS**	**REST (seconds)**
GIANT SET #1	abs — Lying Leg Raise	282	as many as possible	4	No Rest
	abs — Crunch	270	as many as possible	4	No Rest

AEROBIC ACTIVITY
40 minutes of fast walking, stationary biking, or any other type of aerobic activity you enjoy while bringing you to your target heart rate.

14-Day Body Sculpting Workout #3

SPECIAL INSTRUCTIONS FOR WEEKS 1 & 2

Use modified compound supersets. Perform the first exercise, resting for the prescribed rest period, perform the second exercise, rest the prescribed rest period and then go back to the first exercise. Continue in this manner until you have performed all of the prescribed number of sets. Then continue with the next modified compound superset. You will repeat Day 1 on Monday, Day 2 on Wednesday, and Day 3 on Friday.

DAY 1 — MONDAY

	EXERCISE	PAGE NO.	REPS	SETS	REST (seconds)
MODIFIED COMPOUND SUPERSET # 1 — back	Wide Grip Pull-Down	170	12-15	3	90
MODIFIED COMPOUND SUPERSET # 1 — chest	Incline Dumbbell Press	186	12-15	3	90
MODIFIED COMPOUND SUPERSET # 2 — shoulders	Military Press	210	12-15	3	90
MODIFIED COMPOUND SUPERSET # 2 — calves	Multi-Directional Calf Raise	146	15-25	3	90
MODIFIED COMPOUND SUPERSET # 3 — biceps	High Cable Curl	266	12-15	3	90
MODIFIED COMPOUND SUPERSET # 3 — triceps	Triceps Pushdown	242	12-15	3	90
MODIFIED COMPOUND SUPERSET # 4 — thighs	Leg Press	124	12-15	3	90
MODIFIED COMPOUND SUPERSET # 4 — hamstrings	Stiff-Legged Deadlift	142	12-15	3	90

DAY 2 — WEDNESDAY

	EXERCISE	PAGE NO.	REPS	SETS	REST (seconds)
MODIFIED COMPOUND SUPERSET # 1 — thighs	Barbell Squat	110	12-15	3	90
MODIFIED COMPOUND SUPERSET # 1 — hamstrings	Dumbbell Lunge	122	12-15	3	90
MODIFIED COMPOUND SUPERSET # 2 — thighs	Ballet Squat	114	12-15	3	90
MODIFIED COMPOUND SUPERSET # 2 — hamstrings	Standing Hamstring Curl	136	12-15	3	90
MODIFIED COMPOUND SUPERSET # 3 — calves	Seated Machine Calf Raise	148	15-25	3	90
MODIFIED COMPOUND SUPERSET # 3 — shoulders	Bent-Over Lateral Raises on Incline Bench	218	12-15	3	90
MODIFIED COMPOUND SUPERSET # 4 — calves	Standing Calf Raise (two legs)	144	15-25	3	90
MODIFIED COMPOUND SUPERSET # 4 — triceps	Bench Dip	236	12-15	3	90

Weeks 1 & 2

DAY 3				FRIDAY
EXERCISE	**PAGE NO.**	**REPS**	**SETS**	**REST (seconds)**
MODIFIED COMPOUND SUPERSET # 1 · back · Close-Grip Pull-Down (with V-bar)	172	12-15	3	90
chest · Incline Cable Crossover	196	12-15	3	90
MODIFIED COMPOUND SUPERSET # 2 · shoulders · Seated Rear Delt Machine	222	12-15	3	90
calves · Donkey Calf Raise	150	15-25	3	90
MODIFIED COMPOUND SUPERSET # 3 · biceps · Hammer Curl	262	12-15	3	90
triceps · Fixed Bar Bodyweight Triceps Extension	246	12-15	3	90
MODIFIED COMPOUND SUPERSET # 4 · thighs · Leg Extension	126	12-15	3	90
hamstrings · Leg Press	124	12-15	3	90

Cardio and Inner/Outer Thighs, and Abs

			TUESDAY/THURSDAY/SATURDAY	
EXERCISE	**PAGE NO.**	**REPS**	**SETS**	**REST (seconds)**
MODIFIED COMPOUND SUPERSET # 1 · thighs · Adductor Machine	128	15-25	3	90
thighs · Abductor Machine	130	15-25	3	90
MODIFIED COMPOUND SUPERSET # 2 · abs · Lying Leg Raise	282	15-25	3	90
abs · Crunch	270	15-25	3	90

AEROBIC ACTIVITY
20 minutes of fast walking, stationary biking, or any other type of aerobic activity you enjoy while bringing you to your target heart rate.

14-Day Body Sculpting Workout #3

SPECIAL INSTRUCTIONS FOR WEEKS 3 & 4

Use supersets. Perform supersets by pairing exercises with no rest period in between. Only rest after the two exercises have been performed consecutively. Repeat for the prescribed number of sets and then move on to the next pair of exercises. You will repeat Day 1 on Monday, Day 2 on Wednesday, and Day 3 on Friday.

DAY 1   MONDAY

	EXERCISE	PAGE NO.	REPS	SETS	REST (seconds)
SUPERSET #1 — back	Close-Grip Pull-Down (with V-bar)	172	10-12	4	No Rest
SUPERSET #1 — chest	Incline Dumbbell Press	186	10-12	4	60
SUPERSET #2 — shoulders	Front Raise	212	10-12	3	No Rest
SUPERSET #2 — calves	Standing Calf Raise (one leg)	144	15-25	3	60
SUPERSET #3 — biceps	One-Arm Preacher Curl	254	10-12	3	No Rest
SUPERSET #3 — triceps	Overhead Dumbbell Extension	228	10-12	3	60
SUPERSET #4 — thighs	Dumbbell Squat	112	10-12	4	No Rest
SUPERSET #4 — hamstrings	Butt Blaster	132	10-12	4	60

DAY 2   WEDNESDAY

	EXERCISE	PAGE NO.	REPS	SETS	REST (seconds)
SUPERSET #1 — thighs	Hack Squat	118	10-12	4	No Rest
SUPERSET #1 — hamstrings	Seated Leg Curl Machine	134	10-12	4	60
SUPERSET #2 — thighs	Sissy Squat	116	10-12	4	No Rest
SUPERSET #2 — thighs	Step-Up	138	10-12	4	60
SUPERSET #3 — calves	Standing Calf Raise (two legs)	144	15-25	3	No Rest
SUPERSET #3 — shoulders	Two-Arm Cable Lateral Raise	220	10-12	3	60
SUPERSET #4 — calves	Standing Calf Raise (one leg)	144	15-25	3	No Rest
SUPERSET #4 — triceps	Overhead Dumbbell Extension	228	10-12	3	60

Weeks 3 & 4

DAY 3						FRIDAY
EXERCISE			**PAGE NO.**	**REPS**	**SETS**	**REST (seconds)**
SUPERSET #1	back	Two-Arm Row	164	10-12	4	No Rest
	chest	Chest Dip	194	10-12	4	60
SUPERSET #2	shoulders	Bent-Arm Bent-Over Row	216	10-12	3	No Rest
	calves	Tibia Raise	154	15-25	3	60
SUPERSET #3	biceps	Reverse Curl	264	10-12	3	No Rest
	triceps	Lying Dumbbell Extension	230	10-12	3	60
SUPERSET #4	thighs	Front Squat	120	10-12	4	No Rest
	hamstrings	Glute-Ham Raise	140	10-12	4	60

Cardio and Inner/Outer Thighs, and Abs

				TUESDAY/THURSDAY/SATURDAY		
EXERCISE			**PAGE NO.**	**REPS**	**SETS**	**REST (seconds)**
SUPERSET #1	thighs	Adductor Machine	128	15-25	3	No Rest
	thighs	Abductor Machine	130	15-25	3	60
SUPERSET #2	abs	Lying Leg Raise on the Ball	282	15-25	3	No Rest
	abs	Crunch on the Ball	270	15-25	3	60

AEROBIC ACTIVITY
30 minutes of fast walking, stationary biking, or any other type of aerobic activity you enjoy while bringing you to your target heart rate.

14-Day Body Sculpting Workout #3

SPECIAL INSTRUCTIONS FOR WEEKS 5 & 6

Use giant sets. Perform four exercises with no rest period in between. Only rest after the four exercises have been performed consecutively. Repeat for the prescribed number of sets and then move on to the second group of exercises. You will repeat Day 1 on Monday, Day 2 on Wednesday, and Day 3 on Friday.

DAY 1   MONDAY

	EXERCISE	PAGE NO.	REPS	SETS	REST (seconds)
GIANT SET # 1	thighs Dumbbell Lunge	122	8-10	4	No Rest
	hamstrings Seated Leg Curl	134	8-10	4	No Rest
	back Dumbbell One-Arm Row	162	8-10	4	No Rest
	chest Incline Dumbbell Press	186	8-10	4	60
GIANT SET # 2	shoulders Dumbbell Shoulder Press	204	8-10	4	No Rest
	calves Standing Calf Raise (one leg)	144	15-25	4	No Rest
	biceps Concentration Curl	258	8-10	4	No Rest
	triceps Triceps Dip	234	8-10	4	60

DAY 2   WEDNESDAY

	EXERCISE	PAGE NO.	REPS	SETS	REST (seconds)
GIANT SET # 1	thighs Hack Squat	118	8-10	4	No Rest
	hamstrings Leg Press	124	8-10	4	No Rest
	calves Calf Press	152	15-25	4	No Rest
	shoulders Upright Row	214	8-10	4	60
GIANT SET # 2	thighs Barbell Squat	110	8-10	4	No Rest
	hamstrings Lying Leg Curl	134	8-10	4	No Rest
	calves Standing Calf Raise (two legs)	144	15-25	4	No Rest
	triceps Triceps Kickback	244	8-10	4	60

Weeks 5 & 6

DAY 3					FRIDAY
EXERCISE		**PAGE NO.**	**REPS**	**SETS**	**REST (seconds)**
GIANT SET #1	thighs Ballet Squat	114	8-10	4	No Rest
	hamstrings Stiff-Legged Deadlift	142	8-10	4	No Rest
	back Neutral Grip Pull-Up	168	8-10	4	No Rest
	chest Incline Dumbbell Press (palms facing each other)	186	8-10	4	60
GIANT SET #2	shoulders Standing Bent-Over Lateral Raise	208	8-10	4	No Rest
	calves Multi-Directional Calf Raise	146	15-25	4	No Rest
	biceps Incline Hammer Curl	262	8-10	4	No Rest
	triceps Close-Grip Dumbbell Press	240	8-10	4	60

Cardio and Inner/Outer Thighs, and Abs

					TUESDAY/THURSDAY/SATURDAY
EXERCISE		**PAGE NO.**	**REPS**	**SETS**	**REST (seconds)**
GIANT SET #1	thighs Adductor Machine	128	15-25	4	No Rest
	thighs Abductor Machine	130	15-25	4	No Rest
GIANT SET #2	abs Trunk Curl and Crunch	272	15-25	4	No Rest
	abs Crunch/Pelvic Lift Combination	284	15-25	4	No Rest

AEROBIC ACTIVITY
40 minutes of fast walking, stationary biking, or any other type of aerobic activity you enjoy while bringing you to your target heart rate.

WHAT TO DO AFTER WEEK SIX?

By going through all three Body Sculpting Bible Workouts you have learned many useful exercises that target your muscles in a very efficient manner. After week six, you can retain the main structure of the workout but substitute the recommended exercises with similar ones. Don't be afraid to experiment!

Another alternative, if you want to take your body to the next level, is to try out the Advanced Routine. Or, if you want to gain more muscle mass, you may want to try the mass gaining program.

14-Day Rapid Body Sculpting Workout #1

SPECIAL INSTRUCTIONS FOR WEEKS 1 & 2

Use modified compound supersets. Perform modified compound supersets by performing the first exercise, resting for the prescribed rest period, performing the second exercise, resting the prescribed rest period and going back to the first exercise. Continue in this manner until you have performed all of the prescribed number of sets, and then continue with the next modified compound superset. You will repeat Day 1 on Monday, Day 2 on Wednesday, and Day 3 on Friday.

DAY 1 — MONDAY

		EXERCISE	PAGE NO.	REPS	SETS	REST (seconds)
MODIFIED COMPOUND SUPERSET # 1	back	Dumbbell One-Arm Row	162	12-15	2	30
	chest	Push-Up (against the wall if unable to perform on the floor)	198	12-15	2	30
MODIFIED COMPOUND SUPERSET # 2	shoulders	Dumbbell Shoulder Press	204	12-15	2	30
	calves	Standing Calf Raise (one leg)	144	15-25	2	30
MODIFIED COMPOUND SUPERSET # 3	biceps	Dumbbell Curl	250	12-15	2	30
	triceps	Overhead Dumbbell Extension	228	12-15	2	30
MODIFIED COMPOUND SUPERSET # 4	thighs	Dumbbell Squat	112	12-15	2	30
	hamstrings	Stiff-Legged Deadlift	142	12-15	2	30

DAY 2 — WEDNESDAY

		EXERCISE	PAGE NO.	REPS	SETS	REST (seconds)
MODIFIED COMPOUND SUPERSET # 1	thighs	Dumbbell Squat	112	12-15	2	30
	hamstrings	Dumbbell Lunge	122	12-15	2	30
MODIFIED COMPOUND SUPERSET # 2	thighs	Ballet Squat	114	12-15	2	30
	hamstrings	Stiff-Legged Deadlift	142	12-15	2	30
MODIFIED COMPOUND SUPERSET # 3	calves	Standing Calf Raise (one leg)	144	15-25	2	30
	shoulders	Upright Row	214	12-15	2	30
MODIFIED COMPOUND SUPERSET # 4	calves	Standing Calf Raise (two legs)	144	15-25	2	30
	triceps	Triceps Kickback	244	12-15	2	30

Weeks 1 & 2

DAY 3					FRIDAY
EXERCISE	**PAGE NO.**	**REPS**	**SETS**		**REST (seconds)**
MODIFIED COMPOUND SUPERSET # 1 · back · Two-Arm Row	164	12-15	2		30
chest · Flat Dumbbell Fly (lying on the floor)	190	12-15	2		30
MODIFIED COMPOUND SUPERSET # 2 · shoulders · Bent Over Lateral Raise on Incline Bench	218	12-15	2		30
calves · Standing Calf Raise (two legs)	144	15-25	2		30
MODIFIED COMPOUND SUPERSET # 3 · biceps · Hammer Curl	262	12-15	2		30
triceps · Lying Dumbbell Extension	230	12-15	2		30
MODIFIED COMPOUND SUPERSET # 4 · thighs · Ballet Squat	114	12-15	2		30
hamstrings · Dumbbell Lunge	122	12-15	2		30

Cardio and Abs

		TUESDAY/THURSDAY/SATURDAY			
EXERCISE	**PAGE NO.**	**REPS**	**SETS**		**REST (seconds)**
MODIFIED COMPOUND SUPERSET # 1 · lower abs · Lying Leg Raise	282	As many as possible	2		30
upper abs · Crunch	270	As many as possible	2		30

AEROBIC ACTIVITY
15 minutes of fast walking, stationary bike, or any other type of aerobic activity that you enjoy while bringing you to your target heart rate.

14-Day Rapid Body Sculpting Workout #1

SPECIAL INSTRUCTIONS FOR WEEKS 3 & 4

Use supersets. Perform supersets by pairing exercises with no rest period in between. Only rest after the two exercises have been performed consecutively. Repeat for the prescribed number of sets and then move on to the next pair of exercises. You will repeat Day 1 on Monday, Day 2 on Wednesday, and Day 3 on Friday.

DAY 1 — MONDAY

	EXERCISE	PAGE NO.	REPS	SETS	REST (seconds)
SUPERSET # 1 — back	Dumbbell One-Arm Row	162	10-12	3	No Rest
SUPERSET # 1 — chest	Push-Up (against the wall if unable to perform on the floor)	198	10-12	3	30
SUPERSET # 2 — shoulders	Dumbbell Shoulder Press	204	10-12	2	No Rest
SUPERSET # 2 — calves	Standing Calf Raise (one leg)	144	15-25	2	30
SUPERSET # 3 — biceps	Dumbbell Curl	250	10-12	2	No Rest
SUPERSET # 3 — triceps	Overhead Dumbbell Extension	228	10-12	2	30
SUPERSET # 4 — thighs	Dumbbell Squat	112	10-12	3	No Rest
SUPERSET # 4 — hamstrings	Stiff-Legged Deadlift	142	10-12	3	30

DAY 2 — WEDNESDAY

	EXERCISE	PAGE NO.	REPS	SETS	REST (seconds)
SUPERSET # 1 — thighs	Dumbbell Squat	112	10-12	3	No Rest
SUPERSET # 1 — hamstrings	Dumbbell Lunge	122	10-12	3	30
SUPERSET # 2 — thighs	Ballet Squat	114	10-12	2	No Rest
SUPERSET # 2 — hamstrings	Stiff-Legged Deadlift	142	10-12	2	30
SUPERSET # 3 — shoulders/lats	Standing Calf Raise (one leg)	144	15-25	3	No Rest
SUPERSET # 3 — shoulders	Upright Row	214	10-12	3	30
SUPERSET # 4 — calves	Standing Calf Raise (two legs)	144	15-25	2	No Rest
SUPERSET # 4 — triceps	Triceps Kickback	244	10-12	2	30 seconds

Weeks 3 & 4

DAY 3					FRIDAY
EXERCISE		**PAGE NO.**	**REPS**	**SETS**	**REST (seconds)**
SUPERSET # 1	back Two-Arm Row	164	10-12	3	No Rest
	chest Flat Dumbbell Fly (lying on the floor)	190	10-12	3	30
SUPERSET # 2	shoulders Bent Over Lateral Raise on Incline Bench	218	10-12	2	No Rest
	calves Standing Calf Raise (two legs)	144	15-25	2	30
SUPERSET # 3	biceps Hammer Curl	262	10-12	2	No Rest
	triceps Lying Dumbbell Extension	230	10-12	2	30
SUPERSET # 4	thighs Ballet Squat	114	10-12	3	No Rest
	hamstrings Dumbbell Lunge	122	10-12	3	30

Cardio and Abs

					TUESDAY/THURSDAY/SATURDAY
EXERCISE		**PAGE NO.**	**REPS**	**SETS**	**REST (seconds)**
SUPERSET # 1	lower abs Lying Leg Raise	282	As many as possible	3	No Rest
	upper abs Crunch	270	As many as possible	3	30

AEROBIC ACTIVITY
20 minutes of fast walking, stationary bike, or any other type of aerobic activity that you enjoy while bringing you to your target heart rate.

14-Day Rapid Body Sculpting Workout #1

SPECIAL INSTRUCTIONS FOR WEEKS 5 & 6

Use giant sets. Perform four exercises with no rest period in between. Only rest after the four exercises have been performed consecutively. Repeat for the prescribed number of sets and then move on to the second group of exercises. You will repeat Day 1 on Monday, Day 2 on Wednesday, and Day 3 on Friday.

DAY 1 — MONDAY

EXERCISE	PAGE NO.	REPS	SETS	REST (seconds)
GIANT SET #1 thighs Dumbbell Squat	112	8-10	3	No Rest
hamstrings Stiff-Legged Deadlift	142	8-10	3	No Rest
back Dumbbell One-Arm Row	162	8-10	3	No Rest
chest Push-Up (against the wall if unable to perform on the floor)	198	8-10	3	45
GIANT SET #2 shoulders Dumbbell Shoulder Press	204	8-10	3	No Rest
calves Standing Calf Raise (one leg)	144	15-25	3	No Rest
biceps Dumbbell Curl	250	8-10	3	No Rest
triceps Overhead Dumbbell Extension	228	8-10	3	45

DAY 2 — WEDNESDAY

EXERCISE	PAGE NO.	REPS	SETS	REST (seconds)
GIANT SET #1 back Dumbbell Squat	112	8-10	3	No Rest
chest Dumbbell Lunge	122	8-10	3	No Rest
calves Standing Calf Raise (one leg)	144	15-25	3	No Rest
shoulders Upright Row	214	8-10	3	45
GIANT SET #2 thighs Ballet Squat	114	8-10	3	No Rest
hamstrings Stiff-Legged Deadlift	142	8-10	3	No Rest
calves Standing Calf Raise (two legs)	144	15-25	3	No Rest
triceps Triceps Kickback	244	8-10	3	45

Weeks 5 & 6

DAY 3					FRIDAY
EXERCISE		**PAGE NO.**	**REPS**	**SETS**	**REST (seconds)**
GIANT SET #1	thighs Ballet Squat	114	8-10	3	No Rest
	hamstrings Dumbbell Lunge	122	8-10	3	No Rest
	back Two-Arm Row	164	8-10	3	No Rest
	chest Flat Dumbbell Fly (lying on the floor)	190	8-10	3	45
GIANT SET #2	shoulders Bent-Over Lateral Raise on Incline Bench	218	8-10	3	No Rest
	calves Standing Calf Raise (two legs)	144	15-25	3	No Rest
	biceps Hammer Curl	262	8-10	3	No Rest
	triceps Lying Dumbbell Extension	230	8-10	3	45

Cardio and Abs

DAY 1					TUESDAY/THURSDAY/SATURDAY
EXERCISE		**PAGE NO.**	**REPS**	**SETS**	**REST (seconds)**
GIANT SET	lower abs Lying Leg Raise	282	As many as possible	4	No Rest
	upper abs Crunch	270	As many as possible	4	No Rest

AEROBIC ACTIVITY
25 minutes of fast walking, stationary biking, or any other type of aerobic activity that you enjoy while bringing you to your target heart rate.

14-Day Rapid Body Sculpting Workout #2

SPECIAL INSTRUCTIONS FOR WEEKS 1 & 2

Use modified compound supersets. Perform the first exercise, rest for the prescribed rest period, perform the second exercise, rest the prescribed rest period and then go back to the first exercise. Continue in this manner until you have performed all of the prescribed number of sets, and then continue with the next modified compound superset. You will repeat Day 1 on Monday, Day 2 on Wednesday, and Day 3 on Friday.

DAY 1 — MONDAY

	EXERCISE	PAGE NO.	REPS	SETS	REST (seconds)
MODIFIED COMPOUND SUPERSET #1 — back	Dumbbell One-Arm Row	162	12-15	2	30
shoulders	Incline Dumbbell Press	186	12-15	2	30
MODIFIED COMPOUND SUPERSET #2 — shoulders	Dumbbell Shoulder Press	204	12-15	2	30
calves	Standing Calf Raise (one leg)	144	15-25	2	30
MODIFIED COMPOUND SUPERSET #3 — biceps	Dumbbell Curl	250	12-15	2	30
triceps	Overhead Dumbbell Extension	228	12-15	2	30
MODIFIED COMPOUND SUPERSET #4 — thighs	Dumbbell Squat	112	12-15	2	30
hamstrings	Stiff-Legged Deadlift	142	12-15	2	30

DAY 2 — WEDNESDAY

	EXERCISE	PAGE NO.	REPS	SETS	REST (seconds)
MODIFIED COMPOUND SUPERSET #1 — thighs	Dumbbell Squat	112	12-15	2	30
hamstrings	Dumbbell Lunge	122	12-15	2	30
MODIFIED COMPOUND SUPERSET #2 — thighs	Leg Extension	126	12-15	2	30
hamstrings	Lying Leg Curl	134	12-15	2	30
MODIFIED COMPOUND SUPERSET #3 — calves	Standing Calf Raise (one leg)	144	15-25	2	30
shoulders	Upright Row	214	12-15	2	30
MODIFIED COMPOUND SUPERSET #4 — calves	Standing Calf Raise (two legs)	144	15-25	2	30
triceps	Triceps Kickback	244	12-15	2	30

Weeks 1 & 2

DAY 3					FRIDAY
EXERCISE		**PAGE NO.**	**REPS**	**SETS**	**REST (seconds)**
MODIFIED COMPOUND SUPERSET # 1	back — Two-Arm Row	164	12-15	2	30
	chest — Incline Dumbbell Fly	192	12-15	2	30
MODIFIED COMPOUND SUPERSET # 2	shoulders — Bent-Over Lateral Raise on Incline Bench	218	12-15	2	30
	calves — Standing Calf Raise (two legs)	144	15-25	2	30
MODIFIED COMPOUND SUPERSET # 3	biceps — Hammer Curl	262	12-15	2	30
	triceps — Lying Dumbbell Extension	230	12-15	2	30
MODIFIED COMPOUND SUPERSET # 4	thighs — Ballet Squat	114	12-15	2	30
	hamstrings — Dumbbell Lunge	122	12-15	2	30

Cardio and Abs

					TUESDAY/THURSDAY/SATURDAY
EXERCISE		**PAGE NO.**	**REPS**	**SETS**	**REST (seconds)**
MODIFIED COMPOUND SUPERSET # 1	lower abs — Lying Leg Raise	282	As many as possible	2	30 seconds
	upper abs — Crunch	270	As many as possible	2	30 seconds

AEROBIC ACTIVITY
15 minutes of fast walking, stationary biking, or any other type of aerobic activity that you enjoy while bringing you to your target heart rate.

14-Day Rapid Body Sculpting Workout #2

SPECIAL INSTRUCTIONS FOR WEEKS 3 & 4

Use supersets. Perform supersets by pairing exercises with no rest period in between. Only rest after the two exercises have been performed consecutively. Repeat for the prescribed number of sets and then move on to the next pair of exercises. You will repeat Day 1 on Monday, Day 2 on Wednesday, and Day 3 on Friday.

DAY 1 — MONDAY

	EXERCISE	PAGE NO.	REPS	SETS	REST (seconds)
SUPERSET #1	back — Dumbbell One-Arm Row	162	10-12	3	No Rest
	chest — Incline Dumbbell Press	186	10-12	3	30
SUPERSET #2	shoulders — Dumbbell Shoulder Press	204	10-12	2	No Rest
	calves — Standing Calf Raise (one leg)	144	15-25	2	30
SUPERSET #3	biceps — Dumbbell Curl	250	10-12	2	No Rest
	triceps — Overhead Dumbbell Extension	228	10-12	2	30
SUPERSET #4	thighs — Dumbbell Squat	112	10-12	3	No Rest
	hamstrings — Stiff-Legged Deadlift	142	10-12	3	30

DAY 2 — WEDNESDAY

	EXERCISE	PAGE NO.	REPS	SETS	REST (seconds)
SUPERSET #1	thighs — Dumbbell Squat	112	10-12	3	No Rest
	hamstrings — Dumbbell Lunge	122	10-12	3	30
SUPERSET #2	thighs — Leg Extension	126	10-12	2	No Rest
	hamstrings — Lying Leg Curl	134	10-12	2	30
SUPERSET #3	calves — Standing Calf Raise (one leg)	144	15-25	3	No Rest
	shoulders — Upright Row	214	10-12	3	30
SUPERSET #4	calves — Standing Calf Raise (two legs)	144	15-25	2	No Rest
	triceps — Triceps Kickback	244	10-12	2	30 seconds

Weeks 3 & 4

DAY 3					FRIDAY
EXERCISE	**PAGE NO.**	**REPS**	**SETS**	**REST (seconds)**
SUPERSET # 1 — back — Two-Arm Row	164	10-12	3	No Rest
SUPERSET # 1 — chest — Incline Dumbbell Fly	192	10-12	3	30
SUPERSET # 2 — shoulders — Bent Over Lateral Raise on Incline Bench	218	10-12	2	No Rest
SUPERSET # 2 — calves — Standing Calf Raise (two legs)	144	15-25	2	30
SUPERSET # 3 — biceps — Hammer Curl	262	10-12	2	No Rest
SUPERSET # 3 — triceps — Lying Dumbbell Extension	230	10-12	2	30
SUPERSET # 4 — thighs — Ballet Squat	114	10-12	3	No Rest
SUPERSET # 4 — hamstrings — Dumbbell Lunge	122	10-12	3	30

Cardio and Abs

					TUESDAY/THURSDAY/SATURDAY
EXERCISE	**PAGE NO.**	**REPS**	**SETS**	**REST (seconds)**
SUPERSET # 1 — lower abs — Lying Leg Raise	282	As many as possible	3	No Rest
SUPERSET # 1 — upper abs — Crunch	270	As many as possible	3	30

AEROBIC ACTIVITY
20 minutes of fast walking, stationary biking, or any other type of aerobic activity that you enjoy while bringing you to your target heart rate.

14-Day Rapid Body Sculpting Workout #2

SPECIAL INSTRUCTIONS FOR WEEKS 5 & 6

Use giant sets. Perform four exercises with no rest period in between. Only rest after the four exercises have been performed consecutively. Repeat for the prescribed number of sets and then move on to the second group of exercises. You will repeat Day 1 on Monday, Day 2 on Wednesday, and Day 3 on Friday.

DAY 1 — MONDAY

	EXERCISE	PAGE NO.	REPS	SETS	REST (seconds)
GIANT SET # 1 — thighs	Dumbbell Squat	112	8-10	3	No Rest
hamstrings	Stiff-Legged Deadlift	142	8-10	3	No Rest
back	Dumbbell One-Arm Row	162	8-10	3	No Rest
chest	Incline Dumbbell Press	186	8-10	3	45
GIANT SET # 2 — shoulders	Dumbbell Shoulder Press	204	8-10	3	No Rest
calves	Standing Calf Raise (one leg)	144	15-25	3	No Rest
biceps	Dumbbell Curl	250	8-10	3	No Rest
triceps	Overhead Dumbbell Extension	228	8-10	3	45

DAY 2 — WEDNESDAY

	EXERCISE	PAGE NO.	REPS	SETS	REST (seconds)
GIANT SET # 1 — back	Dumbbell Squat	112	8-10	3	No Rest
chest	Dumbbell Lunge	122	8-10	3	No Rest
calves	Standing Calf Raise (one leg)	144	15-25	3	No Rest
shoulders	Upright Row	214	8-10	3	45
GIANT SET # 2 — thighs	Leg Extension	126	8-10	3	No Rest
hamstrings	Lying Leg Curl	134	8-10	3	No Rest
calves	Standing Calf Raise (two legs)	144	15-25	3	No Rest
triceps	Triceps Kickback	244	8-10	3	45

Weeks 5 & 6

DAY 3					FRIDAY
EXERCISE		**PAGE NO.**	**REPS**	**SETS**	**REST (seconds)**
GIANT SET #1	thighs — Ballet Squat	114	8-10	3	No Rest
	hamstrings — Dumbbell Lunge	122	8-10	3	No Rest
	back — Two-Arm Row	164	8-10	3	No Rest
	chest — Incline Dumbbell Fly	192	8-10	3	45
GIANT SET #2	shoulders — Bent-Over Lateral Raise on Incline Bench	218	8-10	3	No Rest
	calves — Standing Calf Raise (two legs)	144	15-25	3	No Rest
	biceps — Hammer Curl	262	8-10	3	No Rest
	triceps — Lying Dumbbell Extension	230	8-10	3	45

Cardio and Abs

					TUESDAY/THURSDAY/SATURDAY
EXERCISE		**PAGE NO.**	**REPS**	**SETS**	**REST (seconds)**
GIANT SET	lower abs — Lying Leg Raise	282	As many as possible	4	No Rest
	upper abs — Crunch	270	As many as possible	4	No Rest

AEROBIC ACTIVITY
20 minutes of fast walking, stationary biking, or any other type of aerobic activity that you enjoy while bringing you to your target heart rate.

Advanced 14-Day Body Sculpting Workout #1

SPECIAL INSTRUCTIONS FOR WEEKS 1 & 2

Use modified compound supersets. Perform the first exercise, resting for the prescribed rest period, perform the second exercise, rest the prescribed rest period and then go back to the first one. Continue in this manner until you have performed all of the prescribed number of sets. Then continue with the next modified compound superset.

DAY 1 — MONDAY/THURSDAY

		EXERCISE	PAGE NO.	REPS	SETS	REST (seconds)
MODIFIED COMPOUND SUPERSET # 1	back	Dumbbell One-Arm Row (alternate with Two-Arm Row, 164)	162	12-15	3	90
	chest	Incline Dumbbell Press (alternate with palms facing each other grip)	186	12-15	3	90
MODIFIED COMPOUND SUPERSET # 2	back	Dumbbell Pullover (alternate with Seated Low-Pulley Row, 174)	176	12-15	3	90
	chest	Chest Dip (alternate with Push-Up, 198)	194	12-15	3	90
MODIFIED COMPOUND SUPERSET # 3	back	Wide Grip Pull-Up to Front (alternate with Straight Arm Pull-Down, 178)	166	12-15	3	90
	chest	Incline Dumbbell Fly (alternate with Incline Cable Crossover, 196)	192	12-15	3	90
MODIFIED COMPOUND SUPERSET # 4	shoulders	Bent-Over Lateral Raise on Incline Bench (alternate with Seated Rear Delt Machine, 222)	218	12-15	3	90
	calves	Seated Machine Calf Raise (alternate with Donkey Calf Raise, 150)	148	15-25	3	90

DAY 2 — TUESDAY/FRIDAY

		EXERCISE	PAGE NO.	REPS	SETS	REST (seconds)
MODIFIED COMPOUND SUPERSET # 1	biceps	Dumbbell Curl (alternate with Incline Dumbbell Curl, 252)	250	12-15	3	90
	triceps	Lying Dumbbell Extension (alternate with Triceps Pushdown, 242)	230	12-15	3	90
MODIFIED COMPOUND SUPERSET # 2	biceps	Concentration Curl (alternate with Hammer Curl, 262)	258	12-15	3	90
	triceps	Triceps Kickback (alternate with Overhead Dumbbell Extension, 228)	244	12-15	3	90
MODIFIED COMPOUND SUPERSET # 3	biceps	Reverse Curl (alternate with One-Arm Preacher Curl, 254)	264	12-15	3	90
	triceps	Triceps Dip (alternate with Close-Grip Dumbbell Press, 240)	234	12-15	3	90
MODIFIED COMPOUND SUPERSET # 4	shoulders	Dumbbell Shoulder Press (alternate with Military Press, 210)	204	12-15	3	90
	shoulders	Upright Row (alternate with Dumbbell Lateral Raise, 206)	214	12-15	3	90

Weeks 1 & 2

DAY 3			WEDNESDAY/SATURDAY
EXERCISE	**PAGE NO.**	**REPS**	**SETS**	**REST (seconds)**
MODIFIED COMPOUND SUPERSET #1 · thighs · Dumbbell Squat (alternate with Ballet Squat, 114)	112	12-15	3	90
hamstrings · Lying Leg Curl (alternate with Dumbbell Lunge, 122)	134	12-15	3	90
MODIFIED COMPOUND SUPERSET #2 · thighs · Hack Squat (alternate with Leg Extension, 126)	118	12-15	3	90
hamstrings · Stiff-Legged Deadlift (alternate with Seated Leg Curl Machine, 134)	142	12-15	3	90
MODIFIED COMPOUND SUPERSET #3 · thighs · Leg Press (alternate with Dumbbell Squat, 112)	124	12-15	3	90
hamstrings · Standing Hamstring Curl (alternate with Lying Leg Curl, 134)	136	12-15	3	90
MODIFIED COMPOUND SUPERSET #4 · calves · Calf Press (alternate with Multi-Directional Calf Raise, 146)	152	15-25	3	90
calves · Standing Calf Raise (one leg) (alternate with Standing Calf Raise (two legs), 144)	144	15-25	3	90

Cardio and Abs

			ALL DAYS
EXERCISE	**PAGE NO.**	**REPS**	**SETS**	**REST (seconds)**
MODIFIED COMPOUND SUPERSET #1 · abs · Lying Leg Raise	282	15-25	3	90
abs · Crunch	270	15-25	3	90
MODIFIED COMPOUND SUPERSET #2 · abs · Knee-In	280	15-25	3	90
abs · Incline Bench Partial Sit-Up	286	15-25	3	90

CARDIO AND ABS
To be performed from Monday through Saturday first thing in the morning on an empty stomach or right after the workout.

AEROBIC ACTIVITY
20 minutes of fast walking, stationary bike, or any other type of aerobic activity that you like at your target heart rate.

Advanced 14-Day Body Sculpting Workout #1

SPECIAL INSTRUCTIONS FOR WEEKS 3 & 4

Use supersets. Perform supersets by pairing exercises with no rest period in between. Only rest after the two exercises have been performed consecutively. Repeat for the prescribed number of sets and then move on to the next pair of exercises. You will repeat Day 1 on Monday, Day 2 on Wednesday, and Day 3 on Friday.

DAY 1 — MONDAY/THURSDAY

	EXERCISE	PAGE NO.	REPS	SETS	REST (seconds)
SUPERSET #1 — back	Dumbbell One-Arm Row (alternate with Two-Arm Row, 164)	162	10-12	4	No Rest
SUPERSET #1 — chest	Incline Dumbbell Press (alternate with palms facing each other grip)	186	10-12	4	60
SUPERSET #2 — back	Dumbbell Pullover (alternate with Seated Low-Pulley Row, 174)	176	10-12	4	No Rest
SUPERSET #2 — chest	Chest Dip (alternate with Push-Up, 198)	194	10-12	4	60
SUPERSET #3 — back	Wide Grip Pull-Up to Front (alternate with Wide Grip Pull-Down, 170)	166	10-12	3	No Rest
SUPERSET #3 — chest	Incline Dumbbell Fly (alternate with Incline Cable Crossover, 196)	192	10-12	3	60
SUPERSET #4 — shoulders	Bent-Over Lateral Raise on Incline Bench (alternate with Seated Rear Delt Machine, 222)	218	10-12	3	No Rest
SUPERSET #4 — calves	Seated Machine Calf Raise (alternate with Donkey Calf Raise, 150)	148	15-25	3	60

DAY 2 — TUESDAY/FRIDAY

	EXERCISE	PAGE NO.	REPS	SETS	REST (seconds)
SUPERSET #1 — biceps	Dumbbell Curl (alternate with Incline Dumbbell Curl, 252)	250	10-12	4	No Rest
SUPERSET #1 — triceps	Lying Dumbbell Extension (alternate with Triceps Pushdown, 242)	230	10-12	4	60
SUPERSET #2 — biceps	Concentration Curl (alternate with Hammer Curl, 262)	258	10-12	4	No Rest
SUPERSET #2 — triceps	Triceps Kickback (alternate with Overhead Dumbbell Extension, 228)	244	10-12	4	60
SUPERSET #3 — biceps	Reverse Curl (alternate with One-Arm Preacher Curl, 254)	264	10-12	3	No Rest
SUPERSET #3 — triceps	Triceps Dip (alternate with Close-Grip Dumbbell Press, 240)	234	10-12	3	60
SUPERSET #4 — shoulders	Dumbbell Shoulder Press (alternate with Military Press, 210)	204	10-12	3	No Rest
SUPERSET #4 — shoulders	Upright Row (alternate with Dumbbell Lateral Raise, 206)	214	10-12	3	60

Weeks 3 & 4

DAY 3					WEDNESDAY/SATURDAY
EXERCISE		**PAGE NO.**	**REPS**	**SETS**	**REST (seconds)**
SUPERSET # 1	thighs — Dumbbell Squat (alternate with Ballet Squat, 114)	112	10-12	4	No Rest
	hamstrings — Lying Leg Curl (alternate with Dumbbell Lunge, 122)	134	10-12	4	60
SUPERSET # 2	thighs — Hack Squat (alternate with Leg Extension, 126)	118	10-12	4	No Rest
	hamstrings — Stiff-Legged Deadlift (alternate with Seated Leg Curl Machine, 134)	142	10-12	4	60
SUPERSET # 3	thighs — Leg Press (alternate with Dumbbell Squat, 112)	124	10-12	3	No Rest
	hamstrings — Standing Hamstring Curl (alternate with Lying Leg Curl, 134)	136	10-12	3	60
SUPERSET # 4	calves — Calf Press (alternate with Multi-Directional Calf Raise, 146)	152	15-25	3	No Rest
	calves — Standing Calf Raise (one leg) (alternate with Standing Calf Raise (two legs), 144)	144	15-25	3	60

Cardio and Abs

					ALL DAYS
EXERCISE		**PAGE NO.**	**REPS**	**SETS**	**REST (seconds)**
SUPERSET # 1	abs — Lying Leg Raise	282	15-25	3	No Rest
	abs — Crunch	270	15-25	3	60
SUPERSET # 2	abs — Knee-In	280	15-25	3	No Rest
	abs — Incline Bench Partial Sit-Up	286	15-25	3	60

CARDIO AND ABS
To be performed from Monday through Saturday first thing in the morning on an empty stomach or right after the workout.

AEROBIC ACTIVITY
30 minutes of fast walking, stationary bike, or any other type of aerobic activity that you like at your target heart rate.

Advanced 14-Day Body Sculpting Workout #1

SPECIAL INSTRUCTIONS FOR WEEKS 5 & 6
Use giant sets. Perform four exercises with no rest period in between. Only rest after the four exercises have been performed consecutively. Repeat for the prescribed number of sets and then move on to the second group of exercises.

DAY 1 — MONDAY/THURSDAY

	EXERCISE	PAGE NO.	REPS	SETS	REST (seconds)
GIANT SET #1	back — Dumbbell One-Arm Row (alternate with Two-Arm Row, 164)	162	8-10	4	No Rest
	chest — Incline Dumbbell Press (alternate with palms facing each other grip)	186	8-10	4	No Rest
	back — Dumbbell Pullover (alternate with Seated Low-Pulley Row, 174)	176	8-10	4	No Rest
	chest — Chest Dip (alternate with Push-Up, 198)	194	8-10	4	60
GIANT SET #2	back — Wide Grip Pull-Up to Front (alternate with Straight Arm Pull-Down, 178)	166	8-10	4	No Rest
	chest — Incline Dumbbell Fly (alternate with Incline Cable Crossover, 196)	192	8-10	4	No Rest
	shoulders — Bent-Over Lateral Raise on Incline Bench (alternate with Seated Rear Delt Machine, 222)	218	8-10	4	No Rest
	calves — Seated Machine Calf Raise (alternate with Donkey Calf Raise, 150)	148	15-25	4	60

DAY 2 — TUESDAY/FRIDAY

	EXERCISE	PAGE NO.	REPS	SETS	REST (seconds)
GIANT SET #1	biceps — Dumbbell Curl (alternate with Incline Dumbbell Curl, 252)	250	8-10	4	No Rest
	triceps — Lying Dumbbell Extension (alternate with Triceps Pushdown, 242)	230	8-10	4	No Rest
	biceps — Concentration Curl (alternate with Hammer Curl, 262)	258	8-10	4	No Rest
	triceps — Triceps Kickback (alternate with Overhead Dumbbell Extension, 228)	244	8-10	4	60
GIANT SET #2	biceps — Reverse Curl (alternate with One-Arm Preacher Curl, 254)	264	8-10	4	No Rest
	triceps — Triceps Dip (alternate with Close-Grip Dumbbell Press, 240)	234	8-10	4	No Rest
	shoulders — Dumbbell Shoulder Press (alternate with Military Press, 210)	204	8-10	4	No Rest
	shoulders — Upright Row (alternate with Dumbbell Lateral Raise, 206)	214	8-10	4	60

Weeks 5 & 6

DAY 3				WEDNESDAY/SATURDAY
EXERCISE	**PAGE NO.**	**REPS**	**SETS**	**REST (seconds)**
GIANT SET #1 — thighs — Dumbbell Squat (alternate with Ballet Squat, 114)	112	8-10	4	No Rest
hamstrings — Lying Leg Curl (alternate with Dumbbell Lunge, 122)	134	8-10	4	No Rest
thighs — Hack Squat (alternate with Leg Extension, 126)	118	8-10	4	No Rest
hamstrings — Stiff-Legged Deadlift (alternate with Seated Leg Curl Machine, 134)	142	8-10	4	60
GIANT SET #2 — thighs — Leg Press (alternate with Dumbbell Squat, 112)	124	8-10	4	No Rest
hamstrings — Standing Hamstring Curl (alternate with Lying Leg Curl, 134)	136	8-10	4	No Rest
calves — Calf Press (alternate with Multi-Directional Calf Raise, 146)	152	8-10	4	No Rest
calves — Standing Calf Raise (one leg) (alternate with two legs, 144)	144	8-10	4	60

Cardio and Abs

				ALL DAYS
EXERCISE	**PAGE NO.**	**REPS**	**SETS**	**REST (seconds)**
GIANT SET #1 — abs — Lying Leg Raise	282	15-25	4	No Rest
abs — Crunch	270	15-25	4	No Rest
abs — Knee-In	280	15-25	4	No Rest
abs — Incline Bench Partial Sit-Up	286	15-25	4	60

CARDIO AND ABS

To be performed from Monday through Saturday first thing in the morning on an empty stomach or right after the workout.

AEROBIC ACTIVITY

40 minutes of fast walking, stationary bike, or any other type of aerobic activity that you like at your target heart rate.

Advanced 14-Day Body Sculpting Workout #2

SPECIAL INSTRUCTIONS FOR WEEKS 1 & 2

Use modified compound supersets. Perform modified compound supersets by performing the first exercise, resting for the prescribed rest period, performing the second exercise, resting the prescribed rest period and going back to the first one. Continue in this manner until you have performed all of the prescribed number of sets.

DAY 1 — MONDAY/THURSDAY

EXERCISE	PAGE NO.	REPS	SETS	REST (seconds)
Two-Arm Row (alternate with Dumbbell One-Arm Row, 162)	164	12-15	3	90
Incline Dumbbell Press (alternate with Incline Barbell Press, 186)	186	12-15	3	90
Dumbbell Pullover (alternate with Neutral Grip Pull-Up, 168)	176	12-15	3	90
Chest Dip (alternate with Flat Dumbbell Press, 188)	194	12-15	3	90
Wide Grip Pull-Down (alternate with Close-Grip Pull-Down, 172)	170	12-15	3	90
Incline Dumbbell Fly (alternate with Incline Cable Crossover, 196)	192	12-15	3	90
Seated Rear Delt Machine (alternate with Bent-Arm Bent-Over Row, 216)	222	12-15	3	90
Seated Machine Calf Raise (alternate with Tibia Raise, 154)	148	15-25	3	90

Modified Compound Superset #1: back, chest; Superset #2: back, chest; Superset #3: back, chest; Superset #4: shoulders, calves

DAY 2 — TUESDAY/FRIDAY

EXERCISE	PAGE NO.	REPS	SETS	REST (seconds)
High Cable Curl (alternate with Concentration Curl, 258)	266	12-15	3	90
Triceps Pushdown (with rope) (alternate with Fixed Bar Bodyweight Triceps Extension, 246)	242	12-15	3	90
Hammer Curl (alternate with E-Z Reverse Preacher Curl, 256)	262	12-15	3	90
E-Z Curl Bar Close-Grip Press (alternate with Overhead Triceps Extension, 228)	238	12-15	3	90
E-Z Preacher Curl (alternate with One-Arm Preacher Curl, 254)	256	12-15	3	90
Bench Dip (alternate with Close-Grip Dumbbell Press, 240)	236	12-15	3	90
Seated Bent-Over Lateral Raise (alternate with Two-Arm Cable Lateral Raise, 220)	208	12-15	3	90
Front Raise (alternate with Dumbbell Shoulder Press, 204)	212	12-15	3	90

Modified Compound Superset #1: biceps, triceps; Superset #2: biceps, triceps; Superset #3: biceps, triceps; Superset #4: shoulders, shoulders

Weeks 1 & 2

DAY 3					WEDNESDAY/SATURDAY
EXERCISE		**PAGE NO.**	**REPS**	**SETS**	**REST** (seconds)
MODIFIED COMPOUND SUPERSET # 1	thighs: Hack Squat (alternate with Leg Extension, 126)	118	12-15	3	90
	hamstrings: Stiff-Legged Deadlift (alternate with Dumbbell Lunge, 122)	142	12-15	3	90
MODIFIED COMPOUND SUPERSET # 2	thighs: Front Squat (alternate with Ballet Squat, 114)	120	12-15	3	90
	hamstrings: Lying Leg Curl (alternate with Seated Leg Curl Machine, 134)	134	12-15	3	90
MODIFIED COMPOUND SUPERSET # 3	thighs: Leg Press (alternate with Barbell Squat, 110)	124	12-15	3	90
	hamstrings: Standing Hamstring Curl (alternate with Step-Up, 138)	136	12-15	3	90
MODIFIED COMPOUND SUPERSET # 4	calves: Calf Press (alternate with Standing Calf Raise (two legs), 144)	152	15-25	3	90
	calves: Standing Calf Raise (one leg) (alternate with Seated Machine Calf Raise, 144)	144	15-25	3	90

Cardio and Abs

					ALL DAYS
EXERCISE		**PAGE NO.**	**REPS**	**SETS**	**REST** (seconds)
MODIFIED COMPOUND SUPERSET # 1	abs: Lying Leg Raise	282	15-25	3	90
	abs: Trunk Curl and Crunch	272	15-25	3	90
MODIFIED COMPOUND SUPERSET # 2	abs: Knee-In	280	15-25	3	90
	abs: Incline Board Partial Sit-Up	286	15-25	3	90

CARDIO AND ABS

To be performed from Monday through Saturday first thing in the morning on an empty stomach or right after the workout.

AEROBIC ACTIVITY

20 minutes of fast walking, stationary bike, or any other type of aerobic activity that you like at your target heart rate.

Advanced 14-Day Body Sculpting Workout #2

DAY 1 — MONDAY/THURSDAY

	EXERCISE	PAGE NO.	REPS	SETS	REST (seconds)
SUPERSET #1	back — Wide Grip Pull-Up to Front (alternate with Close-Grip Pull-Down, 170)	178	10-12	4	No Rest
	chest — Incline Dumbbell Fly (alternate with Incline Cable Crossover, 196)	192	10-12	4	60
SUPERSET #2	back — Close-Grip Pull-Down (alternate with Wide Grip Pull-Down, 170)	170	10-12	4	No Rest
	chest — Incline Dumbbell Press (alternate with Chest Dip, 194)	186	10-12	4	60
SUPERSET #3	back — Seated Low-Pulley Row (alternate with Two-Arm Row, 164)	174	10-12	3	No Rest
	chest — Flat Barbell Press (alternate with Incline Barbell Press, 186)	188	10-12	3	60
SUPERSET #4	shoulders — Seated Rear Delt Machine (alternate with Seated Bent-Over Lateral Raise, 208)	222	10-12	3	No Rest
	calves — Tibia Raise (alternate with Donkey Calf Raise, 150)	154	15-25	3	60

DAY 2 — TUESDAY/FRIDAY

	EXERCISE	PAGE NO.	REPS	SETS	REST (seconds)
SUPERSET #1	biceps — Dumbbell Curl (alternate with Reverse Curl, 264)	250	10-12	4	No Rest
	triceps — Overhead Dumbbell Extension (alternate with Triceps Kickback, 244)	228	10-12	4	60
SUPERSET #2	biceps — E-Z Reverse Preacher Curl (alternate with Hammer Curl, 262)	256	10-12	4	No Rest
	triceps — Fixed Bar Bodyweight Triceps Extension (alternate with Lying E-Z Bar Extension, 232)	246	10-12	4	60
SUPERSET #3	biceps — Reverse Curl (alternate with E-Z Preacher Curl, 256)	264	10-12	3	No Rest
	triceps — Bench Dip (alternate with Close-Grip Dumbbell Press, 240)	236	10-12	3	60
SUPERSET #4	shoulders — Upright Row (alternate with Seated Bent-Over Lateral Raise, 208)	214	10-12	3	No Rest
	shoulders — Rotator Cuff (alternate with Military Press, 210)	224	10-12	3	60

Weeks 3 & 4

DAY 3			WEDNESDAY/SATURDAY		
EXERCISE	PAGE NO.	REPS	SETS	REST (seconds)	
SUPERSET #1	thighs	Dumbbell Squat (alternate with Ballet Squat, 114)	112	10-12	4	No Rest
	hamstrings	Lying Leg Curl (alternate with Leg Press, 124)	134	10-12	4	60
SUPERSET #2	thighs	Hack Squat (alternate with Leg Extension, 126)	118	10-12	4	No Rest
	hamstrings	Stiff-Legged Deadlift (alternate with Seated Leg Curl Machine, 134)	142	10-12	4	60
SUPERSET #3	thighs	Leg Press (alternate with Dumbbell Squat, 112)	124	10-12	3	No Rest
	hamstrings	Standing Hamstring Curl (alternate with Lying Leg Curl, 134)	136	10-12	3	60
SUPERSET #4	calves	Calf Press (alternate with Standing Machine Calf Raise, 148)	152	15-25	3	No Rest
	calves	Standing Calf Raise (one leg) (alternate with two legs, 144)	144	15-25	3	60

Cardio and Abs

EXERCISE			PAGE NO.	REPS	SETS	ALL DAYS REST (seconds)
SUPERSET #1	abs	V-Up	278	15-25	4	No Rest
	abs	Crunch	270	15-25	4	60
SUPERSET #2	abs	Reverse Crunch with Ball	284	15-25	3	No Rest
	abs	Bicycle Crunch	276	15-25	3	60

CARDIO AND ABS

To be performed from Monday through Saturday first thing in the morning on an empty stomach or right after the workout.

AEROBIC ACTIVITY

30 minutes of fast walking, stationary bike, or any other type of aerobic activity that you like at the target heart rate.

Advanced 14-Day Body Sculpting Workout #2

SPECIAL INSTRUCTIONS FOR WEEKS 5 & 6
Use giant sets. Perform giant sets by performing four exercises with no rest period in between. Only rest after the four exercises have been performed consecutively. Repeat for the prescribed number of sets and then move on to the second group of exercises.

DAY 1 — MONDAY/THURSDAY

		EXERCISE	PAGE NO.	REPS	SETS	REST (seconds)
GIANT SET # 1	back	Wide Grip Pull-Up to Front (alternate with Close-Grip Pull-Down, 170)	178	8-10	4	No Rest
	chest	Flat Dumbbell Press (alternate with Incline Dumbbell Press, 186)	188	8-10	4	No Rest
	back	Dumbbell One-Arm Row (alternate with Bent-Over Barbell Row, 160)	162	8-10	4	No Rest
	chest	Push-Up (alternate with Chest Dip, 194)	198	8-10	4	60
GIANT SET # 2	back	Wide Grip Pull-Down (alternate with Straight Arm Pull-Down, 178)	170	8-10	4	No Rest
	chest	Incline Cable Crossover (alternate with Incline Dumbbell Fly, 192)	196	8-10	4	No Rest
	shoulders	Bent-Arm Bent-Over Row (alternate with Seated Rear Delt Machine, 222)	216	8-10	4	No Rest
	calves	Calf Press (alternate with Tibia Raise, 154)	152	15-25	4	60

DAY 2 — TUESDAY/FRIDAY

		EXERCISE	PAGE NO.	REPS	SETS	REST (seconds)
GIANT SET # 1	biceps	E-Z Reverse Preacher Curl (alternate with High Cable Curl, 266)	256	8-10	4	No Rest
	triceps	Triceps Dip (alternate with E-Z Curl Bar Close-Grip Press, 238)	234	8-10	4	No Rest
	biceps	High Cable Curl (alternate with Incline Dumbbell Curl, 252)	266	8-10	4	No Rest
	triceps	Close-Grip Dumbbell Press (alternate with Overhead Dumbbell Extension, 228)	240	8-10	4	60
GIANT SET # 2	biceps	Reverse Curl (alternate with Incline Hammer Curl, 262)	264	8-10	4	No Rest
	triceps	Triceps Pushdown (with rope) (alternate with Triceps Pushdown(with bar))	242	8-10	4	No Rest
	shoulders	Seated Bent-Over Lateral Raise (alternate with Upright Row, 214)	208	8-10	4	No Rest
	shoulders	Dumbbell Shoulder Press (alternate with Military Press, 210)	204	8-10	4	60

Weeks 5 & 6

DAY 3				WEDNESDAY/SATURDAY
EXERCISE	PAGE NO.	REPS	SETS	REST (seconds)
GIANT SET # 1 Dumbbell Squat (alternate with Ballet Squat, 114)	112	8-10	4	No Rest
Lying Leg Curl (alternate with Dumbbell Lunge, 122)	134	8-10	4	No Rest
Leg Press (alternate with Leg Extension, 126)	124	8-10	4	No Rest
Standing Hamstring Curl (alternate with Glute-Ham Raise, 140)	136	8-10	4	60
GIANT SET # 2 Leg Press (alternate with Hack Squat, 126)	124	8-10	4	No Rest
Barbell Stiff-Legged Deadlift (alternate with Seated Leg Curl Machine, 134)	142	8-10	4	No Rest
Calf Press (alternate with Multi-Directional Calf Raise, 146)	152	15-25	4	No Rest
Standing Calf Raise (one leg) (alternate with two legs, 144)	144	15-25	4	60

Cardio and Inner/Outer Thighs, and Abs

				ALL DAYS
EXERCISE	PAGE NO.	REPS	SETS	REST (seconds)
GIANT SET # 1 Hanging Leg Raise	282	15-25	4	No Rest
Crunch on the Ball	270	15-25	4	No Rest
Crunch/Pelvic Lift Combination	284	15-25	4	No Rest
Ab Bench Crunch	288	15-25	4	60

CARDIO AND ABS

To be performed from Monday through Saturday first thing in the morning on an empty stomach or right after the workout.

AEROBIC ACTIVITY

40 minutes of fast walking, stationary bike, or any other type of aerobic activity that you like at your target heart rate.

WHAT TO DO AFTER WEEK SIX OF THE ADVANCED WORKOUT?

After week six, you can start over at week one but substitute the recommended exercises with similar ones. Don't be afraid to experiment! If you are satisfied with your lower body and want to equally emphasize the upper body, then you can adjust the routine to perform chest/back on Monday/Thursday, Shoulders and Arms on Tuesday/Friday, and Legs on Wednesday and Saturday.

Also, if you want to gain additional muscle mass, then feel free to reduce the amount of repetitions in the following manner:

Weeks 1-2: 10-12 reps
Weeks 3-4: 8-10 reps
Weeks 5-6: 6-8 reps

Also, reduce the cardiovascular/abs component of the workout to three days a week instead of six. All other aspects of the program remain the same.

14-Day Body Sculpting Definition Workout

SPECIAL INSTRUCTIONS FOR WEEKS 1 & 2

Use modified compound supersets. Perform these sets by completing the first set of the first exercise, resting for the pre-scribed rest period, performing the first set of the second exercise, resting the prescribed rest period, and then doing the second set of the first exercise. Continue in this manner until you have completed all of the prescribed number of sets for each exercise. Then move on to the next modified compound superset.

DAY 1 — MONDAY/THURSDAY

	EXERCISE	PAGE NO.	REPS	SETS	REST (seconds)
MODIFIED COMPOUND SUPERSET # 1 · back	Dumbbell One-Arm Row	162	10-12	3	90
MODIFIED COMPOUND SUPERSET # 1 · chest	Incline Dumbbell Press	186	10-12	3	90
MODIFIED COMPOUND SUPERSET # 2 · back	Wide Grip Pull-Up to Front	178	10-12	2	90
MODIFIED COMPOUND SUPERSET # 2 · chest	Chest Dip	194	10-12	2	90
MODIFIED COMPOUND SUPERSET # 3 · biceps	Standing E-Z Bar Curl	260	10-12	3	90
MODIFIED COMPOUND SUPERSET # 3 · triceps	Lying E-Z Bar Extension	232	10-12	3	90
MODIFIED COMPOUND SUPERSET # 4 · biceps	Hammer Curl	262	10-12	2	90
MODIFIED COMPOUND SUPERSET # 4 · triceps	Overhead Dumbbell Extension	228	10-12	2	90

DAY 2 — TUESDAY/FRIDAY

	EXERCISE	PAGE NO.	REPS	SETS	REST (seconds)
MODIFIED COMPOUND SUPERSET # 1 · thighs	Dumbbell Squat	112	10-12	3	90
MODIFIED COMPOUND SUPERSET # 1 · hamstrings	Seated Leg Curl Machine	134	10-12	3	90
MODIFIED COMPOUND SUPERSET # 2 · thighs	Dumbbell Lunge	122	10-12	2	90
MODIFIED COMPOUND SUPERSET # 2 · hamstrings	Stiff-Legged Deadlift	142	10-12	2	90
MODIFIED COMPOUND SUPERSET # 3 · calves	Standing Calf Raise (one leg)	144	12-15	3	90
MODIFIED COMPOUND SUPERSET # 3 · shoulders	Dumbbell Shoulder Press	204	10-12	3	90
MODIFIED COMPOUND SUPERSET # 4 · calves	Standing Calf Raise (two legs)	144	12-15	2	90
MODIFIED COMPOUND SUPERSET # 4 · triceps	Bent-Over Lateral Raise on Incline Bench	218	10-12	2	90

Weeks 1 & 2

Cardio and Abs

DAY 3					
EXERCISE		PAGE NO.	REPS	SETS	REST (seconds)
MODIFIED COMPOUND SUPERSET # 1	abs Lying Leg Raise	282	10-12	3	90
	abs Crunch	270	10-12	2	90

AEROBIC ACTIVITY
20 minutes of fast walking, stationary bike, or any other type of aerobic activity that you prefer at the target heart rate.

14-Day Body Sculpting Definition Workout

SPECIAL INSTRUCTIONS FOR WEEKS 3 & 4

Use supersets. Perform these sets by pairing exercises with no rest period in between. Rest only after the two exercises have been performed consecutively. Repeat this routine for the prescribed number of sets before moving on to the next pair of exercises.

DAY 1 — MONDAY/THURSDAY

		EXERCISE	PAGE NO.	REPS	SETS	REST (seconds)
SUPERSET # 1	back	Close-Grip Pull-Down	172	8-10	4	No Rest
	chest	Flat Dumbbell Press	188	8-10	4	60
SUPERSET # 2	back	Bent-Arm Bent-Over Row	216	8-10	3	No Rest
	chest	Incline Dumbbell Press	186	8-10	3	60
SUPERSET # 3	biceps	Incline Dumbbell Curl	252	8-10	4	No Rest
	triceps	Close-Grip Dumbbell Press	240	8-10	4	60
SUPERSET # 4	biceps	Reverse Curl	262	8-10	3	No Rest
	triceps	Triceps Pushdown	242	8-10	3	60

DAY 2 — TUESDAY/FRIDAY

		EXERCISE	PAGE NO.	REPS	SETS	REST (seconds)
SUPERSET # 1	thighs	Barbell Squat	110	8-10	4	No Rest
	hamstrings	Lying Leg Curl	134	8-10	4	60
SUPERSET # 2	thighs	Leg Extension	126	8-10	3	No Rest
	hamstrings	Leg Press	124	8-10	3	60
SUPERSET # 3	calves	Standing Machine Calf Raise	148	12-15	4	No Rest
	shoulders	Upright Row	214	8-10	4	60
SUPERSET # 4	calves	Seated Machine Calf Raise	148	12-15	3	No Rest
	shoulders	Bent-Over Lateral Raise on Incline Bench	218	8-10	3	60

Weeks 3 & 4

Cardio and Abs

DAY 3					WEDNESDAY/SATURDAY
EXERCISE		PAGE NO.	REPS	SETS	REST (seconds)
SUPERSET # 1	abs Lying Leg Raise	282	10-12	4	No Rest
	abs Crunch	270	10-12	3	60

AEROBIC ACTIVITY
25 minutes of fast walking, stationary bike, or any other type of aerobic activity that you prefer at your target heart rate.

14-Day Body Sculpting Definition Workout

> **SPECIAL INSTRUCTIONS FOR WEEKS 5 & 6**
>
> Use giant sets. Perform these sets by doing four exercises with no rest periods in between. Rest only after the four exercises have been performed consecutively. Repeat for the prescribed number of sets before moving on to the next group of exercises.

DAY 1 — MONDAY/THURSDAY

	EXERCISE	PAGE NO.	REPS	SETS	REST (seconds)
GIANT SET #1	back — Close-Grip Pull-Down	172	6-8	4	No Rest
	chest — Incline Dumbbell Press	186	6-8	4	No Rest
	back — Dumbbell One-Arm Row	162	6-8	4	No Rest
	chest — Flat Dumbbell Press	188	6-8	4	60
GIANT SET #2	triceps — One-Arm Preacher Curl	254	8-10	4	No Rest
	triceps — Triceps Dip	234	8-10	4	No Rest
	biceps — Reverse Curl	264	8-10	4	No Rest
	triceps — E-Z Curl Bar Close-Grip Press	238	8-10	4	60

DAY 2 — TUESDAY/FRIDAY

	EXERCISE	PAGE NO.	REPS	SETS	REST (seconds)
GIANT SET #1	thighs — Barbell Squat	110	6-8	4	No Rest
	hamstrings — Barbell Lunge	122	6-8	4	No Rest
	thighs — Ballet Squat	114	6-8	4	No Rest
	hamstrings — Barbell Stiff-Legged Deadlift	142	6-8	4	60
GIANT SET #2	calves — Calf Press	152	6-8	4	No Rest
	shoulders — Military Press	210	6-8	4	No Rest
	calves — Donkey Calf Raise	150	6-8	4	No Rest
	shoulders — Seated Rear Delt Machine	222	6-8	4	60

Cardio and Abs

DAY 3					WEDNESDAY/SATURDAY
EXERCISE		**PAGE NO.**	**REPS**	**SETS**	**REST (seconds)**
GIANT SET # 1 — abs	Lying Leg Raise	282	10-12	4	No Rest
— abs	Crunch	270	10-12	4	No Rest

AEROBIC ACTIVITY

30 minutes of fast walking, stationary bike, or any other type of aerobic activity that you prefer at your target heart rate.

NOTES ON REPETITIONS

Continue until you complete all four sets of each exercise. Don't worry if the first few times that you perform this abdominal workout you are not able to perform all of the recommended reps. As you get used to this rigorous workout, your body will adapt and become stronger.

14-Day Bodyweight Body Sculpting Workout

SPECIAL INSTRUCTIONS FOR WEEKS 1 & 2

Use modified compound supersets. Perform modified compound supersets by performing the first exercise, resting for the prescribed rest period, performing the second exercise, resting the prescribed rest period, and going back to the first exercise. Continue in this manner until you have performed all of the prescribed number of sets. Then continue with the next modified compound superset. You will repeat Day 1 on Monday, Day 2 on Wednesday, and Day 3 on Friday. You will then perform Cardio on Tuesday, Thursday, and Saturday.

DAY 1 — MONDAY

	EXERCISE	PAGE NO.	REPS	SETS	REST (seconds)
MODIFIED COMPOUND SUPERSET # 1 — back	Close-Grip Pull-Up	168	As many as possible	2	60
MODIFIED COMPOUND SUPERSET # 1 — chest	Push-Up (feet on floor)	198	As many as possible	2	60
MODIFIED COMPOUND SUPERSET # 2 — abs	Bicycle Crunch	276	As many as possible	2	60
MODIFIED COMPOUND SUPERSET # 2 — calves	Standing Calf Raise (one leg)	144	As many as possible	2	60
MODIFIED COMPOUND SUPERSET # 3 — biceps	Close-Grip Pull-Up (emphasize biceps)	168	As many as possible	2	60
MODIFIED COMPOUND SUPERSET # 3 — triceps	Bench Dip	236	As many as possible	2	60
MODIFIED COMPOUND SUPERSET # 4 — thighs	Dumbbell Lunge (bodyweight only; one leg at a time; press with toes)	122	As many as possible	2	60
MODIFIED COMPOUND SUPERSET # 4 — hamstrings	Dumbbell Lunge (bodyweight only; press with heels; alternate with legs in a walking motion)	122	As many as possible	2	60

DAY 2 — WEDNESDAY

	EXERCISE	PAGE NO.	REPS	SETS	REST (seconds)
MODIFIED COMPOUND SUPERSET # 1 — thighs	Dumbbell Lunge (bodyweight only; one leg at a time; press with toes)	122	As many as possible	2	60
MODIFIED COMPOUND SUPERSET # 1 — hamstrings	Dumbbell Lunge (bodyweight only; press with heels; alternate with legs in a walking motion)	122	As many as possible	2	60
MODIFIED COMPOUND SUPERSET # 2 — thighs	Sissy Squat	116	As many as possible	2	60
MODIFIED COMPOUND SUPERSET # 2 — hamstrings	Dumbbell Lunge (bodyweight only; press with heels; alternate with legs in a walking motion)	122	As many as possible	2	60
MODIFIED COMPOUND SUPERSET # 3 — calves	Standing Calf Raise (one leg)	144	As many as possible	2	60
MODIFIED COMPOUND SUPERSET # 3 — calves	Standing Calf Raise (two legs)	144	As many as possible	2	60
MODIFIED COMPOUND SUPERSET # 4 — abs	Lying Leg Raise	282	As many as possible	2	60
MODIFIED COMPOUND SUPERSET # 4 — abs	Crunch	270	As many as possible	2	60

Weeks 1 & 2

DAY 3				FRIDAY
EXERCISE	**PAGE NO.**	**REPS**	**SETS**	**REST (seconds)**
MODIFIED COMPOUND SUPERSET # 1 — back — Wide-Grip Pull-Up to Front	178	As many as possible	2	60
chest — Push-Up (feet on raised surface)	198	As many as possible	2	60
MODIFIED COMPOUND SUPERSET # 2 — abs — V-Up	278	As many as possible	2	60
calves — Standing Raise (two legs)	144	As many as possible	2	60
MODIFIED COMPOUND SUPERSET # 3 — biceps — Neutral Grip Chin-Up (emphasize biceps)	168	As many as possible	2	60
triceps — Push-Up (narrow hand-width)	198	As many as possible	2	60
MODIFIED COMPOUND SUPERSET # 4 — thighs — Ballet Squat (bodyweight only; press with ball of foot)	114	As many as possible	2	60
hamstrings — Dumbbell Lunge (bodyweight only; press with heels; alternate with legs in a walking motion)	122	As many as possible	2	60

	TUESDAY/THURSDAY/SATURDAY
AEROBIC ACTIVITY	
25 minutes of fast walking, stationary biking, or any other type of aerobic activity that you enjoy while bringing you to your target heart rate.	

14-Day Bodyweight Body Sculpting Workout

DAY 1 — MONDAY

	EXERCISE	PAGE NO.	REPS	SETS	REST (seconds)
SUPERSET #1	back — Close-Grip Pull-Up	168	As many as possible	3	No Rest
	chest — Push-Up (feet on floor)	198	As many as possible	3	60
SUPERSET #2	shoulders — Bicycle Crunch	276	As many as possible	3	No Rest
	abs — Standing Calf Raise (one leg)	144	As many as possible	3	6
SUPERSET #3	calves — Close-Grip Pull-Up (emphasize biceps)	168	As many as possible	3	No Rest
	biceps — Bench Dip	236	As many as possible	3	60
SUPERSET #4	thighs — Dumbbell Lunge (bodyweight only; one leg at a time; press with toes)	122	As many as possible	3	No Rest
	hamstrings — Dumbbell Lunge (bodyweight only; press with heels; alternate with legs in a walking motion)	122	As many as possible	3	60

DAY 2 — WEDNESDAY

	EXERCISE	PAGE NO.	REPS	SETS	REST (seconds)
SUPERSET #1	thighs — Dumbbell Lunge (bodyweight only; one leg at a time; press with toes)	122	As many as possible	3	No Rest
	hamstrings — Dumbbell Lunge (bodyweight only; press with heels; alternate with legs in a walking motion)	122	As many as possible	3	60
SUPERSET #2	thighs — Sissy Squat	116	As many as possible	3	No Rest
	hamstrings — Dumbbell Lunge (bodyweight only; press with heels; alternate with legs in a walking motion)	122	As many as possible	3	60
SUPERSET #3	calves — Standing Calf Raise (one leg)	144	As many as possible	3	No Rest
	calves — Standing Calf Raise (two legs)	144	As many as possible	3	6
SUPERSET #4	abs — Lying Leg Raise	282	As many as possible	3	No Rest
	abs — Crunch	270	As many as possible	3	60

Weeks 3 & 4

DAY 1					FRIDAY
EXERCISE		**PAGE NO.**	**REPS**	**SETS**	**REST (seconds)**
SUPERSET #1 · back	Wide-Grip Pull-Up to Front	178	As many as possible	3	No Rest
SUPERSET #1 · chest	Push-Up (feet on raised surface)	198	As many as possible	3	60
SUPERSET #2 · abs	V-Up	278	As many as possible	3	No Rest
SUPERSET #2 · calves	Standing Calf Raise (two legs)	144	As many as possible	3	60
SUPERSET #3 · biceps	Neutral Grip Chin-Up (emphasize biceps)	168	As many as possible	3	No Rest
SUPERSET #3 · triceps	Push-Up (narrow hand-width)	198	As many as possible	3	60
SUPERSET #4 · thighs	Ballet Squat (bodyweight only; press with ball of foot)	114	As many as possible	3	No Rest
SUPERSET #4 · hamstrings	Dumbbell Lunge (bodyweight only; press with heels; alternate with legs in a walking motion)	122	As many as possible	3	60

	TUESDAY/THURSDAY/SATURDAY
AEROBIC ACTIVITY	
30 minutes of fast walking, stationary biking, or any other type of aerobic activity that you enjoy while bringing you to your target heart rate.	

14-Day Bodyweight Body Sculpting Workout

SPECIAL INSTRUCTIONS FOR WEEKS 5 & 6

Use giant sets. Perform giant sets by performing four exercises with no rest in between. Only rest after the four exercises have been performed consecutively. Repeat for the prescribed number of sets and then move on to the second group of exercises. You will repeat Day 1 on Monday, Day 2 on Wednesday, and Day 3 on Friday. You will then perform Cardio on Tuesday, Thursday, and Saturday.

DAY 1 — MONDAY

	EXERCISE	PAGE NO.	REPS	SETS	REST (seconds)
GIANT SET #1	back Close-Grip Pull-Up	168	As many as possible	4	No Rest
	chest Push-Up (feet on floor)	198	As many as possible	4	No Rest
	abs Bicycle Crunch	276	As many as possible	4	No Rest
	calves Standing Calf Raise (one leg)		As many as possible	4	60
GIANT SET #2	biceps Close-Grip Pull-Up (emphasize biceps)	168	As many as possible	4	No Rest
	triceps Bench Dip	236	As many as possible	4	No Rest
	thighs Dumbbell Lunge (bodyweight only; one leg at a time; press with toes)	122	As many as possible	4	No Rest
	hamstrings Dumbbell Lunge (bodyweight only; press with heels; alternate with legs in a walking motion)	122	As many as possible	4	60

DAY 2 — WEDNESDAY

	EXERCISE	PAGE NO.	REPS	SETS	REST (seconds)
GIANT SET #1	thighs Dumbbell Lunge (bodyweight only; one leg at a time; press with toes)	122	As many as possible	4	No Rest
	hamstrings Dumbbell Lunge (bodyweight only; press with heels; alternate with legs in a walking motion)	122	As many as possible	4	No Rest
	thighs Sissy Squat	116	As many as possible	4	No Rest
	hamstrings Dumbbell Lunge (bodyweight only; press with heels; alternate with legs in a walking motion)	122	As many as possible	4	60
GIANT SET #2	calves Standing Calf Raise (one leg)	144	As many as possible	4	No Rest
	calves Standing Calf Raise (two legs)	144	As many as possible	4	No Rest
	abs Lying Leg Raise	282	As many as possible	4	No Rest
	abs Crunch	270	As many as possible	4	60

DAY 3

	EXERCISE	PAGE NO.	REPS	SETS	REST (seconds)
GIANT SET #1	back — Wide-Grip Pull-Up to Front	178	As many as possible	4	No Rest
	chest — Push-Up (feet on raised surface)	198	As many as possible	4	No Rest
	abs — V-Up	278	As many as possible	4	No Rest
	calves — Standing Calf Raise (two legs)	144	As many as possible	4	60
GIANT SET #2	biceps — Neutral Grip Chin-Up (emphasize biceps)	168	As many as possible	4	No Rest
	triceps — Push-Up (narrow hand-width)	198	As many as possible	4	No Rest
	thighs — Ballet Squat (bodyweight only; press with ball of foot)	114	As many as possible	4	No Rest
	hamstrings — Dumbbell Lunge (bodyweight only; press with heels; alternate with legs in a walking motion)	122	As many as possible	4	60

TUESDAY/THURSDAY/SATURDAY

AEROBIC ACTIVITY

40 minutes of fast walking, stationary biking, or any other type of aerobic activity that you enjoy while bringing you to your target heart rate.

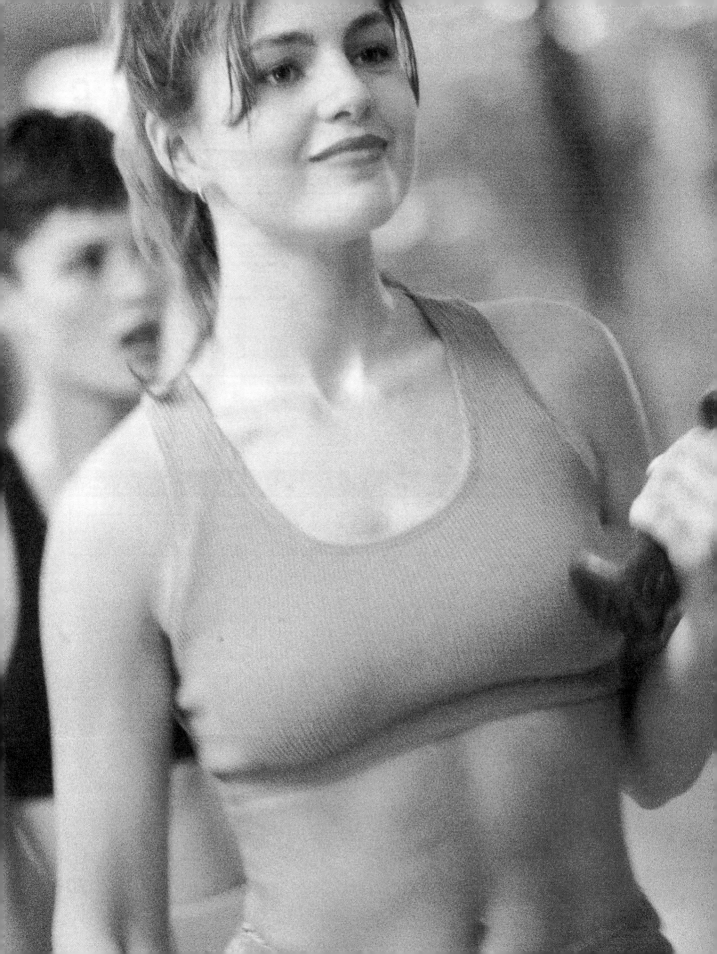

THE EXPRESS WORKOUTS: FOR THOSE ON THE GO!

The Body Sculpting Bible *EXPRESS* program offers three workouts. One is the all-dumbbell workout that can be performed either in the comfort of your home, or at a gym, with an adjustable bench and a set of dumbbells. The second workout is one that makes use of selectorized weight machine equipment (or weight stack machines). This is a good workout to use while on vacation at a hotel gym that does not offer dumbbells. The third is an overall body workout using the combination exercises.

These workouts are designed to be done three days each week within a 21-minute limit. They are fast-paced, providing good cardiovascular conditioning as well as toning and strengthening. On the days off you can perform some abdominal work in the comfort of your home along with some optional cardiovascular exercise.

For the fastest results, you are encouraged to use the dumbbell workout in addition to adding the optional cardiovascular exercise component on your days off.

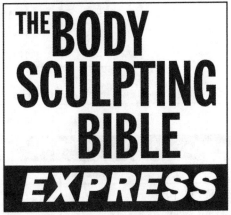

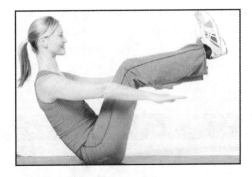

MONDAY	TUESDAY	WEDNESDAY	THURSDAY	FRIDAY	SATURDAY	SUNDAY
Day 1	Abs/Cardio	Day 2	Abs/Cardio	Day 3	Abs/Cardio	Off
Day 1	Abs/Cardio	Day 2	Abs/Cardio	Day 3	Abs/Cardio	Off

Three days a week weight training with three different routines each week.
Three days of abdominals with optional cardiovascular exercise.

Workout #1: Dumbbell Only

SPECIAL INSTRUCTIONS: Use Modified Compound Supersets. Perform Modified Compound Supersets by doing the exercises and resting the prescribed amount of time until you have completed a circuit. Then start at the beginning and repeat for the recommended number of times before moving on to the next modified compound superset.

ABS AND CARDIO				
EXERCISE	**PAGE NO.**	**REPS**	**SETS**	**REST**
MODIFIED COMPOUND SUPERSET # 1				
Lower Abs: Lying Leg Raises	282	12-15	2	30 seconds
Upper Abs: Crunches	270	12-15	2	30 seconds
Obliques: Bicycle	276	12-15	2	30 seconds
Aerobic Activity				
15 minutes of fast paced walking, stationary bike, or any other type of aerobic activity that you like.				

DAY 1				
EXERCISE	**PAGE NO.**	**REPS**	**SETS**	**REST**
MODIFIED COMPOUND SUPERSET # 1				
Back: One-Arm Rows (Palms facing Torso)	162	12-15	2	30 seconds
Chest: Incline Dumbbell Bench Press	186	12-15	2	30 seconds
Thighs: Dumbbell Squats	112	12-15	2	30 seconds
Hamstrings: Dumbbell Stiff-Legged Deadlifts	142	12-15	2	30 seconds
MODIFIED COMPOUND SUPERSET # 2				
Biceps: Dumbbell Curls	250	12-15	2	30 seconds
Triceps: Lying Dumbbell Triceps Extensions	230	12-15	2	30 seconds
Shoulders: Dumbbell Upright Rows	214	12-15	2	30 seconds
Calves: Two-Legged Dumbbell Calf Raises	144	12-15	2	30 seconds

Weeks 1 & 2

DAY 2				
EXERCISE	**PAGE NO.**	**REPS**	**SETS**	**REST**
MODIFIED COMPOUND SUPERSET # 1	112			
Thighs: Dumbbell Squats		12-15	2	30 seconds
Hamstrings: Static Dumbbell Lunges (Press with Heels)	122	12-15	2	30 seconds
Thighs: Wide-Stance Dumbbell Squats	114	12-15	2	30 seconds
Hamstrings: Dumbbell Stiff-Legged Deadlifts	142	12-15	2	30 seconds
MODIFIED COMPOUND SUPERSET # 2	144			
Calves: One-Legged Dumbbell Calf Raises		12-15	2	30 seconds
Shoulders: Bent-Over Lateral Raises	208	12-15	2	30 seconds
Calves: Two-Legged Dumbbell Calf Raises	144	12-15	2	30 seconds
Triceps: Lying Dumbbell Triceps Extension	230	12-15	2	30 seconds

DAY 3				
EXERCISE	**PAGE NO.**	**REPS**	**SETS**	**REST**
FULL BODY COMBINATION WORKOUT # 1	292			
Back and Thighs: Squats with Dumbbell Rows		12-15	2	30 seconds
Chest and Core: Push-Ups with Side Rotation	304	12-15	2	30 seconds
Shoulders and Thighs: Upright Rows with Side-to-Side Lunges	300	12-15	2	30 seconds
Hamstrings and Back: Deadlift/Row Combo	306	12-15	2	30 seconds
FULL BODY COMBINATION WORKOUT # 2				
Biceps and Thighs: Knee-Ups into Back Lunge with Bicep Curl	298	12-15	2	30 seconds
Triceps and Thighs: Plié Squats with Triceps Extension	296	12-15	2	30 seconds
Shoulders and Thighs: Lunges with Overhead Press	294	12-15	2	30 seconds
Thighs: Squat with Alternating Leg Kick	302	12-15	2	30 seconds

Workout #1: Dumbbell Only

SPECIAL INSTRUCTIONS: Use Supersetting. Perform two exercises with no rest period in between. Rest for 30 seconds and then perform another two exercises with no rest in between. Repeat for the prescribed number of sets and then continue with the next group of exercises.

ABS AND CARDIO

EXERCISE	PAGE NO.	REPS	SETS	REST
MODIFIED COMPOUND SUPERSET # 1				
Lower Abs: Lying Leg Raises	282	10-12	3	0 seconds
Upper Abs: Crunches	270	10-12	3	0 seconds
Obliques: Bicycle	276	10-12	2	30 seconds
Aerobic Activity				
15 minutes of fast paced walking, stationary bike, or any other type of aerobic activity that you like.				

DAY 1

EXERCISE	PAGE NO.	REPS	SETS	REST
MODIFIED COMPOUND SUPERSET # 1				
Back: One-Arm Rows (Palms facing Torso)	162	10-12	3	0 seconds
Chest: Incline Dumbbell Bench Press	186	10-12	3	30 seconds
Thighs: Dumbbell Squats	112	10-12	3	0 seconds
Hamstrings: Dumbbell Stiff-Legged Deadlifts	142	10-12	3	30 seconds
MODIFIED COMPOUND SUPERSET # 2				
Biceps: Dumbbell Curls	250	10-12	3	0 seconds
Triceps: Lying Dumbbell Triceps Extensions	230	10-12	3	30 seconds
Shoulders: Dumbbell Upright Rows	214	10-12	3	0 seconds
Calves: Two-Legged Dumbbell Calf Raises	144	10-12	3	30 seconds

Weeks 3 & 4

DAY 2

EXERCISE	PAGE NO.	REPS	SETS	REST
MODIFIED COMPOUND SUPERSET # 1				
Thighs: Dumbbell Squats	112	10-12	3	0 seconds
Hamstrings: Static Dumbbell Lunges (Press with Heels)	122	10-12	3	30 seconds
Thighs: Wide Stance Dumbbell Squats	114	10-12	3	0 seconds
Hamstrings: Dumbbell Stiff-Legged Deadlifts	142	10-12	3	30 seconds
MODIFIED COMPOUND SUPERSET # 2				
Calves: One-Legged Dumbbell Calf Raises	144	10-12	3	0 seconds
Shoulders: Bent-Over Lateral Raises	208	10-12	3	30 seconds
Calves: Two-Legged Dumbbell Calf Raises	144	10-12	3	0 seconds
Triceps: Lying Dumbbell Triceps Extension	230	10-12	3	30 seconds

DAY 3

EXERCISE	PAGE NO.	REPS	SETS	REST
FULL BODY COMBINATION WORKOUT # 1				
Back and Thighs: Squats with Dumbbell Rows	292	10-12	3	0 seconds
Chest and Core: Push-Ups with Side Rotation	304	10-12	3	30 seconds
Shoulders and Thighs: Upright Rows with Side-to-Side Lunges	300	10-12	3	0 seconds
Hamstrings and Back: Deadlift/Row Combo	306	10-12	3	30 seconds
FULL BODY COMBINATION WORKOUT # 2				
Biceps and Thighs: Knee-Ups into Back Lunge with Bicep Curl	298	10-12	3	0 seconds
Triceps and Thighs: Plié Squats with Triceps Extension	296	10-12	3	30 seconds
Shoulders and Thighs: Lunges with Overhead Press	294	10-12	3	0 seconds
Thighs: Squat with Alternating Leg Kick	302	10-12	3	30 seconds

Workout #1: Dumbbell Only

SPECIAL INSTRUCTIONS: Use Giant Sets. Perform four exercises with no rest period in between. Only rest after the four exercises have been performed consecutively. Repeat for the prescribed number of sets and then continue with the next group of exercises.

ABS AND CARDIO

EXERCISE	PAGE NO.	REPS	SETS	REST
GIANT SET # 1				
Lower Abs: Lying Leg Raises	282	8-10	3	0 seconds
Upper Abs: Crunches	270	8-10	3	0 seconds
Obliques: Bicycle	276	8-10	2	30 seconds
Aerobic Activity				
15 minutes of fast paced walking, stationary bike, or any other type of aerobic activity that you like.				

DAY 1

EXERCISE	PAGE NO.	REPS	SETS	REST
GIANT SET # 1				
Back: One-Arm Rows (Palms facing Torso)	162	8-10	3	0 seconds
Chest: Incline Dumbbell Bench Press	186	8-10	3	0 seconds
Thighs: Dumbbell Squats	112	8-10	3	0 seconds
Hamstrings: Dumbbell Stiff-Legged Deadlifts	142	8-10	3	30 seconds
GIANT SET # 2				
Biceps: Dumbbell Curls	250	8-10	3	0 seconds
Triceps: Lying Dumbbell Triceps Extensions	230	8-10	3	0 seconds
Shoulders: Dumbbell Upright Rows	214	8-10	3	0 seconds
Calves: Two-Legged Dumbbell Calf Raises	144	8-10	3	30 seconds

Weeks 5 & 6

DAY 2

EXERCISE	PAGE NO.	REPS	SETS	REST
GIANT SET # 1				
Thighs: Dumbbell Squats	112	8-10	3	0 seconds
Hamstrings: Static Dumbbell Lunges (Press with Heels)	122	8-10	3	0 seconds
Thighs: Wide-Stance Dumbbell Squats	114	8-10	3	0 seconds
Hamstrings: Dumbbell Stiff-Legged Deadlifts	142	8-10	3	30 seconds
GIANT SET # 2				
Calves: One-Legged Dumbbell Calf Raises	144	8-10	3	0 seconds
Shoulders: Bent-Over Lateral Raises	208	8-10	3	0 seconds
Calves: Two-Legged Dumbbell Calf Raises	144	8-10	3	0 seconds
Triceps: Lying Dumbbell Triceps Extension	230	8-10	3	30 seconds

DAY 3

EXERCISE	PAGE NO.	REPS	SETS	REST
FULL BODY COMBINATION GIANT SET # 1 (HEAVIER WEIGHTS)				
Back and Thighs: Squats with Dumbbell Rows	292	8-10	3	0 seconds
Chest and Core: Push-Ups with Side Rotation	304	8-10	3	0 seconds
Shoulders and Thighs: Upright Rows with Side-to-Side Lunges	300	8-10	3	0 seconds
Hamstrings and Back: Deadlift/Row Combo	306	8-10	3	30 seconds
FULL BODY COMBINATION GIANT SET # 1 (HEAVIER WEIGHTS)				
Biceps and Thighs: Knee-Ups into Back Lunge with Bicep Curl	298	8-10	3	0 seconds
Triceps and Thighs: Plié Squats with Triceps Extension	296	8-10	3	0 seconds
Shoulders and Thighs: Lunges with Overhead Press	294	8-10	3	0 seconds
Thighs: Squat with Alternating Leg Kick	302	8-10	3	30 seconds

Workout #2: Machine Only

SPECIAL INSTRUCTIONS: Use Modified Compound Supersets. Perform Modified Compound Supersets by doing the exercises and, resting the prescribed amount of time until you have completed a circuit. Then start at the beginning and repeat for the recommended number of times before moving on to the next modified compound superset.

ABS AND CARDIO				
EXERCISE	**PAGE NO.**	**REPS**	**SETS**	**REST**
MODIFIED COMPOUND SUPERSET # 1				
Lower Abs: Lying Leg Raises	282	12-15	2	30 seconds
Upper Abs: Crunches	270	12-15	2	30 seconds
Obliques: Bicycle	276	12-15	2	30 seconds
Aerobic Activity				
15 minutes of fast paced walking, stationary bike, or any other type of aerobic activity that you like.				

DAY 1				
EXERCISE	**PAGE NO.**	**REPS**	**SETS**	**REST**
MODIFIED COMPOUND SUPERSET # 1				
Back: Two-Arm Row Machine	164	12-15	2	30 seconds
Chest: Bench Press Machine	201	12-15	2	30 seconds
Thighs: Leg Press Machine	124	12-15	2	30 seconds
Hamstrings: Lying Leg Curl Machine	134	12-15	2	30 seconds
MODIFIED COMPOUND SUPERSET # 2				
Biceps: Biceps Curl Machine	268	12-15	2	30 seconds
Triceps: Triceps Extension Machine	248	12-15	2	30 seconds
Shoulders: Lateral Raise Machine	218	12-15	2	30 seconds
Calves: Calf Raise Machine	152	12-15	2	30 seconds

Weeks 1 & 2

DAY 2

EXERCISE	PAGE NO.	REPS	SETS	REST
MODIFIED COMPOUND SUPERSET # 1				
Thighs: Leg Press Machine	124	12-15	2	30 seconds
Hamstrings: Lying Leg Curl Machine	134	12-15	2	30 seconds
Thighs: Leg Extension Machine	126	12-15	2	30 seconds
Hamstrings: Wide-Stance Leg Press (Press with Heels)	124	12-15	2	30 seconds
MODIFIED COMPOUND SUPERSET # 2				
Calves: Calf Raise Machine	148	12-15	2	30 seconds
Bent Over Lateral Raise on Incline Bench	218	12-15	2	30 seconds
Calves: Calf Press	152	12-15	2	30 seconds
Triceps: Triceps Pushdowns	242	12-15	2	30 seconds

DAY 3

EXERCISE	PAGE NO.	REPS	SETS	REST
FULL BODY MODIFIED COMPOUND SUPERSET # 1				
Back: Wide Grip Pulldowns to Front	170	12-15	2	30 seconds
Chest: Peck Deck Machine	202	12-15	2	30 seconds
Thighs: Leg Extension Machine	126	12-15	2	30 seconds
Hamstrings: Wide-Stance Leg Press (Press with Heels)	124	12-15	2	30 seconds
FULL BODY MODIFIED COMPOUND SUPERSET # 2				
Biceps: High Pulley Cable Curls on Pulldown Machine	266	12-15	2	30 seconds
Triceps: Triceps Pushdowns	242	12-15	2	30 seconds
Shoulders: Reverse Fly Machine	226	12-15	2	30 seconds
Calves: Calf Raise Machine	148	12-15	2	30 seconds

Workout #2: Machine Only

Special Instructions: Use Supersetting. Perform two exercises with no rest period in between. Rest for 30 seconds and then perform another two exercises with no rest in between. Repeat for the prescribed number of sets and then continue with the next group of exercises.

ABS AND CARDIO

EXERCISE	PAGE NO.	REPS	SETS	REST
MODIFIED COMPOUND SUPERSET # 1				
Lower Abs: Lying Leg Raises	282	10-12	3	0 seconds
Upper Abs: Crunches	270	10-12	3	0 seconds
Obliques: Bicycle	276	10-12	2	30 seconds
Aerobic Activity				
15 minutes of fast paced walking, stationary bike, or any other type of aerobic activity that you like.				

DAY 1

EXERCISE	PAGE NO.	REPS	SETS	REST
MODIFIED COMPOUND SUPERSET # 1				
Back: Two-Arm Row Machine	164	10-12	3	0 seconds
Chest: Bench Press Machine	201	10-12	3	30 seconds
Thighs: Leg Press Machine	124	10-12	3	0 seconds
Hamstrings: Lying Leg Curl Machine	134	10-12	3	30 seconds
MODIFIED COMPOUND SUPERSET # 2				
Biceps: Biceps Curl Machine	268	10-12	3	0 seconds
Triceps: Triceps Extension Machine	248	10-12	3	30 seconds
Shoulders: Lateral Raise Machine	218	10-12	3	0 seconds
Calves: Calf Raise Machine	152	10-12	3	30 seconds

Weeks 3 & 4

DAY 2

EXERCISE	PAGE NO.	REPS	SETS	REST
MODIFIED COMPOUND SUPERSET # 1				
Thighs: Leg Press Machine	124	10-12	3	0 seconds
Hamstrings: Lying Leg Curl Machine	134	10-12	3	30 seconds
Thighs: Leg Extension Machine	126	10-12	3	0 seconds
Hamstrings: Wide-Stance Leg Press (Press with Heels)	124	10-12	3	30 seconds
MODIFIED COMPOUND SUPERSET # 2				
Calves: Calf Raise Machine	148	10-12	3	0 seconds
Bent Over Lateral Raise on Incline Bench	218	10-12	3	30 seconds
Calves: Calf Press	152	10-12	3	0 seconds
Triceps: Triceps Pushdowns	242	10-12	3	30 seconds

DAY 3

EXERCISE	PAGE NO.	REPS	SETS	REST
GIANT SET # 1				
Back: Wide Grip Pulldowns to Front	170	10-12	3	0 seconds
Chest: Peck Deck Machine	202	10-12	3	30 seconds
Thighs: Leg Extension Machine	126	10-12	3	0 seconds
Hamstrings: Wide-Stance Leg Press (Press with Heels)	124	10-12	3	30 seconds
GIANT SET # 2				
Biceps: High Pulley Cable Curls on Pulldown Machine	266	10-12	3	0 seconds
Triceps: Triceps Pushdowns	242	10-12	3	30 seconds
Shoulders: Reverse Fly Machine	226	10-12	3	0 seconds
Calves: Calf Raise Machine	148	10-12	3	30 seconds

Workout #2: Machine Only

SPECIAL INSTRUCTIONS: Use Giant Sets. Perform four exercises with no rest period in between. Only rest after the four exercises have been performed consecutively. Repeat for the prescribed number of sets and then continue with the next group of exercises.

ABS AND CARDIO

EXERCISE	PAGE NO.	REPS	SETS	REST
GIANT SET # 1				
Lower Abs: Lying Leg Raises	282	10-12	3	0 seconds
Upper Abs: Crunches	270	10-12	3	0 seconds
Obliques: Bicycle	276	12-15	2	30 seconds
Aerobic Activity				
15 minutes of fast paced walking, stationary bike, or any other type of aerobic activity that you like.				

DAY 1

EXERCISE	PAGE NO.	REPS	SETS	REST
GIANT SET # 1				
Back: Two-Arm Row Machine	164	10-12	3	0 seconds
Chest: Bench Press Machine	201	10-12	3	0 seconds
Thighs: Leg Press Machine	124	10-12	3	0 seconds
Hamstrings: Lying Leg Curl Machine	134	10-12	3	30 seconds
GIANT SET # 1				
Biceps: Biceps Curl Machine	268	10-12	3	0 seconds
Triceps: Triceps Extensions Machine	248	10-12	3	0 seconds
Shoulders: Lateral Raise Machine	218	10-12	3	0 seconds
Calves: Calf Press	152	10-12	3	30 seconds

Weeks 5 & 6

DAY 2

EXERCISE	PAGE NO.	REPS	SETS	REST
GIANT SET # 1				
Thighs: Leg Press Machine	124	10-12	3	0 seconds
Hamstrings: Lying Leg Curl Machine	134	10-12	3	0 seconds
Thighs: Leg Extension Machine	126	10-12	3	0 seconds
Hamstrings: Wide-Stance Leg Press (Press with Heels)	124	10-12	3	30 seconds
GIANT SET # 2				
Calves: Calf Raise Machine	148	10-12	3	0 seconds
Bent Over Lateral Raise on Incline Bench	218	10-12	3	0 seconds
Calves: Calf Press	152	10-12	3	0 seconds
Triceps: Triceps Pushdowns	242	10-12	3	30 seconds

DAY 3

EXERCISE	PAGE NO.	REPS	SETS	REST
GIANT SET # 1				
Back: Wide Grip Pulldowns to Front	170	10-12	3	0 seconds
Chest: Peck Deck Machine	202	10-12	3	0 seconds
Thighs: Leg Extension Machine	126	10-12	3	0 seconds
Hamstrings: Wide-Stance Leg Press (Press with Heels)	124	10-12	3	30 seconds
GIANT SET # 2				
Biceps: High Pulley Cable Curls on Pulldown Machine	266	10-12	3	0 seconds
Triceps: Triceps Pushdowns	242	10-12	3	0 seconds
Shoulders: Reverse Fly Machine	226	10-12	3	0 seconds
Calves: Calf Raise Machine	148	10-12	3	30 seconds

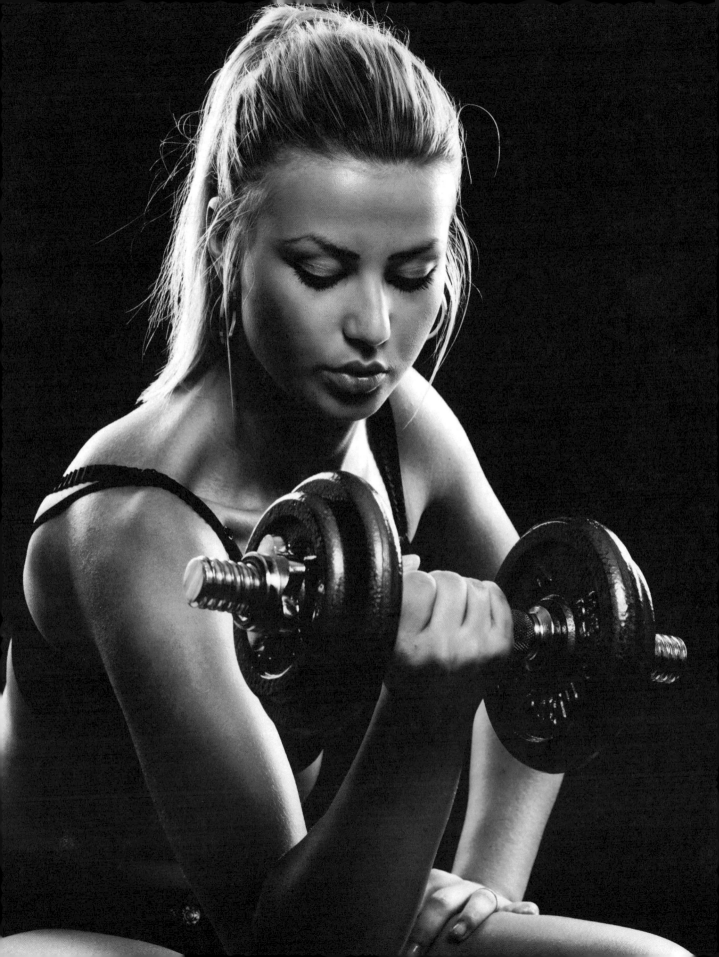

Appendix A
Glossary

A

THE **BODY**
SCULPTING
BIBLE
FOR**WOMEN**

Aerobic Exercise: Constant moderate intensity work that uses oxygen at a rate in which the cardio respiratory system can replenish oxygen in the working muscles. Examples of such activity are stationary bike riding or walking. It is a good activity for fat loss when done in the right amounts but highly catabolic if done in excess.

Anaerobic Exercise: Exercise in which oxygen is used more quickly than the body is able to replenish it inside the working muscle. Weight training is an example of such an activity. It is highly anabolic in nature but also highly catabolic if done in excess.

Anabolic State: Favorable state in the body created by a combination of good training, nutrition and rest that leads to favorable changes in body composition.

Anabolic Steroids: Synthetic (man-made) hormones that simulate the effects of the male hormone testosterone.

Anti-catabolic Properties: Properties provided by certain nutrients that protect the muscle mass in the body from being broken down.

Anti-lypolitic Properties: Properties provided by certain nutrients that prevent the body from turning calories into fat.

Antioxidant Properties: Properties provided by certain nutrients that protect the body from disease.

Basic Exercises: Exercise movement that involves a large number of muscles in the body. They are generally multi-joint movements that target the larger muscles of the body (such as chest, back and thighs) but also involve the smaller muscles as well (such as shoulders,

arms, calves and abs) as auxiliary muscles. Examples of such movements are chin-ups, pull-ups, dips, bench presses, squats, and lunges.

Bulk Minerals: Minerals which the body needs in great quantities (in the order of grams) such as calcium, magnesium, potassium, sodium and phosphorus.

Carbohydrates: Macronutrient used by the body as its main source of energy. Carbohydrates are divided into complex carbs and simple carbs. The complex carbs give you sustained energy ("timed release") while the simple carbs give you immediate energy. This macronutrient can be found in rice (complex, starchy), pasta (complex, starchy), breads (complex, starchy), fruits (simple), sugars (simple), fruit juices (simple), dairy products (simple), and vegetables (complex, fibrous).

Catabolic State: Unfavorable state in the body created by a combination of too much training, lack of good nutrition and lack of rest that leads to muscle loss and fat accumulation.

Cortisol: Catabolic hormone secreted by the adrenal glands in situations of stress (both physical and mental), lack of calories/nutrients and lack of sleep. This hormone is associated with loss of muscle mass, loss of strength, and fat accumulation. An excess of it over long periods of time may also contribute to hardening of the arteries; leading to heart disease.

Diuretics: Drugs used to remove excess water from the body. There are two versions: the drug version (can only be prescribed by a physician), and the herbal version. Excessive use of the drug version has as side effects muscle cramps and harsh arrhythmia. The herbal version, while safer than the drug version, can lead to potassium loss and excessive use puts stress on the kidneys.

Dumbbell: A short-handled barbell 10-12 inches long that can be carried in one hand. Dumbbells allow flexibility in the execution of a movement and full range of motion.

Endorphins: Hormones that make us feel good and happy. The production of these hormones is stimulated by exercise.

Essential Fatty Acids (EFAs): Fats that have anti-catabolic, anti-lypolitic and antioxidant properties. These fats affect good cholesterol in a positive way. In addition, these fats aid in the muscle-building, fat-loss process. The Omega 3 Fatty Acids found in fats such as fish oils and flaxseed oil are a good source of EFAs.

Estrogen: Female hormone that regulates and sustains female sexual development and reproductive function. An excess of this hormone appears to be related to heart disease and cancer. In addition, when this hormone is in excess, it causes fat gain and water retention. Estrogen deficits, on the other hand, cause memory problems, trouble finding words, inability to pay attention, mood swings and irritability. Exercise helps reduce the risk of these diseases and conditions by helping to balance the levels of this hormone.

Exercise Volume: The amount of work performed in an exercise session defined by the product resulting from the amount of weight lifted, multiplied by the number of sets and multiplied by the number of repetitions. For example, if you had a workout that consisted of 10 sets of dumbbell curls, and for each set you used 30 pounds and performed 10 repetitions, then your biceps routine volume equals 10 x 10 x 30 = 3000 pounds. Too much volume leads to overtraining.

Fats: Macronutrient needed by the body in order to manufacture hormones and sustain cell metabolism. All the cells in the body have some fat in them. Hormones are manufactured from fats. Also, fats lubricate your joints. If you eliminate the fat from your diet, your hormonal production will go down and a whole array of chemical reactions will be interrupted. There are three types of fats: saturated, polyunsaturated and monounsaturated.

Fat Soluble Vitamins: Vitamins stored in fat that if taken in excessive amounts will become toxic. They include vitamins A, D, E, and K.

Giant Set: Giant Sets are four exercises done one after the other with no rest in between sets. Again, there are two ways to implement this. You can either use four exercises for the same muscle group or perform 2 pairs of opposing muscle group exercises. For the purposes of this manual, whenever we do Giant Sets, we will perform two pairs of opposing muscle group exercises with no rest. The exception is when we do abs in which we will alternate between lower abs and upper abs.

Growth Hormone: Hormone secreted by the pituitary gland that aids in fat loss and muscle building.

Hormones: Fats similar to, and usually synthesized from, cholesterol, starting with Acetyl-CoA, moving through squalene, lanosterol, cholesterol, and, in the gonads and adrenal cortex, a number of steroid hormones. Because they stimulate cell growth, either by changing the internal structure or increasing the rate of proliferation, they are often called anabolic steroids.

Hypertrophy: Scientific term for describing an increase in muscle mass and strength caused by the stimulation of the muscles.

Intensity: Intensity has two definitions in the weight-training world. (1) Relative term that indicates the level of effort exerted during the performance of an exercise. (2) In strength training circles, intensity refers to the amount of weight used on a specific exercise.

Insulin: Hormone secreted by the pancreas responsible for carbohydrate metabolism. This hormone determines if carbohydrates are to be used for energy, storage inside the muscle cells as glycogen, or converting and storing the carbohydrates as fats when they are found in excess in the bloodstream.

Isolation Exercises: Exercise movements that are generally single jointed and serve to isolate a single area of the body. Examples of such are dumbbell flys, concentration curls, triceps kickbacks, leg extensions, and leg curls.

Lactic Acid: By-product created by a lack of oxygen flow to the working muscles. Lactic acid is created by anaerobic activities such as weight training exercises. It is believed that its presence causes a surge in growth hormone levels.

Macronutrient: One of the three major nutrients that the body needs for survival. These nutrients are carbohydrates, proteins and fats.

Metabolism: The rate at which the body utilizes calories and nutrients in order to sustain its daily activities.

Minerals: Minerals are inorganic compounds (not produced by animals or vegetables) whose main function is to assure that your brain receives the correct signals from the body, as well as to ensure balance of fluids, make muscular contractions possible and allow energy production, as well as building muscle and bones. There are two types of minerals: bulk and trace minerals.

Modified Compound Superset: In a modified compound set, you pair exercises for opposing muscle groups or for opposing muscle movements (e.g. Push vs. Pull). First you perform one exercise, rest the recommended amount of seconds and then perform the second exercise (for instance, first do biceps, rest, then do triceps). You then rest the prescribed amount of time again and go back to the first exercise. Using this technique of pairing exercises in a modified superset fashion not only saves time and keeps the body warm, but allows for faster recovery of the nervous system between sets. This will allow the person to lift heavier weights than possible if she just stayed idle for 2-3 minutes waiting to recover.

Monounsaturated Fats: Fats that have a positive effect on good cholesterol levels. These fats are usually high in essential fatty acids and may have antioxidant properties. Sources of these fats are fish oils, virgin olive oil, canola oil, and flaxseed oil.

Muscle Failure: Point during the exercise at which it becomes impossible to perform another repetition in good form. This point is reached due to the lack of oxygen reaching the working muscles and the increased levels of lactic acid.

Overtraining: Condition caused by an excess of volume in a training routine that leads to muscle loss, strength loss and fat accumulation. Symptoms include depression, insomnia, lethargy and lack of energy.

Polyunsaturated Fats: Fats that do not have an effect on cholesterol levels. Most of the fats in vegetable oils, such as corn, cottonseed, safflower, soybean, and sunflower oil are polyunsaturated.

Protein: Every tissue in your body is made from protein (i.e. muscle, hair, skin, nails). Proteins are the building blocks of muscle tissue. This macronutrient can be found in poultry, meats, and dairy products.

Repetitions: The amount of times you perform an exercise. For instance, pretend that you are performing a bench press. You pick up the bar, lower it, pause and lift it up. That action of executing the movement for one time counts for one repetition. If you perform that same movement a second time, then that is your second repetition, and so on.

Rest Interval: The amount of time a person rests between sets. For instance, a rest interval of 60 seconds means that after you finish your first set, you will remain idle for 60 seconds before going on to the next set.

Saturated Fats: Saturated fats are associated with heart disease and high cholesterol levels. They are found to a large extent in products of animal origin. However, some vegetable fats are altered in a way that increases the amount of saturated fats in them by a chemical process known as hydrogenation. Hydrogenated vegetable oils are generally found in packaged foods. In addition, coconut oil, palm oil, and palm kernel oil, which are also frequently used in packaged foods and non-dairy creamers are also highly saturated.

Sets: A set is a collection of repetitions that culminates in the muscle reaching muscular failure.

Supersets: A superset is a combination of exercises performed right after each other with no rest in between. There are two ways to implement a superset. The first way is to do two exercises for the same muscle group at once; for example dumbbell curls immediately followed by concentration curls. The drawback to this technique is that you will not be as strong as you usually are on the second exercise. The second and best way to superset is by pairing exercises of opposing muscle groups or different muscle movements such as back and chest, thighs and hamstrings, biceps and triceps, shoulders and calves, upper abs and lower abs. When pairing antagonistic exercises, there is no drop of strength once your cardiovascular system is well conditioned.

Trace Minerals: Minerals which are needed by the body in minute amounts, usually in the order of micrograms, such as chromium, copper, cobalt, silicon, selenium, iron and zinc.

Testosterone: Hormone responsible for increasing muscle size. Even though this hormone is predominantly present in males, it is also present in women to a lesser degree. It is believed that this hormone also aids in fat loss to a lesser degree.

Vitamins: Vitamins are organic compounds (produced by both animals and vegetables) whose function is to enhance the actions of proteins that cause chemical reactions such as muscle building, fat burning and energy production. There are two types of vitamins: fat-soluble and water-soluble.

Water Soluble Vitamins: Vitamins that are not stored in the body, such as B-Complex vitamins and vitamin C. Therefore, they need to be taken on a frequent basis.

Appendix B
Table of Food Values

B

THE **BODY SCULPTING BIBLE** FOR **WOMEN**

Nutrition Chart and Glycemic Index

STARCHY CARBOHYDRATES			
Eat with all 5-6 meals throughout the day. Around 25-27 grams of carbohydrates per serving. 1 serving per meal.			
FOOD ITEM	**SERVING SIZE (MEASURE DRY)**	**GLYCEMIC INDEX**	**DESIRABLE**
Old Fashioned Oats	1/2 cup dry	Low	Highly
Cream of Rice	1/4 cup dry	High	Good After Workout Only
Cream of Wheat	4 tablespoons dry	Medium	Good
Baked Potatoes	4 ounce cooked	Medium	Good
Sweet Potatoes	4 ounce cooked	Medium	Good
Rice (Brown Whole Grain)	1/2 cup cooked	Medium	Good
White Rice	1/2 cup cooked	High	Good After Workout Only
Spaghetti	4 oz cooked	Low	Good in GI but too many carbs for a small serving.
Whole wheat flour bread	2 slices	High	Not a great choice but ok in moderation.
Corn	3/4 cup	Medium	Good
Peas	1 cups	Medium	Good
Low GI=1-55 Medium GI=56-69 High GI=70-100			

SIMPLE CARBOHYDRATES

If you must, eat 1 serving with Breakfast and 1 after workout as even though they are low to medium in GI, too many simple sugars from fruits in the diet throughout the day can prevent fat loss. If your post workout meal is breakfast, then just consume 1 serving per day of fruits.

Around 10 grams of carbohydrates per serving. If breakfast is the post workout meal: 1 serving per day with post workout meal. If post workout meal is not breakfast: 1 serving with breakfast and 1 serving with post workout meal.

FOOD ITEM	SERVING SIZE	GLYCEMIC INDEX	DESIRABLE
Apples	1/2	Low	Good
Oranges	1/2	Low	Good
Grapefruit	1/2	Low	Good
Cherries	7	Low	Good
Pears	1/3	Low	Good
Bananas	1/3	Medium	After Workout Only
Lemons	1	Low	Good
Cantaloupe	1/4 melon	High	After Workout Only
Strawberries	1 cup	1 cup	Good
Apricots	3	Medium	After Workout Only
Grapes	1/2 cup	Low	Good
Mango	1/3 cup	Medium	After Workout Only
Papaya	1/2 cup	Medium	After Workout Only

Low GI=1-55 Medium GI=56-69 High GI=70-100Low GI=1-55 Medium GI=56-69 High GI=70-100

FIBROUS CARBOHYDRATES

Eat at least 1 serving with lunch and 1 serving with dinner though more can be consumed if desired; consider these free foods as they do not get absorbed.

Around 10 grams of carbohydrates per serving. At least 1 serving at lunch and 1 serving at dinner.

FOOD ITEM	SERVING SIZE (MEASURE COOKED)	GLYCEMIC INDEX	DESIRABLE
Broccoli	1 cup	Low	Good
Green Beans	1 cup	Low	Good
Asparagus	12 spears or 1 cup	Low	Good
Lettuce	1 head raw	Low	Good
Tomatoes	2 cups chopped	Low	Good
Green Peppers (chopped)	1-1/2 cup raw	Low	Good
Onions	1/2 cup	Low	Good
Mushrooms	1 cup	Low	Good
Cucumber sliced	3 cups	Low	Good
Cauliflower	2 cups	Low	Good
Spinach	4 cups	Low	Good
Cabbage	2 cups	Low	Good
Carrots	1/2 cup sliced	High	After Workout

Low GI=1-55 Medium GI=56-69 High GI=70-100

PROTEINS

Eat with all 5-6 meals throughout the day. Around 20-23 grams of protein per serving. 1 serving per meal.

FOOD ITEM	SERVING SIZE (MEASURE COOKED)	GLYCEMIC INDEX	DESIRABLE
Chicken breast (skinless)	3 ounces	Low	Good
Turkey	3 ounces	Low	Good
Veal	3 ounces	Low	Good
Top Sirloin	3 ounces	Low	Good
Tuna	3 ounces	Low	Good
Wild Alaskan Salmon	3 ounces	Low	Good
Egg Whites (in carton)	1 cup	Low	Good
Whey Protein	1 scoop	Low	Good
Orange Roughy	3 ounces	Low	Good

GOOD FATS

Around 5 grams of fats per serving. 1 serving at lunch, dinner, and any other meal except post workout meal.

FOOD ITEM	SERVING SIZE	GLYCEMIC INDEX	DESIRABLE
Fish Oils	1 teaspoon	Low	Good
Flax Oils	1 teaspoon	Low	Good
Extra Virgin Olive Oil	1 teaspoon	Low	Good
Natural Peanut Butter	2 teaspoons	Low	Good

All fats are low in glycemic index and by combining a carbohydrate with a protein the combined glycemic index of the whole meal goes down. The fats included here were selected due to their high essential fatty acids content and their health properties.

NOTES: Avoid cooking with flax oil as the heat degrades the oil. Bake and broil instead of frying. Also, if eating salmon, eliminate 2 servings of good fats as salmon is high on EFAs.

The complete list of the glycemic index and glycemic load for 750 foods can be found in the article "International tables of glycemic index and glycemic load values: 2002," by Kaye Foster-Powell, Susanna H.A. Holt, and Janette C. Brand-Miller in the July 2002 American Journal of Clinical Nutrition, Vol. 62, pages 5–56. <http://www.ajcn.org/cgi/content/full/76/1/5>

Now that you know your approved list of foods, simply use the following guidelines to create your meal plan.

For sample diets that use these exact measurements, please see Appendix C.

WEEKS 1-2: CALORIES:LOW (Approximately 1200 calories)

Around 120 grams of carbohydrates (mostly complex with simple carbs being saved for after the workout)

Around 120 grams of protein

Around 26 grams of fats

MEAL #1 (7:30 AM) BREAKFAST (POST-WORKOUT)

Choose 1 serving of Proteins
Choose 1 serving of Starchy Carbs
Optionally, you may choose to add 1 serving of Simple Carbs in the form of Fruit, if you can't live without them.

MEAL #2 (10:30 AM) MORNING BREAK SNACK

Choose 1 serving of Proteins
Choose 1 serving of Starchy Carbs
Choose 1 serving of Good Fats

MEAL #3 (1:30 PM) LUNCH TIME

Choose 1 serving of Proteins
Choose 1 serving of Starchy Carbs
Choose 1 serving of Fibrous Carbs
Choose 1 serving of Good Fats

MEAL #4 (3:30 PM) AFTERNOON BREAK SNACK

Choose 1 serving of Proteins
Choose 1 serving of Starchy Carbs

MEAL #5 (6:30 PM) DINNER

Choose 1 serving of Proteins
Choose 1/2 serving of Starchy Carbs
Choose 1 serving of Fibrous Carbs
Choose 1 serving of Good Fats

WEEKS 3-4 CALORIES: HIGH (Approximately 1500 calories)

150 grams of carbohydrates (mostly complex with simple carbs being saved for after the workout)

150 grams of protein

33 grams of fats

MEAL #1 (7:30 AM) BREAKFAST (POST-WORKOUT)

Choose 1 serving of Proteins
Choose 1 serving of Starchy Carbs
Optionally, you may choose to add 1 serving of Simple Carbs in the form of Fruit, if you can't live without them.

MEAL #2 (10:30 AM) MORNING BREAK SNACK

Choose 1 serving of Proteins
Choose 1 serving of Starchy Carbs

MEAL #3 (1:30 PM) LUNCH TIME

Choose 1 serving of Proteins
Choose 1 serving of Starchy Carbs
Choose 1 serving of Fibrous Carbs
Choose 1 serving of Good Fats

MEAL #4 (3:30 PM) AFTERNOON BREAK SNACK

Choose 1 serving of Proteins
Choose 1 serving of Starchy Carbs

MEAL #5 (6:30 PM) DINNER

Choose 1 serving of Proteins
Choose 1/2 serving of Starchy Carbs
Choose 1 serving of Fibrous Carbs
Choose 1 serving of Good Fats

MEAL #6 (8:30 PM) LATE SNACK

Choose 1 serving of Proteins
Choose 1/2 serving of Starchy Carbs
Choose 1 serving of Fibrous Carbs
Choose 1 serving of Good Fats

NOTES:

- While the foods above contain trace amounts of other macronutrients in them (for example, skinless chicken breasts contain 2.5 to 5 grams of fat), for the purposes of our calculations we will assume that these foods contain only the macronutrient under which they are listed.

- If you choose to include **skim milk** in your diet, remember that it not only has protein (8-9 grams for every 8 ounces of milk) but also simple carbs (12-13 grams for every 8 ounces of milk). Therefore, count milk as both. Note that since the carbs in milk are simple carbs, this food item ideally should only be used in the post workout meal. However, if due to schedule you need to include more protein shakes throughout the day, and the carbs that you will rely on are those found in skim milk, ensure that you add a teaspoon of flaxseed oil to it as the oil will slow down the release of the simple carbs into the blood stream. Women interested in competing should however eliminate any dairy products from the diet as these products tend to make you retain water and the lactose in them makes it harder to get to the desired low body fat percentage required for the contest.

- If you use **flaxseed oil** as your Essential Fatty Acids supplement, remember to count these as fat grams. Each teaspoon contains approximately 5 grams of good fats.

- If you use **fish oil** capsules as your Essential Fatty Acids supplement, count each capsule as 1 gram of good fat.

- Remember that carbohydrates have 4 calories per gram. Therefore, a 6-ounce banana has 27 grams of carbs x 4 = 108 calories.

- Remember that protein has 4 calories per gram. Therefore, a 3.5-ounce chicken breast has 35 grams of protein x 4 = 140 calories.

- Remember that fat has 9 calories per gram. Therefore, a teaspoon of flaxseed oil has 5 grams of fat x 9 = 45 calories.

Appendix C
Sample Diets

C

THE **BODY**
SCULPTING
BIBLE
FOR**WOMEN**

These diets were created using the Appendix B menu charts. These diets are samples of what you can eat on a daily basis. Remember that you don't have to be stuck to just what is written here. You can vary your daily plan by using the food tables from Appendix B in conjunction with the daily menus. Also remember that these diets are samples of the normal Body Sculpting Bible diet program. For the advanced carb cycling program, follow the recommendations on that section of the Nutrition chapter.

WEEKS 1-2: CALORIES:LOW (Approximately 1200 calories)

Around 120 grams of carbohydrates (mostly complex with simple carbs being saved for after the workout)

Around 120 grams of protein

Around 26 grams of fats

MEAL #1 (7:30 AM) BREAKFAST (POST-WORKOUT)
Choose 1 serving of Proteins
Choose 1 serving of Starchy Carbs
Optionally, you may choose to add 1 serving of Simple Carbs in the form of Fruit, if you can't live without them.

MEAL #2 (10:30 AM) MORNING BREAK SNACK
Choose 1 serving of Proteins
Choose 1 serving of Starchy Carbs
Choose 1 serving of Good Fats

MEAL #3 (1:30 PM) LUNCH TIME
Choose 1 serving of Proteins
Choose 1 serving of Starchy Carbs
Choose 1 serving of Fibrous Carbs
Choose 1 serving of Good Fats

MEAL #4 (3:30 PM) AFTERNOON BREAK SNACK
Choose 1 serving of Proteins
Choose 1 serving of Starchy Carbs

MEAL #5 (6:30 PM) DINNER
Choose 1 serving of Proteins
Choose 1/2 serving of Starchy Carbs
Choose 1 serving of Fibrous Carbs
Choose 1 serving of Good Fats

WEEKS 3-4 CALORIES: HIGH (Approximately 1500 calories)

150 grams of carbohydrates (mostly complex with simple carbs being saved for after the workout)

150 grams of protein

33 grams of fats

MEAL #1 (7:30 AM) BREAKFAST (POST-WORKOUT)
Choose 1 serving of Proteins
Choose 1 serving of Starchy Carbs
Optionally, you may choose to add 1 serving of Simple Carbs in the form of Fruit, if you can't live without them.

MEAL #2 (10:30 AM) MORNING BREAK SNACK
Choose 1 serving of Proteins
Choose 1 serving of Starchy Carbs

MEAL #3 (1:30 PM) LUNCH TIME
Choose 1 serving of Proteins
Choose 1 serving of Starchy Carbs
Choose 1 serving of Fibrous Carbs
Choose 1 serving of Good Fats

MEAL #4 (3:30 PM) AFTERNOON BREAK SNACK
Choose 1 serving of Proteins
Choose 1 serving of Starchy Carbs

MEAL #5 (6:30 PM) DINNER
Choose 1 serving of Proteins
Choose 1/2 serving of Starchy Carbs
Choose 1 serving of Fibrous Carbs
Choose 1 serving of Good Fats

MEAL #6 (8:30 PM) LATE SNACK
Choose 1 serving of Proteins
Choose 1/2 serving of Starchy Carbs
Choose 1 serving of Fibrous Carbs
Choose 1 serving of Good Fats

SAMPLE 14-DAY LOW-CALORIE MILK-FREE DIET

(THIS DIET IS GOOD FOR THOSE WHO WANT TO ELIMINATE MILK PRODUCTS FROM THEIR PROGRAM.)

MEAL #	FOOD	SERVING SIZE
MEAL 1 BREAKFAST (POST-WORKOUT) 7:30 AM	WHEY PROTEIN BANANA CREAM OF RICE	1 SCOOP 1/3 BANANA 1/4 CUP DRY
MEAL 2 10:30 AM	WHEY PROTEIN OLD-FASHIONED OATS FLAXSEED OIL	1 SCOOP 1/2 CUP (MEASURED DRY) 1 TEASPOON
MEAL 3 1:30 PM	BROWN RICE GREEN BEANS CHICKEN BREAST EXTRA-VIRGIN OLIVE OIL	1/2 CUP COOKED 1 CUP 3 OUNCES 1 TEASPOON
MEAL 4 3:30 PM	WHEY PROTEIN OLD-FASHIONED OATS	1 SCOOP 1/2 CUP (MEASURED DRY)
MEAL 5 6:30 PM	WILD ALASKAN SALMON SWEET POTATOES BROCCOLI	3 OUNCES 2 OUNCES COOKED 1 CUP

SAMPLE 14-DAY HIGH-CALORIE MILK-FREE DIET

(THIS DIET IS GOOD FOR THOSE WHO WANT TO ELIMINATE MILK PRODUCTS FROM THEIR PROGRAM.)

MEAL #	FOOD	SERVING SIZE
MEAL 1 BREAKFAST (POST-WORKOUT) 7:30 AM	WHEY PROTEIN BANANA CREAM OF RICE	1 SCOOP 1/3 BANANA 1/4 CUP DRY
MEAL 2 10:30 AM	WHEY PROTEIN OLD-FASHIONED OATS FLAXSEED OIL	1 SCOOP 1/2 CUP (MEASURED DRY) 1 TEASPOON
MEAL 3 1:30 PM	BROWN RICE GREEN BEANS CHICKEN BREAST EXTRA-VIRGIN OLIVE OIL	1/2 CUP COOKED 1 CUP 3 OUNCES 1 TEASPOON
MEAL 4 3:30 PM	WHEY PROTEIN OLD-FASHIONED OATS	1 SCOOP 1/2 CUP (MEASURED DRY)
MEAL 5 6:30 PM	WILD ALASKAN SALMON SWEET POTATOES BROCCOLI	3 OUNCES 2 OUNCES COOKED 1 CUP
MEAL 6 8:30 PM	ORANGE ROUGHY BAKED POTATOES ASPARAGUS FLAXSEED OIL	3 OUNCES 2 OUNCES 1 CUP 1 TEASPOON

SAMPLE 14-DAY LOW-CALORIE DIET WITH MILK PRODUCTS

MEAL #	FOOD	SERVING SIZE
MEAL 1 BREAKFAST (POST-WORKOUT) 7:30 AM	WHEY PROTEIN SKIM MILK CREAM OF RICE	1/2 SCOOP 8 OUNCES 1/4 CUP DRY
MEAL 2 10:30 AM	WHEY PROTEIN OLD-FASHIONED OATS SKIM MILK FLAXSEED OIL	1/2 SCOOP 1/4 CUP (MEASURED DRY) 8 OUNCES 1 TEASPOON
MEAL 3 1:30 PM	BROWN RICE GREEN BEANS CHICKEN BREAST EXTRA-VIRGIN OLIVE OIL	1/2 CUP COOKED 1 CUP 3 OUNCES 1 TEASPOON
MEAL 4 3:30 PM	WHEY PROTEIN OLD-FASHIONED OATS	1 SCOOP 1/2 CUP (MEASURED DRY)
MEAL 5 6:30PM	WILD ALASKAN SALMON SWEET POTATOES BROCCOLI	3 OUNCES 2 OUNCES COOKED 1 CUP

SAMPLE 14-DAY HIGH-CALORIE DIET WITH MILK PRODUCTS

MEAL #	FOOD	SERVING SIZE
MEAL 1 BREAKFAST (POST-WORKOUT) 7:30 AM	WHEY PROTEIN SKIM MILK CREAM OF RICE	1/2 SCOOP 8 OUNCES 1/4 CUP DRY
MEAL 2 10:30 AM	WHEY PROTEIN OLD-FASHIONED OATS SKIM MILK FLAXSEED OIL	1/2 SCOOP 1/4 CUP (MEASURED DRY) 8 OUNCES 1 TEASPOON
MEAL 3 1:30 PM	BROWN RICE GREEN BEANS CHICKEN BREAST EXTRA-VIRGIN OLIVE OIL	1/2 CUP COOKED 1 CUP 3 OUNCES 1 TEASPOON
MEAL 4 3:30 PM	WHEY PROTEIN OLD-FASHIONED OATS	1 SCOOP 1/2 CUP (MEASURED DRY)
MEAL 5 6:30 PM	WILD ALASKAN SALMON SWEET POTATOES BROCCOLI	3 OUNCES 2 OUNCES COOKED 1 CUP
MEAL 6 8:30 PM	ORANGE ROUGHY BAKED POTATOES ASPARAGUS FLAXSEED OIL	3 OUNCES 2 OUNCES COOKED 1 CUP 1 TEASPOON

SAMPLE 14-DAY LOW-CALORIE OVO-LACTO VEGETARIAN DIET

MEAL #	FOOD	SERVING SIZE
MEAL 1 BREAKFAST (POST-WORKOUT) 7:30 AM	WHEY PROTEIN SKIM MILK CREAM OF RICE	1/2 SCOOP 8 OUNCES 1/4 CUP DRY
MEAL 2 10:30 AM	WHEY PROTEIN OLD-FASHIONED OATS SKIM MILK FLAXSEED OIL	1/2 SCOOP 1/4 CUP (MEASURED DRY) 8 OUNCES 1 TEASPOON
MEAL 3 1:30 PM	BROWN RICE GREEN BEANS EGG WHITES EXTRA-VIRGIN OLIVE OIL	1/2 CUP COOKED 1 CUP 1 CUP 1 TEASPOON
MEAL 4 3:30 PM	WHEY PROTEIN OLD-FASHIONED OATS	1 SCOOP 1/2 CUP (MEASURED DRY)
MEAL 5 6:30 PM	EGG WHITES SWEET POTATOES BROCCOLI	1 CUP 2 OUNCES COOKED 1 CUP

SAMPLE 14-DAY HIGH-CALORIE OVO-LACTO VEGETARIAN DIET

MEAL #	FOOD	SERVING SIZE
MEAL 1 BREAKFAST (POST-WORKOUT) 7:30 AM	WHEY PROTEIN SKIM MILK CREAM OF RICE	1/2 SCOOP 8 OUNCES 1/4 CUP DRY
MEAL 2 10:30 AM	WHEY PROTEIN OLD-FASHIONED OATS SKIM MILK FLAXSEED OIL	1/2 SCOOP 1/4 CUP (MEASURED DRY) 8 OUNCES 1 TEASPOON
MEAL 3 1:30 PM	BROWN RICE GREEN BEANS EGG WHITES EXTRA-VIRGIN OLIVE OIL	1/2 CUP COOKED 1 CUP 1 CUP 1 TEASPOON
MEAL 4 3:30 PM	WHEY PROTEIN OLD-FASHIONED OATS	1 SCOOP 1/2 CUP (MEASURED DRY)
MEAL 5 6:30PM	EGG WHITES SWEET POTATOES BROCCOLI	1 CUP 2 OUNCES COOKED 1 CUP
MEAL 6 8:30 PM	EGG WHITES BAKED POTATOES ASPARAGUS FLAXSEED OIL	1 CUP 2 OUNCES COOKED 1 CUP 1 TEASPOON

Appendix D
Recipes

THE **BODY**
SCULPTING
BIBLE
FOR**WOMEN**

D

A Note from Chef Marie

Following are 60 Breakfast, Lunch, Dinner and Dessert recipes. All of these recipes meet the requirements for nutritious, low-fat weight loss and, when used in conjunction with the 21-Day *EXPRESS* Body Sculpting program, are guaranteed to produce results.

How to Begin

At the start of each week, use the Daily Nutrition Journal in Appendix B to outline your meal plans. You can pick and choose your weekly meals from each category; just be sure that your daily caloric requirement is within the right range for weight loss (1200-1500).

Also, as explained on page 25, keep in mind that, during the first two weeks of your workout, you should aim to consume 1200 calories, and then increase your caloric intake to 1500 calories for the last 2 weeks. This will help your body gain muscle and lose fat more efficiently.

If you prefer to prepare your meals entirely on your own, consult the nutrition guidelines and use the food group charts in Appendix B as a guide.

A Note on Sunday Rewards

If you've stayed true to your diet all week, you deserve a reward. Treat yourself to one "cheat meal" per week. As described on pages 31-32, this can include an appetizer, main meal, and dessert. But be sure not to go overboard, or you'll run the risk of going backwards.

A Note on Times to Eat and Frequency of Meals

To help boost your metabolism, you should try to eat five or six small meals throughout the day, which amounts to approximately every 2-3 hours. This will make it easier for your body to get the energy it needs to build muscle and burn fat.

Choosing Healthier Food for Better Health

You should always try to use fresh and organic products. Limiting the amount of chemicals, colorings, preservatives, and additives in your food will benefit your body and decrease the chances of food allergies, sensitivities, and diseases.

Use canola oil, olive oil, and grapeseed oil (a great substitution to butter because of its buttery flavor) which are the healthiest fats for cooking. Those oils, plus flaxseed oil, fish oil, and walnut oil should be used for salads or cold applications. Remember that these are still fats, and you should use as little as possible which is already done in these recipes.

Reduce animal proteins and increase plant proteins such as beans or tofu. Quickly par-boil or steam vegetables to preserve their vitamins and minerals, which will also limit the addition of calories that are often found in casseroles or other vegetable dishes.

Use low-sodium and low-fat broth/stock for light sauces rather than using fats such as butter, cream, or beurre manié (butter and flour combination). Thicken sauces with cornstarch/arrowroot or waxy maze (for frozen dishes as it won't separate) instead of using flour or a flour-butter mixture. As many of these recipes are low in fat, which we know contributes to flavor, try adding flavor with fresh herbs, spices, and vegetable-concentrated broth/stock. Remember that a pinch of salt can go a long way. Way too many recipes use too much salt, which is harmful to your health because it increases blood pressure, and isn't necessary to obtain a well-balanced recipe. ∎

Chef Marie-Annick Courtier is a native of Paris, France, where she learned about gourmet foods and wine in the French tradition. Chef Marie holds a Culinary Arts Degree, has worked with many world renowned chefs, and runs her own personal chef service. A Certified Fitness Nutritionist and Professional Food Manager, she also teaches cooking and created the new Certified Personal Fitness Chef Program. Chef Marie lives in Orange County, California.

One of the most important (and most commonly overlooked) aspects of a healthy diet is proper hydration. As explained on page 30, you can use the formula (0.66 x body weight) to figure out how many ounces of water you need to drink throughout the day.

Breakfast

You have probably heard the phrase "breakfast is the most important meal of the day" many times. With the hectic pace of life today, stopping to eat on your way out the door can seem like a chore. But if you don't take the time to eat first thing in the morning, you will throw off your eating regimen for the rest of the day, and risk undoing all your hard work at the gym!

Be sure to eat breakfast no later than 30 minutes after you wake up. The recipes below are designed to kickstart your day and provide you with the physical and mental energy you will need to get through the morning. Stick to it and you will notice that the first part of your day is a lot easier to handle when you provide your body with the nutrients it needs. Your energy boost is sure to increase your productivity—and encourage your metabolism to work fast, so that the pounds come off easier.

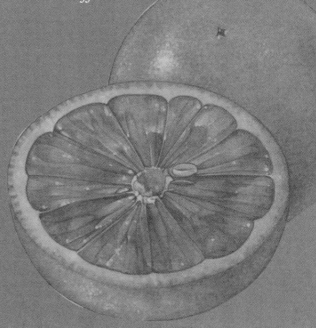

Oatmeal with Mango and Kiwi

Yield: 1 serving

1/2 cup to 3/4 cup oatmeal
1 cup to 1½ cup low-fat milk, hot
1 teaspoon almonds
1/4 mango, diced
1 kiwi, diced

Mix the oatmeal with the hot milk until the liquid is incorporated. Add in the almonds, mango, kiwi, and serve immediately.

Option: Add 1 scoop protein powder which adds 100 calories

Per Serving (1/2 cup oatmeal): 356 Cal (18% from Fat, 15% from Protein, 67% from Carb); 14 g Protein; 7 g Tot Fat; 3 g Sat Fat; 2 g Mono Fat; 63 g Carb; 9 g Fiber; 29 g Sugar; 340 mg Calcium; 2 mg Iron; 105 mg Sodium; 20 mg Cholesterol
Per Serving (3/4 cup oatmeal): 483 Cal (18% from Fat, 16% from Protein, 66% from Carb); 21 g Protein; 10 g Tot Fat; 5 g Sat Fat; 3 g Mono Fat; 84 g Carb; 11 g Fiber; 35 g Sugar; 490 mg Calcium; 2 mg Iron; 156 mg Sodium; 29 mg Cholesterol

Homemade Granola with Berries

Yield: 7 to 10 servings

1/4 cup honey
1/4 cup vegetable oil
1 teaspoon vanilla extract
3 ½ cup old fashioned oats, uncooked
1/4 cup sliced almonds
1/4 cup pumpkin seeds
1/4 cup raisins
1/4 cup cranberries
2 teaspoons cinnamon

Preheat the oven to 350°F.
In a bowl, mix the honey, oil, vanilla extract, and cinnamon. Stir in the oats, almonds, pumpkin seeds, raisins, and cranberries. Mix well and spread over a greased cookie sheet. Bake for 10 minutes. Stir and continue to bake for another 10 minutes or until golden brown. Cool completely and break apart.

Option: Add 1 scoop protein powder which adds 100 calories

Per Serving (1/2 cup homemade granola 1/2 cup low-fat milk, 1/4 cup mixed fresh berries, and 1 teaspoon freshly grinded flaxseeds): 424 Cal (30% from Fat, 14% from Protein, 56% from Carb); 15 g Protein; 15 g Tot Fat; 3 g Sat Fat; 4 g Mono Fat; 61 g Carb; 10 g Fiber; 19 g Sugar; 202 mg Calcium; 3 mg Iron; 54 mg Sodium; 10 mg Cholesterol
Per Serving (3/4 cup homemade granola, 3/4 cup low-fat milk, 1/4 cup mixed fresh berries, and 1 teaspoon freshly grinded flaxseeds): 604 Cal (30% from Fat, 14% from Protein, 56% from Carb); 22 g Protein; 20 g Tot Fat; 5 g Sat Fat; 6 g Mono Fat; 87 g Carb; 13 g Fiber; 28 g Sugar; 295 mg Calcium; 5 mg Iron; 80 mg Sodium; 15 mg Cholesterol

Kashi Flakes with Apples and Walnuts

Yield: 1 serving

1/2 to 3/4 cup Kashi Seven Whole Grains Flakes
1/2 to 3/4 cup low-fat milk, hot or cold
1/4 cup apples
1   tablespoon walnuts
1   teaspoon flaxseeds
Cinnamon to taste

In a bowl mix the cereal with the milk and cinnamon. Top with the apples and walnuts. Sprinkle the freshly ground flaxseeds and serve immediately.

Option: Add 1 scoop protein powder which adds 100 calories

Per Serving (1/2 cup Kashi and 1/2 cup low-fat milk): 228 Cal (33% from Fat, 15% from Protein, 53% from Carb); 9 g Protein; 9 g Tot Fat; 2 g Sat Fat; 2 g Mono Fat; 32 g Carb; 2 g Fiber; 12 g Sugar; 158 mg Calcium; 2 mg Iron; 126 mg Sodium; 10 mg Cholesterol
Per Serving (3/4 cup Kashi and 3/4 cup low-fat milk): 303 Cal (29% from Fat, 15% from Protein, 56% from Carb); 12 g Protein; 10 g Tot Fat; 3 g Sat Fat; 2 g Mono Fat; 45 g Carb; 2 g Fiber; 16 g Sugar; 229 mg Calcium; 3 mg Iron; 189 mg Sodium; 15 mg Cholesterol

Fennel, Leek, and Spinach Omelette

Yield: 1 serving

1/2 teaspoon canola oil
2 to 3 eggs (or 1/2 cup to 3/4 cup egg beaters)
1   tablespoon low-fat milk
3   ounces leek, white part only and thinly sliced
3   ounces fennel bulb, thinly sliced (about 1/2 small bulb)
1/4 cup spinach, thinly sliced
Pinch nutmeg
Salt and pepper to taste

Heat the oil in a nonstick pan over medium heat. Add the leek, fennel, and sauté until tender, about 3 minutes. Add the spinach, lightly season, and sauté another minute or two.

Meanwhile, beat the eggs in a bowl and lightly season to taste. Mix in the nutmeg and pour the mixture into a nonstick pan. Cook until the base of the omelette has set and spread over the cooked vegetables evenly. Reduce heat and continue to cook until almost completely set, about 2 to 3 minutes. Fold over in half, cook for another minute, and serve immediately.

Per Serving (2 eggs): 280 Cal (47% from Fat, 25% from Protein, 29% from Carb); 18 g Protein; 15 g Tot Fat; 4 g Sat Fat; 6 g Mono Fat; 20 g Carb; 4 g Fiber; 5 g Sugar; 179 mg Calcium; 5 mg Iron; 236 mg Sodium; 492 mg Cholesterol
Per Serving (3 eggs): 365 Cal (50% from Fat, 27% from Protein, 23% from Carb); 25 g Protein; 20 g Tot Fat; 6 g Sat Fat; 8 g Mono Fat; 21 g Carb; 4 g Fiber; 6 g Sugar; 210 mg Calcium; 6 mg Iron; 317 mg Sodium; 737 mg Cholesterol

Scrambled Eggs with Tomatoes & Onions

Yield: 1 serving

1   teaspoon olive oil
3   ounces yellow onion, chopped (about 1/2 medium onion)
4   ounces plum tomatoes; peeled, seeded, and chopped (about 1 large tomato)
3   ounces eggplant, skin removed and diced (about 1/2 medium eggplant)
1   garlic clove, minced
1   tablespoon freshly minced basil
2 to 3 eggs (or 1/2 cup to 3/4 cup egg beaters)
Salt and pepper to taste

Heat the oil in a nonstick pan over medium heat. Add the onion and sauté until translucent. Add the tomatoes, eggplant, garlic, and cook until all liquid evaporates.

Beat the eggs in a bowl with the basil and season to taste. Pour the eggs over the vegetables. Cook over medium heat, stirring and scraping the bottom and sides of the pan constantly with a wooden spoon. As soon as the eggs begin to set, remove from heat, continue to stir for a few seconds, and serve immediately.

Per Serving (2 eggs): 292 Cal (50% from Fat, 23% from Protein, 27% from Carb); 17 g Protein; 17 g Tot Fat; 4 g Sat Fat; 8 g Mono Fat; 20 g Carb; 6 g Fiber; 10 g Sugar; 108 mg Calcium; 3 mg Iron; 173 mg Sodium; 491 mg Cholesterol
Per Serving (3 eggs): 377 Cal (53% from Fat, 26% from Protein, 21% from Carb); 25 g Protein; 22 g Tot Fat; 6 g Sat Fat; 10 g Mono Fat; 20 g Carb; 6 g Fiber; 10 g Sugar; 139 mg Calcium; 4 mg Iron; 254 mg Sodium; 736 mg Cholesterol

Poached Eggs over Bell Peppers and Spinach

Yield: 1 serving

2 to 3 eggs
1   teaspoon olive oil
3   ounces onion, thinly sliced (about 1/2 medium onion)
1   garlic clove, minced
3   ounces red bell peppers, seeded, ribs removed, and thinly sliced
    (about 1/2 medium bell pepper)
3   ounces fresh spinach, thinly sliced
1   pinch nutmeg
Salt and pepper to taste

Grease an elongated casserole with olive oil and set aside.

Heat the oil in a nonstick pan over medium heat. Add the onion and sauté until translucent. Add the garlic, bell peppers, and cook for 2 minutes. Add the spinach, nutmeg, and season to taste.

Meanwhile, bring a pan filled with water to boil. Reduce the heat under the boiling water to a point where the water barely bubbles. Break the eggs and slide them one by one into the simmering water. Make sure the eggs do not touch.

Spread the vegetables on the casserole. Using a slotted spoon carefully transfer the eggs to the prepared casserole, sprinkle pepper, and serve immediately.

Per Serving (2 eggs): 309 Cal (47% from Fat, 25% from Protein, 28% from Carb); 20 g Protein; 17 g Tot Fat; 4 g Sat Fat; 8 g Mono Fat; 22 g Carb; 5 g Fiber; 9 g Sugar; 196 mg Calcium; 5 mg Iron; 236 mg Sodium; 491 mg Cholesterol
Per Serving (3 eggs): 394 Cal (50% from Fat, 27% from Protein, 23% from Carb); 27 g Protein; 23 g Tot Fat; 6 g Sat Fat; 10 g Mono Fat; 23 g Carb; 5 g Fiber; 9 g Sugar; 227 mg Calcium; 6 mg Iron; 318 mg Sodium; 736 mg Cholesterol

Cottage Cheese and Fruits

Yield: 1 serving

1/2 cup cottage cheese
1/4 cup pineapple, diced
1/4 cup nectarine, diced
1/4 cup berries
1 teaspoon flaxseeds

Mix the cottage cheese with the flaxseeds. Add in the fruits and refrigerate to chill before use.

Option: Add 1 scoop protein powder which adds 100 calories

Per Serving: 167 Cal (19% from Fat, 40% from Protein, 41% from Carb); 17 g Protein; 4 g Tot Fat; 2 g Sat Fat; 1 g Mono Fat; 17 g Carb; 4 g Fiber; 8 g Sugar; 99 mg Calcium; 1 mg Iron; 461 mg Sodium; 9 mg Cholesterol

Bell Peppers and Turkey Roll

Yield: 1 serving

3 ounces yellow squash, cut into strips (about 1/2 squash)
3 ounces bell peppers, seeded, ribs removed, and cut into strips
(about 1/2 bell pepper)
1 tablespoon sun-dried tomatoes, minced
3 to 4 ounces turkey slices (about 1 ounce each or 3 to 4 slices)
3 to 4 tablespoons eggplant spread
6 to 8 basil leaves
Salt and pepper to taste

Mix the sun-dried tomatoes and eggplant spread in a bowl. Lay each turkey slice on a large cutting board. Spread 1 tablespoon of the prepared mixture and 2 basil leaves over each turkey slice. Divide the bell peppers and zucchini strips equally and season to taste. Roll up each turkey slice and serve immediately.

Per Serving (3 turkey slices): 180 Cal (31% from Fat, 34% from Protein, 34% from Carb); 17 g Protein; 7 g Tot Fat; 1 g Sat Fat; 1 g Mono Fat; 17 g Carb; 3 g Fiber; 7 g Sugar; 32 mg Calcium; 2 mg Iron; 1210 mg Sodium; 35 mg Cholesterol
Per Serving (4 turkey slices): 224 Cal (32% from Fat, 36% from Protein, 32% from Carb); 22 g Protein; 9 g Tot Fat; 1 g Sat Fat; 1 g Mono Fat; 19 g Carb; 3 g Fiber; 8 g Sugar; 35 mg Calcium; 2 mg Iron; 1604 mg Sodium; 46 mg Cholesterol

Chicken and Vegetables Roll

Yield: 1 serving

3 to 4 ounces zucchini, cut into strips (about 1/2 zucchini)
3 to 4 ounces red bell peppers, seeded, ribs removed, and cut
    into strips (about 1/2 bell pepper)
3 to 4 ounces chicken breast slices (about 1 ounce each or 3 to 4 slices)
3 to 4 tablespoons tapenade
Salt and pepper to taste

Lay each chicken slice on a large cutting board. Spread 1 tablespoon of tapenade over each chicken slice. Divide the zucchini and bell pepper strips equally among the chicken slice. Season to taste, roll and serve immediately or refrigerate until needed.

Per Serving (3 chicken slices): 225 Cal (49% from Fat, 28% from Protein, 23% from Carb); 16 g Protein; 13 g Tot Fat; 2 g Sat Fat; 0 g Mono Fat; 13 g Carb; 2 g Fiber; 5 g Sugar; 26 mg Calcium; 1 mg Iron; 1325 mg Sodium; 31 mg Cholesterol
Per Serving (4 chicken slices): 299 Cal (49% from Fat, 28% from Protein, 23% from Carb); 21 g Protein; 17 g Tot Fat; 2 g Sat Fat; 0 g Mono Fat; 18 g Carb; 3 g Fiber; 7 g Sugar; 34 mg Calcium; 1 mg Iron; 1766 mg Sodium; 41 mg Cholesterol

Smoked Salmon Roll

Yield: 1 serving

3 to 4 ounces smoked salmon (about 4 to 5 ½ slices)
12 to 16 asparagus, trimmed (about 12 ounces to 1 pound asparagus)
4 to 5 ½ tablespoons Boursin Light Cheese
Pepper to taste

Preheat a steamer over high heat. Add the asparagus, reduce heat, and cook until desired doneness. Remove from the steamer and blanch in ice cold water to stop the cooking process.

Lay each smoked salmon slice on a large cutting board. Spread 1 tablespoon of Boursin over each slice. Add 3 asparagus per slice, sprinkle pepper to taste, and roll over. For the half salmon slice use one asparagus. Serve immediately or refrigerate until needed.

Per Serving: 264 Cal (33% from Fat, 45% from Protein, 22% from Carb); 31 g Protein; 10 g Tot Fat; 5 g Sat Fat; 2 g Mono Fat; 15 g Carb; 7 g Fiber; 6 g Sugar; 91 mg Calcium; 8 mg Iron; 986 mg Sodium; 32 mg Cholesterol

Fish/Seafood Entrees

A healthy diet should include plenty of fish and some shellfish, good sources of protein, fats, vitamins, and minerals, as well as many essential amino acids. In addition, one of the best sources for Omega-3 are oily fish like cod, tuna, salmon, sardines, herring, mackerel, trout, and anchovies—which are all easier to digest than meat.

You may have already heard about the health benefits of Omega-3 fatty acids, which help promote weight loss while still having a positive effect on the metabolizing of muscle proteins. Keep in mind that the protein levels of shellfish are usually a little lower than fish and, from a nutrition standpoint, can result in higher cholesterol. So be sure not to indulge on shellfish. Cooking fish and shellfish requires particular attention, as the flesh tends to be rather delicate. It is recommended that you use healthier cooking techniques such as steaming, baking, broiling, barbecuing, or sautéing in a nonstick pan with very little oil.

Shrimp with Basil and Garlic

Yield: 2 servings

2 tablespoons olive oil
6 to 8 ounces shrimps, shelled
   and deveined
1 cup onions, sliced (about 1 large onion)
1 cup bell peppers, seeded, ribs removed,
   and sliced (about 2 medium bell peppers)

2 large garlic cloves, minced
1/2 lemon, juiced
2 tablespoons fresh basil, minced
4 to 6 ounces whole wheat pasta
Salt and pepper to taste

Cook the pasta according to package directions.
   Heat 1 tablespoon of oil and the garlic in a large pan over medium heat. Add the shrimp and cook for 1 minute stirring occasionally. In another pan, heat the remaining oil. Add the onion and sauté until translucent. Add the bell pepper and sauté for another couple of minutes. Combine the lemon juice, basil, shrimp and pasta. Season to taste. Mix and continue to sauté for 1 to 2 minutes. Serve immediately.

Per Serving (3 ounces shrimp and 4 ounces cooked pasta): 483 Cal (29% from Fat, 22% from Protein, 49% from Carb); 28 g Protein; 16 g Tot Fat; 2 g Sat Fat; 10 g Mono Fat; 63 g Carb; 4 g Fiber; 5 g Sugar; 138 mg Calcium; 5 mg Iron; 139 mg Sodium; 129 mg Cholesterol
Per Serving (4 ounces shrimp and 6 ounces cooked pasta): 611 Cal (24% from Fat, 24% from Protein, 52% from Carb); 38 g Protein; 17 g Tot Fat; 2 g Sat Fat; 10 g Mono Fat; 84 g Carb; 4 g Fiber; 5 g Sugar; 164 mg Calcium; 7 mg Iron; 183 mg Sodium; 172 mg Cholesterol

Spicy Tuna with Avocado Spread

Yield: 2 servings

2 teaspoons olive oil
Two 3 to 4-ounce tuna fillets
4 ounces red onions, diced (about 1/2 large
   onion)
1 large Roma tomato, peeled and diced
6 ounces yellow bell peppers, seeded, ribs
   removed, and diced (about 1 medium bell
   pepper)

1 jalapeno, seeded and diced
1/2 avocado, puréed
2 tablespoons low-fat yogurt
1 tablespoon cilantro
1/4 lime, juiced
Tabasco
Cajun spices
Salt to taste

Mix the avocado with the lime juice. Mix in the yogurt, jalapeno chiles, cilantro, and season to taste. Add tabasco to taste and refrigerate until needed.
   Preheat the broiler. Sprinkle Cajun spices on both sides of the fillets. Place the fillets on a greased baking sheet and broil for 2 to 3 minutes. Turnover and continue to cook for 3 to 4 minutes or until the fish flesh starts to flake. You may slightly salt before serving.
   Meanwhile, heat the remaining oil in a large pan over medium heat. Add the onion and sauté until translucent. Add the yellow bell peppers and continue to sauté for 2 minutes. Mix in the tomatoes and cook for 2 more minutes. Add a little Cajun spices and lightly salt.
   Plate the vegetables, top with the tuna, avocado spread, and serve immediately.

Per Serving (3 ounces tuna fillet): 279 Cal (40% from Fat, 32% from Protein, 27% from Carb); 24 g Protein; 13 g Tot Fat; 2 g Sat Fat; 8 g Mono Fat; 20 g Carb; 6 g Fiber; 6 g Sugar; 71 mg Calcium; 2 mg Iron; 51 mg Sodium; 40 mg Cholesterol
Per Serving (4 ounces tuna fillet): 309 Cal (37% from Fat, 38% from Protein, 25% from Carb); 30 g Protein; 13 g Tot Fat; 2 g Sat Fat; 8 g Mono Fat; 20 g Carb; 6 g Fiber; 6 g Sugar; 75 mg Calcium; 2 mg Iron; 61 mg Sodium; 53 mg Cholesterol

Sea Scallops with Mandarin Wedges

Yield: 2 servings

2   teaspoons grapeseed oil
6 to 8 ounces sea scallops
2   scallions, chopped
1/2 cup fresh squeezed orange juice
1   teaspoon orange zest

1   mandarin, wedged
1/2 teaspoon rosemary, minced
4   ounces baby carrots
12 ounces zucchini (about 2
    medium zucchini)
Salt and pepper to taste

Pat dry the sea scallops and sprinkle a little pepper on both sides.
   Preheat a steamer over high heat. Add the carrots and cook until barely tender. Add the zucchini and steam for a minute.

   Meanwhile, heat the oil in a large nonstick pan over medium heat. Add the scallops and cook until golden brown, about a minute or so. Turn and continue to cook for 1 to 2 minutes or until cooked through. Do not overcook as the scallops will become tough. Transfer the scallops to a serving platter and cover with aluminum foil to keep warm. Add the scallions and sauté quickly. Add the orange juice, orange zest, rosemary, and bring to a boil. Reduce by half; add the mandarin wedges, parsley, and sauté quickly. Pour over the sea scallops and serve immediately with the steamed carrots and zucchini.

Per Serving (3 ounces sea scallops): 221 Cal (23% from Fat, 31% from Protein, 46% from Carb); 18 g Protein; 6 g Tot Fat; 1 g Sat Fat; 1 g Mono Fat; 27 g Carb; 5 g Fiber; 15 g Sugar; 93 mg Calcium; 2 mg Iron; 198 mg Sodium; 28 mg Cholesterol
Per Serving (4 ounces sea scallops): 246 Cal (22% from Fat, 36% from Protein, 43% from Carb); 23 g Protein; 6 g Tot Fat; 1 g Sat Fat; 1 g Mono Fat; 27 g Carb; 5 g Fiber; 15 g Sugar; 100 mg Calcium; 2 mg Iron; 243 mg Sodium; 37 mg Cholesterol

Broiled Salmon with Pesto

Yield: 2 servings

2   tablespoons olive oil
4   tablespoons basil
2   tablespoons almonds
1   large garlic clove
1   teaspoon fresh thyme
1   teaspoon lemon zest
1   teaspoon lemon juice

Two 3 to 4-ounces salmon fillets
1   cup broccoli
1   cup cherry tomatoes
2   tablespoons Italian breadcrumbs
1/2 lemon cut into 2 wedges
Salt and pepper to taste

In a food processor puree the basil, almonds, garlic, thyme, lemon zest, lemon juice, and olive oil. Season to taste and set aside.

   Preheat the oven to 400° F. Spread the pesto over the salmon fillets and top with Italian breadcrumbs. Grease a baking sheet and add the fillets. Bake for 7 to 8 minutes or until the flesh starts to flake. Time may vary based on the thickness of the fish.

   Meanwhile preheat a steamer over high heat. Turn the broiler on and brown the fish breadcrumbs until golden brown, about 2 minutes. Steam the broccoli for 1 minute. Add the tomatoes and continue to steam for 1 minute. Serve the fillets with the broccoli, tomatoes, and lemon wedges.

Per Serving (3 ounces salmon fillet): 360 Cal (53% from Fat, 25% from Protein, 22% from Carb); 24 g Protein; 22 g Tot Fat; 3 g Sat Fat; 14 g Mono Fat; 21 g Carb; 5 g Fiber; 4 g Sugar; 328 mg Calcium; 3 mg Iron; 136 mg Sodium; 33 mg Cholesterol
Per Serving (4 ounces salmon fillet): 400 Cal (51% from Fat, 29% from Protein, 20% from Carb); 30 g Protein; 24 g Tot Fat; 4 g Sat Fat; 14 g Mono Fat; 21 g Carb; 5 g Fiber; 4 g Sugar; 398 mg Calcium; 3 mg Iron; 157 mg Sodium; 44 mg Cholesterol

Steamed Salmon with Fennel

Yield: 2 servings

Two 3 to 4-ounce salmon fillets
2   ounces leeks, white part only and julienned (about 1/2 leek)
2   ounces carrots, julienned (about 1/2 small carrot)
12 ounces fennel bulbs, julienned (about 1 large bulb)
1   garlic clove, minced
2   tablespoons Pastis or anisette (You may substitute vegetable stock)
2   pinches Herbs de Provence
1   teaspoon fennel seeds
Salt and pepper to taste

Preheat the oven to 400° F.
   Prepare two aluminum foil packets. Place the vegetables in the center of the foil, spread the fennel seeds, and season to taste. Top with the seasoned fish and sprinkle the Herbs de Provence. Fold the aluminum foil a bit; add the Pastis, and close tightly. Place on a baking dish and bake for 10 to 12 minutes or until the salmon starts to flake. Transfer each foil to a serving plate, open carefully, and serve immediately.

Per Serving (3 ounces salmon fillet): 233 Cal (20% from Fat, 37% from Protein, 42% from Carb); 22 g Protein; 5 g Tot Fat; 1 g Sat Fat; 2 g Mono Fat; 25 g Carb; 7 g Fiber; 3 g Sugar; 360 mg Calcium; 3 mg Iron; 273 mg Sodium; 33 mg Cholesterol
Per Serving (4 ounces salmon fillet): 273 Cal (23% from Fat, 41% from Protein, 37% from Carb); 28 g Protein; 7 g Tot Fat; 2 g Sat Fat; 2 g Mono Fat; 25 g Carb; 7 g Fiber; 3 g Sugar; 430 mg Calcium; 3 mg Iron; 294 mg Sodium; 44 mg Cholesterol

Cod Fish with Jicama & Red Bell Pepper Slaw

Yield: 2 servings

1   teaspoon olive oil
Two 3 to 4-ounce cod fillets
6   ounces Jicama, julienned (about 1 medium Jicama)
6   ounces red bell peppers, seeded, ribs removed and julienned (about 1 medium red bell pepper)
4   ounces carrots, julienned (about 1 small carrot)
1   green onion, julienned
2   tablespoons olive oil
2   tablespoons lime juice
2   tablespoon fresh parsley, minced
3   pinches ground cumin
Salt and pepper to taste

Place the julienned Jicama, red bell peppers, carrots, and green onions in a bowl. Whisk 2 tablespoons olive oil, lime juice, parsley, and two pinches ground cumin. Add the dressing to the vegetables, season to taste, mix well, and set aside.

   Sprinkle pepper and ground cumin over both sides of the fish. Heat 1 teaspoon olive oil in nonstick pan over medium heat. Add the fish and sauté until golden brown, about 2 minutes. Turnover and continue to cook until the fish starts to flake.

   Meanwhile, quickly sauté the prepared slaw in a nonstick pan over medium heat. Lightly season the cod fillets with salt, if desired.

   Transfer the slaw to two serving plates, top with the cod fillets, and serve immediately.

Per Serving (3 ounces cod fillet): 297 Cal (50% from Fat, 23% from Protein, 27% from Carb); 18 g Protein; 17 g Tot Fat; 2 g Sat Fat; 12 g Mono Fat; 21 g Carb; 8 g Fiber; 8 g Sugar; 65 mg Calcium; 2 mg Iron; 95 mg Sodium; 37 mg Cholesterol
Per Serving (4 ounces cod fillet): 320 Cal (47% from Fat, 28% from Protein, 25% from Carb); 23 g Protein; 17 g Tot Fat; 2 g Sat Fat; 12 g Mono Fat; 21 g Carb; 8 g Fiber; 8 g Sugar; 70 mg Calcium; 2 mg Iron; 110 mg Sodium; 49 mg Cholesterol

Jamaican Red Snapper

Yield: 2 servings

Two 3 to 4-ounce red snapper fillets
5   ounces carrots cut into thin diagonal
    slices (about 1 medium carrot)
5   ounces yellow squash cut into thin diago-
    nal slices (about 1 medium squash)
6   ounces pea pods
1   large garlic clove, minced

1   tablespoon fresh ginger, minced
1   teaspoon low-sodium soy sauce
2   tablespoons chives, chopped
2   teaspoons sesame oil
Jamaican jerk spices or rub
Salt and pepper to taste

Preheat a pan with water. Parboil each vegetable (carrots, squash, and pea pods) separately and until barely tender. Blanch immediately in ice cold water to stop the cooking process.

Preheat the broiler with the rack five inches away from the broiler. Spread the spices over the fillets and place them on a greased cookie sheet. Broil for a few minutes or until the fillets starts to flake. Time may vary based on thickness.

Meanwhile, heat the oil in a large nonstick pan over medium heat. Sauté the ginger and garlic quickly. Add the vegetables and sauté for another minute. Add the soy sauce, chives, and season with pepper. Bring to a boil and serve immediately with the red snapper fillets.

Per Serving (3 ounces red snapper fillet): 227 Cal (24% from Fat, 39% from Protein, 37% from Carb); 23 g Protein; 6 g Tot Fat; 1 g Sat Fat; 2 g Mono Fat; 21 g Carb; 6 g Fiber; 8 g Sugar; 127 mg Calcium; 3 mg Iron; 263 mg Sodium; 31 mg Cholesterol
Per Serving (4 ounces red snapper fillet): 255 Cal (23% from Fat, 44% from Protein, 33% from Carb); 28 g Protein; 7 g Tot Fat; 1 g Sat Fat; 2 g Mono Fat; 21 g Carb; 6 g Fiber; 8 g Sugar; 136 mg Calcium; 3 mg Iron; 281 mg Sodium; 42 mg Cholesterol

Ahi Tartar

Yield: 2 servings

Two 3 to 4-ounce Ahi fillets
2   tablespoons shallots, chopped
4   ounces cucumbers (about 1/3
    large cucumber)
1   lemon
1   lime
3   ounces red bell peppers, seeded and ribs
    removed, diced (about1/2 medium
    red bell pepper)

1   jalapeno chile, seeded and diced
1   sage leaf
2   tablespoons basil, chopped
1/2 teaspoon green tea
1/2 teaspoon honey
2   tablespoons olive oil
1   cup baby lettuce mix
Salt and pepper to taste

Take nice strips of the lemon and lime zests. Mince and set aside. Juice the lemon, lime, and set aside. Cut the cucumber in half and remove seeds. Cut into half again and dice. Warm up on low heat the lemon juice, lime juice, tea powder, and sage until the honey is well incorporated. Remove and cool down. Refrigerate to get cold.

Dice the Ahi, place it into a soup plate and season to taste. Mix in the shallot, cucumber, red bell pepper, jalapeno chiles, and basil. Drizzle half of the olive oil, add the cold marinade, and refrigerate for 20 to 30 minutes.

Equally divide the baby greens among two ice cold plates. With a slotted spoon, scoop out the Ahi Tartar. Drizzle a little bit of the marinade, the remaining olive oil, and serve immediately.

Per Serving (3 ounces Ahi): 298 Cal (51% from Fat, 28% from Protein, 21% from Carb); 22 g Protein; 18 g Tot Fat; 3 g Sat Fat; 11 g Mono Fat; 17 g Carb; 5 g Fiber; 5 g Sugar; 74 mg Calcium; 2 mg Iron; 42 mg Sodium; 32 mg Cholesterol
Per Serving (4 ounces Ahi): 339 Cal (49% from Fat, 32% from Protein, 19% from Carb); 29 g Protein; 20 g Tot Fat; 3 g Sat Fat; 12 g Mono Fat; 17 g Carb; 5 g Fiber; 5 g Sugar; 76 mg Calcium; 2 mg Iron; 53 mg Sodium; 43 mg Cholesterol

Meat / Poultry Entrees

I t is important to your health that you choose a good source of protein and make sure you get the right amount. You may already know that animal protein is not as healthy for you as the protein from fresh fruits and vegetables; this is because meat can raise cholesterol levels. To minimize cholesterol, look for lean protein sources. Additionally, seek out organic meat. This is healthier for you, due to the animal's natural diet.

Here are some good general rules for selecting meat: choose venison or ostrich over beef, and choose white meat such as chicken or turkey breast over darker meat. Note that lamb and pork, which are higher in fat, should be eaten sparingly, (this is why you will find only one recipe for each in this section.) When you do eat pork, choose pork loin tender cuts and employ healthy cooking techniques, such as those described on the following pages, which will limit the addition of fat and calories during preparation while also preserving the succulent flavor of the meat.

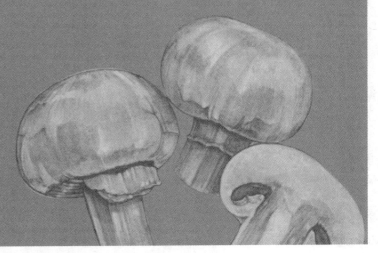

Chicken Burgers with Lettuce Wraps

Yield: 2 servings

Two 3 to 4-ounce chicken burgers
2   garlic cloves, minced
2   tablespoons low-cal Caesar dressing
1   white anchovy fillet

8   lettuce leaves
2   tablespoons Parmesan Cheese
Canola oil
Salt and pepper to taste

In a food processor, puree the anchovy fillet with the dressing. Add a little water to thin out. Lightly season the burgers and shape them to fit in the lettuce leaves. Do not allow the meat to touch the leaves. Heat up 2 tablespoons olive oil with the minced garlic. Remove at the first boil and set aside.

Preheat the grill on medium high heat. Don't forget to grease the grill before adding the burgers. Cook them for 3 to 5 minutes on each side or until cooked through. Meanwhile, carefully brush the garlic oil over the lettuce leaves.

Place two leaves on a plate, top with one burger, spread 1 tablespoon Caesar dressing, sprinkle cheese and fold a bit over the top. Top with 2 more leaves and tuck underneath to seal. Serve immediately with your favorite accompaniment. You may use toothpick to hold for presentation.

Suggestion: Serve with Eggplant Mediterranean

Per Serving (3 ounces chicken burger): 334 Cal (52% from Fat, 37% from Protein, 11% from Carb); 31 g Protein; 19 g Tot Fat; 4 g Sat Fat; 12 g Mono Fat; 9 g Carb; 1 g Fiber; 3 g Sugar; 131 mg Calcium; 2 mg Iron; 408 mg Sodium; 80 mg Cholesterol
Per Serving (4 ounces chicken burger): 381 Cal (49% from Fat, 42% from Protein, 9% from Carb); 40 g Protein; 20 g Tot Fat; 4 g Sat Fat; 12 g Mono Fat; 9 g Carb; 1 g Fiber; 3 g Sugar; 135 mg Calcium; 2 mg Iron; 429 mg Sodium; 104 mg Cholesterol

Lamb Chops with Garlic Spread

Yield: 2 servings

3   teaspoons olive oil
Two 3 to 4-ounce loin lamb chops
1   tablespoon minced garlic
1   teaspoon parsley
1   teaspoon minced rosemary
1/4 teaspoon dry crushed red pepper
2   cups green beans
Salt and pepper to taste

Bring to a boil enough water to cover the green beans. Add 1 teaspoon of salt, the green beans, and bring to boil. Reduce heat and simmer until tender. Drain and transfer to a serving bowl. Add 1 teaspoon olive oil, season to taste, and mix well.

Mix 1 teaspoon olive oil, garlic, parsley, rosemary, and dry crushed red pepper in a bowl. Rub the garlic spread over the lamb chops.

Heat the remaining olive oil in a nonstick pan over medium heat. Add the lamb chops and cook for 3 to 4 minutes on each side or until desired. Serve immediately with the prepared green beans.

Per Serving (3 ounces lamb chops): 213 Cal (46% from Fat, 36% from Protein, 17% from Carb); 20 g Protein; 11 g Tot Fat; 3 g Sat Fat; 7 g Mono Fat; 9 g Carb; 4 g Fiber; 2 g Sugar; 58 mg Calcium; 3 mg Iron; 62 mg Sodium; 54 mg Cholesterol
Per Serving (4 ounces lamb chops): 250 Cal (45% from Fat, 40% from Protein, 15% from Carb); 25 g Protein; 12 g Tot Fat; 3 g Sat Fat; 7 g Mono Fat; 9 g Carb; 4 g Fiber; 2 g Sugar; 60 mg Calcium; 4 mg Iron; 81 mg Sodium; 73 mg Cholesterol

New York Steaks with Mushrooms and Onions

Yield: 2 servings

Two 3 to 4-ounce New York steaks
2 teaspoons olive oil
8 ounces onions, sliced (about 1 large onion)
8 ounces mushrooms, sliced
1 garlic clove, minced
1 tablespoon parsley, minced
2 tablespoons Dijon mustard
Salt and pepper to taste

Preheat the broiler. Brush a little olive oil over the steaks and season with pepper. Broil for 3 to 5 minutes on each side or until desired. Sprinkle a little salt before serving.

Meanwhile, heat 1 teaspoon olive oil in a nonstick pan over medium heat. Add the onions and slightly brown. Add the mushrooms, garlic, and continue to cook until the mushrooms are barely tender. Add the parsley and season to taste.

Plate the vegetables in the center of a serving platter and top with the steaks. Serve with Dijon mustard on the side.

Per Serving (3 ounces New York Steak): 340 Cal (42% from Fat, 34% from Protein, 24% from Carb); 29 g Protein; 16 g Tot Fat; 5 g Sat Fat; 8 g Mono Fat; 21 g Carb; 4 g Fiber; 8 g Sugar; 88 mg Calcium; 3 mg Iron; 235 mg Sodium; 57 mg Cholesterol
Per Serving (4 ounces New York Steak): 405 Cal (44% from Fat, 36% from Protein, 21% from Carb); 37 g Protein; 20 g Tot Fat; 6 g Sat Fat; 10 g Mono Fat; 21 g Carb; 4 g Fiber; 8 g Sugar; 94 mg Calcium; 3 mg Iron; 251 mg Sodium; 76 mg Cholesterol

Chicken Breasts with Tomato Sauce

Yield: 2 servings

1 teaspoon olive oil
Two 3 to 4-ounce chicken breasts
4 small Roma tomatoes (about 1 pound)
3/4 cup pearl onions

1/4 cup dry white wine
1 pinch Italian herbs
1 tablespoon fresh basil, minced
Salt and pepper to taste

Par-boil the pearl onions for a couple of minutes. Remove the pearl onions from the water and let cool. Peel them and set aside.

Make a small X incision into the tops of the tomatoes. Heat some water over high heat and bring to boil. Blanch the tomatoes for 15 to 20 seconds. Remove and place in ice-cold water to stop the cooking process. Peel, seed, and dice the tomatoes.

Heat the oil in a large saucepan. Add the chicken and sauté until golden brown. Turnover and continue to cook for 2 minutes. Deglaze the pan with the wine and reduce a little. Add the tomatoes, pearl onions, Italian herbs, and season to taste. Reduce heat and cook for 10 minutes or until the chicken is cooked through. Add the basil and cook for another minute. Transfer to a serving platter and serve immediately.

Suggestion: Serve with wild rice and mushrooms

Per Serving (3 ounces chicken breast): 211 Cal (18% from Fat, 46% from Protein, 36% from Carb); 23 g Protein; 4 g Tot Fat; 1 g Sat Fat; 2 g Mono Fat; 17 g Carb; 4 g Fiber; 10 g Sugar; 64 mg Calcium; 2 mg Iron; 71 mg Sodium; 49 mg Cholesterol
Per Serving (4 ounces chicken breast): 242 Cal (17% from Fat, 52% from Protein, 31% from Carb); 29 g Protein; 4 g Tot Fat; 1 g Sat Fat; 2 g Mono Fat; 17 g Carb; 4 g Fiber; 10 g Sugar; 67 mg Calcium; 2 mg Iron; 89 mg Sodium; 66 mg Cholesterol

Chicken Breasts with Spinach and Pepper Jack

Yield: 2 servings

1   teaspoon olive oil
Two 3 to 4-ounce chicken breasts
2   pepper jack cheese slices
8   spinach leaves, cleaned and pat dry
1   shallot, minced
1/4 cup chicken stock

Italian herbs
2   cups fresh spinach, cleaned and pat dry
1   lemon
Salt and pepper to taste
Twine

Place the chicken breasts between two plastic wrap sheets. Flatten with a mallet until fairly thin. Sprinkle pepper and Italian herbs. Add one slice of pepper jack cheese and the spinach leaves. Roll tightly making sure the cheese has no way out and secure with twine.

Heat the oil in a sauté pan over high heat. Add the chicken rolls, placing the folded side down first. Brown and turn over. Once browned, add the shallot, stock, a teaspoon lemon juice, a pinch of Italian herbs, and bring to boil. Reduce heat, cover, and continue to cook for 10 minutes.

Meanwhile, preheat a steamer. Add the spinach and cook for a minute or until barely wilted. Serve immediately with the chicken rolls and lemon wedges.

Per Serving (3 ounces chicken breast): 265 Cal (42% from Fat, 41% from Protein, 17% from Carb); 29 g Protein; 13 g Tot Fat; 6 g Sat Fat; 5 g Mono Fat; 12 g Carb; 4 g Fiber; 1 g Sugar; 288 mg Calcium; 3 mg Iron; 368 mg Sodium; 76 mg Cholesterol
Per Serving (4 ounces chicken breast): 297 Cal (39% from Fat, 46% from Protein, 15% from Carb); 35 g Protein; 13 g Tot Fat; 6 g Sat Fat; 5 g Mono Fat; 12 g Carb; 4 g Fiber; 1 g Sugar; 291 mg Calcium; 3 mg Iron; 386 mg Sodium; 93 mg Cholesterol

Roasted Cornish Hen with Chinese Five Spices Blend

Yield: 2 servings

1 Cornish hen
1 teaspoon sesame oil
1 tablespoon honey
1 teaspoon Oriental hot mustard
1 teaspoon ginger, minced
1 teaspoon garlic, minced
1 teaspoon Chinese Five Spices Blend
Salt and pepper to taste

Preheat the oven to 350°F.

Wash and pat dry the hen. Combine the honey, mustard, ginger, garlic, and spices. Brush the mixture over the hen. Roast for an hour or until the juices come out clear. Time may vary based on the hen size. Cut the hen in half and transfer to a serving platter. Drizzle sesame oil and serve immediately.

Suggestion: Serve with Snap Peas with Garlic

Per Serving (1/2 Cornish hen): 393 Cal (60% from Fat, 30% from Protein, 10% from Carb); 29 g Protein; 26 g Tot Fat; 7 g Sat Fat; 11 g Mono Fat; 9 g Carb; 0 g Fiber; 9 g Sugar; 23 mg Calcium; 1 mg Iron; 103 mg Sodium; 170 mg Cholesterol

Venison with Spicy Raspberry Sauce

Yield: 2 servings

2   teaspoons grapeseed oil
Two 3 to 4-ounce venison steaks
1   small shallot, minced
1/4 to 1/2 teaspoon black peppercorns,
    crushed (based on how spicy you like)
1   pinch dry thyme
2   tablespoons aged balsamic vinegar

1/2 cup Cabernet Sauvignon
1/2 cup raspberries
2   tablespoons demi-glace (if not available,
    substitute brown sauce)
1   tablespoon freshly minced parsley
Salt and pepper to taste

Puree half the raspberries in a food processor. Pass through a sieve and set aside.
    Heat the oil in a nonstick pan over medium-high heat. Add the venison steaks and sauté until golden brown. Turnover and continue to cook for 2 to 3 minutes. Transfer the steaks to a plate and cover with aluminum foil to keep warm. Add the shallots, peppercorns, thyme, vinegar, wine, raspberry sauce, and deglaze the pan. Bring to a boil and reduce liquid by half. Add demi-glace, steaks juices, season to taste, and bring to a boil. Add the steaks, remaining raspberries, and continue to simmer for a minute. Serve immediately.

Serve with Green Beans and Almonds

Per Serving (3 ounces venison loin): 216 Cal (35% from Fat, 47% from Protein, 19% from Carb); 21 g Protein; 7 g Tot Fat; 1 g Sat Fat; 1 g Mono Fat; 8 g Carb; 2 g Fiber; 2 g Sugar; 28 mg Calcium; 4 mg Iron; 99 mg Sodium; 72 mg Cholesterol
Per Serving (4 ounces venison loin): 250 Cal (32% from Fat, 52% from Protein, 16% from Carb); 27 g Protein; 8 g Tot Fat; 2 g Sat Fat; 2 g Mono Fat; 8 g Carb; 2 g Fiber; 2 g Sugar; 29 mg Calcium; 5 mg Iron; 113 mg Sodium; 96 mg Cholesterol

Turkey Breast with Italian Herbs

Yield: 8 to 10 servings

1 tablespoon olive oil
2 pounds turkey breast (with skin)
4 teaspoons Italian herbs
A bunch of fresh basil leaves
1/4 cup chicken stock
Salt and pepper to taste

Preheat the oven to 350° F.
    Mix 1 tablespoon of Italian herbs with a little pepper. Spread all over the turkey breast under its skin. Add as many basil leaves as you can fit under the skin without breaking it. Brush olive oil over the skin.
    Place the turkey breast skin side up in a roasting pan. Pour 1/4 cup of chicken stock in the pan, add the remaining Italian herbs, and bake for an hour or until a meat thermometer registers 180° F. Keep moistening with chicken stock. Do not allow the pan to get dry in order to keep the turkey breast moist. Transfer the turkey breast to a platter and let cool before slicing.

Great way to prepare your own turkey breast meat for salads, sandwiches, rolls, etc....

Per Serving (10 servings of 3 ounces): 159 Cal (46% from Fat, 52% from Protein, 2% from Carb); 20 g Protein; 8 g Tot Fat; 2 g Sat Fat; 3 g Mono Fat; 1 g Carb; 0 g Fiber; 0 g Sugar; 21 mg Calcium; 2 mg Iron; 95 mg Sodium; 59 mg Cholesterol
Per Serving (8 servings of 4 ounces): 199 Cal (46% from Fat, 52% from Protein, 2% from Carb); 25 g Protein; 10 g Tot Fat; 2 g Sat Fat; 4 g Mono Fat; 1 g Carb; 0 g Fiber; 0 g Sugar; 26 mg Calcium; 2 mg Iron; 119 mg Sodium; 74 mg Cholesterol

Pork Loin with Figs

Yield: 2 servings

8 to 10 ounces pork loin
1   teaspoon olive oil
4   figs
1/2 orange
1/4 cup Chardonnay wine
1   tablespoon honey

1/2 cup veal stock
1   fresh rosemary branch
1   acorn squash, halved and seeded
2   teaspoons sliced almonds
Salt and pepper to taste

Preheat the broiler. Cover a baking sheet with parchment paper. Spread over the almonds and brown under the broiler. Remove from the pan and set aside for later use.

Preheat the oven to 350° F.

Place the loin in a roasting pan, rub with a little oil, and sprinkle pepper. Bake until the inside temperature reaches 185° F.

Make an X incision into the top of the figs. Place the figs and the acorn squash (cut side down) into a baking pan. Bring to a boil the orange juice, wine, and honey in a saucepan over high heat. Mix well and pour over the figs and acorn squash. Bake for 30 minutes at 350° F spooning the sauce over every 10 minutes.

Remove the roast from the pan and set aside in a plate. Sprinkle salt to taste. Cover with aluminum foil to keep warm. Allow 10 to 15 minutes before slicing.

Deglaze the pan with the stock and scrape out all the particles in the bottom and side of the pan. Add the rosemary branch and pour in the sauce rendered by the acorn and figs. Bring to boil and reduce to concentrate flavors. If necessary, thicken with a little cornstarch water mixture and bring to a boil. Add the parsley, any rendered meat juices, and bring to a boil. Adjust seasonings and pour over the loin. Serve immediately with the figs and acorn squash.

Per Serving (3 ounces pork loin): 434 Cal (16% from Fat, 26% from Protein, 58% from Carb); 29 g Protein; 8 g Tot Fat; 2 g Sat Fat; 4 g Mono Fat; 63 g Carb; 9 g Fiber; 30 g Sugar; 165 mg Calcium; 4 mg Iron; 187 mg Sodium; 74 mg Cholesterol
Per Serving (4 ounces pork loin): 468 Cal (17% from Fat, 29% from Protein, 54% from Carb); 35 g Protein; 9 g Tot Fat; 2 g Sat Fat; 5 g Mono Fat; 63 g Carb; 9 g Fiber; 30 g Sugar; 166 mg Calcium; 5 mg Iron; 201 mg Sodium; 92 mg Cholesterol

Soups/Salads

Soups and salads are very versatile and can be served as an appetizer, main course, side dish, or even dessert. They're quick and healthy meal options, and can be a great way to use left-overs. In addition, salad recipes don't require much cooking knowledge, as the techniques used here are very basic.

Here are a few important things to keep in mind whenever you prepare soup or a salad. First, stay away from croutons in soups and avoid unhealthy salad dressings. Healthy dressing choices include oil and vinegar or citrus juice with fresh herbs, and apple cider vinegar can be beneficial to your health due to its cleansing and healing properties. Be careful not to overcook the vegetables you add to soup bases as they will lose their nutrients. This can be tricky because a soup's ingredients will continue to cook as long as the soup is hot, even after you've taken the soup off the stove. Try to undercook the vegetables to allow for that extra time and to preserve their nutritive values. Use dry herbs at first and finish with fresh herbs (using fresh herbs at the beginning will only be a waste of money, as the flavors will evaporate during the cooking process.) For balanced nutrition, be sure to include lean proteins, complex carbohydrates, and vegetables in your soups and salads.

Beans, Vegetables, and Avocado Salad

Yield: 7 to 10 servings.

4 ounces garbanzos
4 ounces black beans
4 ounces red beans
4 ounces green beans, trimmed and cut into
    bite sized pieces
1 ounce red onions, diced (about
    1/4 small onion)
8 ounces tomatoes, diced (about
    2 small tomatoes)

1 garlic clove, minced
2 tablespoons olive oil
1/4 cup white balsamic vinegar
1 ½ tablespoons freshly minced salad herbs
1 avocado, diced
Salt and pepper to taste

In a bowl mix the garlic, oil, vinegar, and herbs.
   Cook the beans separately following the packages instructions. Generally, it takes about 30 to 45 minutes to cook these types of beans.

   Place the green beans with a little salt in a pan and bring to a boil over high heat. Cook to desired. Strain and place immediately in ice-cold water to stop the cooking process. Strain and pat dry.

   Place all the beans and red onions in a large bowl. Add the tomatoes and dressing. Season to taste and refrigerate for an hour. Before serving, add the avocado.

Per Serving (3 ounces): 184 Cal (30% from Fat, 17% from Protein, 53% from Carb); 8 g Protein; 6 g Tot Fat; 1 g Sat Fat; 4 g Mono Fat; 26 g Carb; 8 g Fiber; 3 g Sugar; 57 mg Calcium; 3 mg Iron; 10 mg Sodium; 0 mg Cholesterol
Per Serving (4 ounces): 246 Cal (30% from Fat, 17% from Protein, 53% from Carb); 11 g Protein; 9 g Tot Fat; 1 g Sat Fat; 5 g Mono Fat; 34 g Carb; 11 g Fiber; 4 g Sugar; 76 mg Calcium; 3 mg Iron; 14 mg Sodium; 0 mg Cholesterol

Beets and Chicken Salad

Yield: 2 servings

10 ounces cooked beets, trimmed and diced
4   ounces Romaine heart leaves
1/3 small onion, diced
1/4 cup walnuts
1   small apple, diced and mixed with a little lemon juice (about 4 ounces)
Two 3 to 4-ounce cooked chicken breasts, diced
2   tablespoons vinaigrette
Salt and pepper to taste

Place the beets, romaine leaves, red onion, and chicken in a large bowl. Mix in the vinaigrette and adjust seasoning. Equally divide the salad in two plates. Top with the diced apple, walnut, and serve immediately.

Option: Add 2 tablespoons feta cheese

Per Serving (3 ounces chicken breast): 311 Cal (40% from Fat, 24% from Protein, 36% from Carb); 20 g Protein; 15 g Tot Fat; 2 g Sat Fat; 2 g Mono Fat; 30 g Carb; 7 g Fiber; 18 g Sugar; 69 mg Calcium; 3 mg Iron; 1283 mg Sodium; 31 mg Cholesterol
Per Serving (4 ounces chicken breast): 334 Cal (37% from Fat, 28% from Protein, 35% from Carb); 25 g Protein; 15 g Tot Fat; 2 g Sat Fat; 2 g Mono Fat; 31 g Carb; 7 g Fiber; 19 g Sugar; 71 mg Calcium; 3 mg Iron; 1592 mg Sodium; 41 mg Cholesterol
Per Serving (feta cheese): 25 Cal (72% from Fat, 21% from Protein, 6% from Carb); 1 g Protein; 2 g Tot Fat; 1 g Sat Fat; 0 g Mono Fat; 0 g Carb; 0 g Fiber; 0 g Sugar; 46 mg Calcium; 0 mg Iron

Grapefruit and Crabmeat Salad

Yield: 2 servings

1 large pink grapefruit (about 16 ounces grapefruit)
Two 3 to 4-ounce crabmeat portions (without excess water)
2 tablespoons low-fat canola mayonnaise
1 cup lettuce, shredded
1 tablespoon freshly minced cilantro
Chili powder to taste
Salt and pepper to taste

Place the crabmeat in a bowl.
Cut the grapefruit in half. Insert a thin knife all around the skin to loosen up the flesh. Separate the flesh from the skin and place the flesh on a cutting board. Dice the flesh small and transfer to the crabmeat bowl. Add mayonnaise, chili powder, cilantro, and season to taste. Cover with plastic wrap and refrigerate for half an hour.
Equally divide the lettuce in two plates and top with the prepared grapefruit crabmeat salad.

Per Serving (3 ounces crabmeat): 192 Cal (19% from Fat, 37% from Protein, 43% from Carb); 18 g Protein; 4 g Tot Fat; 1 g Sat Fat; 1 g Mono Fat; 21 g Carb; 3 g Fiber; 16 g Sugar; 88 mg Calcium; 1 mg Iron; 936 mg Sodium; 48 mg Cholesterol
Per Serving (4 ounces crabmeat): 219 Cal (19% from Fat, 43% from Protein, 38% from Carb); 24 g Protein; 5 g Tot Fat; 1 g Sat Fat; 1 g Mono Fat; 21 g Carb; 3 g Fiber; 16 g Sugar; 105 mg Calcium; 1 mg Iron; 1240 mg Sodium; 63 mg Cholesterol

---

Salmon and Vegetables Carpaccio

Yield: 2 servings

6 to 8 ounces smoked salmon thin slices
8 ounces cucumber, peeled (about 1 medium cucumber)
8 ounces yellow squash, peeled (about 1 large yellow squash)
2 green onions, minced
2 teaspoons fresh dill, minced
4 tablespoons olive oil
1 lemon
Salt and pepper to taste

Remove a couple of zest strips from the lemon and mince. Juice the lemon and set aside in a bowl. Add the olive oil, 1 teaspoon dill, half of the prepared zest, and season to taste.
Thinly slice the cucumber and the zucchini. Refrigerate until use.
Equally divide the salmon in two plates, season to taste, and sprinkle dill. Pour half the dressing over and refrigerate for 20 minutes. In the center of the salmon slices and in a round formation, alternate the cucumber and zucchini slices. Season lightly and garnish with the green onions, remaining zest and dill. Pour over the remaining dressing and serve immediately.

Per Serving (3 ounces smoked salmon): 388 Cal (69% from Fat, 18% from Protein, 13% from Carb); 19 g Protein; 31 g Tot Fat; 5 g Sat Fat; 22 g Mono Fat; 14 g Carb; 5 g Fiber; 4 g Sugar; 104 mg Calcium; 3 mg Iron; 687 mg Sodium; 20 mg Cholesterol
Per Serving (4 ounces smoked salmon): 421 Cal (66% from Fat, 22% from Protein, 12% from Carb); 24 g Protein; 33 g Tot Fat; 5 g Sat Fat; 22 g Mono Fat; 14 g Carb; 5 g Fiber; 4 g Sugar; 107 mg Calcium; 3 mg Iron; 910 mg Sodium; 26 mg Cholesterol

Calamari Salad

Yield: 2 to 4 servings

8 to 10 ounces Calamari or squids
1 garlic clove, minced
2 tablespoons olive oil
1/2 lemon, juiced
4 ounces baby greens
6 ounces red bell peppers, chopped (about 1 medium red bell pepper)
4 ounces tomatoes, sliced (about 1 small tomato)
2 ounces red onions, sliced (about 1/2 small onion)
1 tablespoon freshly minced basil
Salt and pepper to taste

Clean and then cut the calamari into bite size pieces. Boil the calamari in water for 20 minutes or until tender. Drain and transfer to a serving bowl. Add the garlic, olive oil, lemon juice, half the basil, and season to taste. Refrigerate for a few hours to allow marinade to flavor the calamari.

Dress up four plates with lettuce and top with the marinated calamari. Equally divide the red bell pepper, tomato, red onion among the four plates. Sprinkle a little more fresh basil and serve immediately.

Option: You may substitute frozen, cleaned calamari.

Per Serving (4 ounces calamari): 298 Cal (45% from Fat, 27% from Protein, 28% from Carb); 21 g Protein; 16 g Tot Fat; 2 g Sat Fat; 10 g Mono Fat; 22 g Carb; 5 g Fiber; 5 g Sugar; 121 mg Calcium; 2 mg Iron; 76 mg Sodium; 264 mg Cholesterol
Per Serving (5 ounces calamari): 324 Cal (43% from Fat, 30% from Protein, 27% from Carb); 26 g Protein; 16 g Tot Fat; 2 g Sat Fat; 10 g Mono Fat; 23 g Carb; 5 g Fiber; 5 g Sugar; 130 mg Calcium; 3 mg Iron; 88 mg Sodium; 330 mg Cholesterol

Seared Ahi Salad

Yield: 2 servings

Two 3 to 4-ounce Ahi fillets, Sushi grade
4 ounces mixed greens
6 cherry tomatoes
4 ounces carrots, sliced diagonally
2 ounces daikon, sliced
2 ounces sugar snap peas
1 teaspoon sesame oil

1 teaspoon soy sauce
1 tablespoon lime juice
4 teaspoons olive oil
1 teaspoon ginger, minced
1 lime
Salt and pepper to taste

Mix the sesame oil, soy sauce, lime juice, 1 tablespoon olive oil, and ginger together in a bowl. Season with pepper.

Par-boil the carrot and sugar snap peas to desired tenderness. Transfer to an ice-cold water bath to stop the cooking process. Pat dry and set aside.

Mix the greens, carrots, daikon, and sugar snap peas in a bowl with the prepared dressing. Equally divide among two plates and refrigerate until use.

Preheat 1 teaspoon olive oil in a nonstick pan over high heat. Season the fish with pepper and light salt. Sear the fish for 2 minutes on both sides. You may sear longer, if you want the center of the fish more cooked.

Slice the fish and spread over the top of the prepared salad. Serve immediately with lime wedges.

Per Serving (3 ounces Ahi): 306 Cal (46% from Fat, 30% from Protein, 24% from Carb); 24 g Protein; 16 g Tot Fat; 3 g Sat Fat; 9 g Mono Fat; 19 g Carb; 6 g Fiber; 6 g Sugar; 68 mg Calcium; 2 mg Iron; 237 mg Sodium; 32 mg Cholesterol
Per Serving (4 ounces Ahi): 347 Cal (45% from Fat, 34% from Protein, 21% from Carb); 30 g Protein; 17 g Tot Fat; 3 g Sat Fat; 9 g Mono Fat; 19 g Carb; 6 g Fiber; 6 g Sugar; 70 mg Calcium; 3 mg Iron; 248 mg Sodium; 43 mg Cholesterol

Greek Salad

Yield: 2 servings

3 ounces mixed greens	6 white anchovy fillets
2 ounces red onions, sliced (about 1/2 small onion)	Two 3 to 4-ounce chicken breasts
	1 tablespoon wine vinegar
3 ounces cucumbers, sliced (about 1/2 medium cucumber)	2 tablespoons olive oil
	1/2 tablespoon flaxseed oil
3 ounces red bell peppers, sliced (about 1/2 medium red bell pepper)	1 teaspoon garlic cloves, minced
	1 tablespoon low-fat yogurt
6 ounces tomatoes, sliced (about 1 large tomato)	1 teaspoon freshly minced oregano
	1 tablespoon freshly minced parsley
4 teaspoons feta cheese crumbled	Salt and pepper to taste
2 tablespoons black olives	

In a bowl, mix the vinegar, oils, and garlic. Blend in the yogurt. Add the oregano, parsley, and season to taste. In a large bowl, place the lettuce, red onions, cucumbers, bell peppers, and tomatoes. Add the dressing and mix well. Divide equally among two plates. Top with the olives, feta cheese, anchovy fillets, and serve immediately.

Per Serving (3 ounces chicken breast): 324 Cal (57% from Fat, 26% from Protein, 17% from Carb); 21 g Protein; 21 g Tot Fat; 4 g Sat Fat; 12 g Mono Fat; 14 g Carb; 3 g Fiber; 7 g Sugar; 131 mg Calcium; 2 mg Iron; 1534 mg Sodium; 47 mg Cholesterol
Per Serving (4 ounces chicken breast): 346 Cal (54% from Fat, 29% from Protein, 17% from Carb); 26 g Protein; 21 g Tot Fat; 4 g Sat Fat; 12 g Mono Fat; 15 g Carb; 3 g Fiber; 7 g Sugar; 133 mg Calcium; 2 mg Iron; 1842 mg Sodium; 57 mg Cholesterol

---

Fish Soup

Yield: 4 servings

1 teaspoon olive oil	4 cups fish stock (low-sodium)
5 ounces onions, diced (about 1 medium onion)	1 bouquet garni
	6 ounces tomatoes (about 1 large tomato)
3 ounces carrots, diced (about 1 small carrot)	3 tablespoons parsley, minced
1 tablespoon minced garlic	1 strip orange zest
4 ounces Chardonnay wine	1 teaspoon fennel seeds
3 pounds fish steaks and fillets	Salt and pepper to taste

Make a small X incision on the top and bottom of the tomato. Blanch the tomato for 15 to 20 seconds. Remove and place the tomato in ice-cold water to stop the cooking process. Peel, seed, and dice the tomatoes. Set aside.

Heat the oil in a large pan over high heat. Add the onions and sauté until translucent. Add the carrots, garlic, and sauté for 2 minutes. Add the white wine and reduce the liquid by half. Add the stock, bouquet garni, tomatoes, parsley, orange zest, saffron, fennel seeds, and bring to a boil. Reduce heat, add the fish, and simmer until the fish starts to flake. Remove the bouquet garni and orange zest. Skim the surface, adjust seasonings, and serve immediately.

For this soup, these fish work best: cod, sea-bream, eel, haddock, hake, mackerel, monkfish, perch, red snapper, or white fish. Remember the total calories will vary depending on the fish selected.

This soup can be refrigerated for 2 days, and can be frozen up to 1 month.

Per Serving: 447 Cal (16% from Fat, 74% from Protein, 10% from Carb); 76 g Protein; 7 g Tot Fat; 2 g Sat Fat; 2 g Mono Fat; 10 g Carb; 2 g Fiber; 3 g Sugar; 215 mg Calcium; 2 mg Iron; 1017 mg Sodium; 126 mg Cholesterol

---

White Beans and Chard Soup

Yield: 4 servings

2   teaspoons olive oil
6   ounces onions, chopped (about 1 medium onion)
4   ounces carrots, chopped (about 1 small carrot)
4   ounces celery, chopped (about 2 celery stalks)
4   ounces red bell peppers; seeded, ribs removed and chopped (about 1 small bell pepper)
4   ounces yellow bell peppers; seeded, ribs removed and chopped (about 1 small bell pepper)
1   chard head, chopped
4   cups chicken or vegetable stock (low-fat and low-sodium)
12 ounces organic can cooked white beans
2   tablespoons freshly minced Italian herbs
Salt and pepper to taste

Heat the oil in a large pan over medium heat. Add the onions and sauté until slightly browned. Add the bell peppers and cook for 2 minutes. Add the chard and sauté until the chard is wilted. Add stock, beans, and herbs. Bring to a boil, adjust seasoning, and serve immediately.

Per Serving: 243 Cal (17% from Fat, 16% from Protein, 67% from Carb); 10 g Protein; 5 g Tot Fat; 1 g Sat Fat; 3 g Mono Fat; 43 g Carb; 8 g Fiber; 9 g Sugar; 154 mg Calcium; 6 mg Iron; 898 mg Sodium; 0 mg Cholesterol

Vegetable Soup

Yield: 4 servings

2   teaspoons olive oil
8   ounces onions, diced (about 1 large onion)
6   ounces carrots, diced (about 1 medium carrot)
4   ounces celery stalks, diced (about 2 celery stalks)
6   ounces turnips, diced (about 1 medium turnip)
6   ounces red bell-peppers, diced (about 1 medium red bell pepper)

2   garlic cloves, minced
6   cups chicken or vegetable stock
1   bouquet garni
6   ounces fresh tomatoes peeled, seeded, and diced (about 1 large tomato)
3   ounces frozen peas
2   tablespoons fresh parsley, minced
Salt and pepper to taste

Make a small X incision on the top and bottom of the tomato. Blanch the tomato for 15 to 20 seconds. Place in ice-cold water to stop the cooking process. Peel, seed, and chop the tomato.

Heat the oil in a large pan over high heat. Add the onions and sauté until translucent. Add the carrots, celery stalks, bell peppers, and sauté rapidly. Add the turnips, garlic, stock, bouquet garni, and bring to a boil over high heat. Reduce heat and simmer until barely tender. Add the peas, tomatoes, and simmer for a minute. Finish with the parsley and adjust seasonings.

Option: Add whole wheat pasta, brown rice, or quinoa. You can also add chicken, turkey, venison, or buffalo meat.

Per Serving: 249 Cal (20% from Fat, 11% from Protein, 69% from Carb); 7 g Protein; 6 g Tot Fat; 1 g Sat Fat; 3 g Mono Fat; 45 g Carb; 8 g Fiber; 15 g Sugar; 115 mg Calcium; 3 mg Iron; 1312 mg Sodium; 0 mg Cholesterol

Turkey Chili

Yield: 4 servings

1   teaspoon canola oil
8   ounces onions, diced (about 1 large onion)
6   ounces yellow bell pepper; seeded, ribs removed, and diced (about 1 medium yellow bell pepper)
2   garlic cloves, minced
1   pound ground turkey meat
1   can (15 ounces) diced tomatoes
2   ounces tomato paste

1 ¼ cup beef stock
12 ounces cooked kidney beans or pinto beans
1   teaspoon thyme
1   teaspoon oregano
2   teaspoons cumin
2   tablespoons chili powder
1/4 teaspoon cayenne pepper
Salt to taste

Heat the oil in a deep pan over high heat. Add the meat and brown slightly. Remove the excess fat rendered by the meat. Add the onion, pepper, garlic, and mix well. Stir in the tomatoes, tomato paste, stock, herbs, and spices. Bring to a boil and reduce heat. Simmer uncovered for 50 minutes to an hour. Stir occasionally. Add the beans and bring to a simmer. Adjust seasonings and serve immediately.

Per Serving: 352 Cal (15% from Fat, 41% from Protein, 44% from Carb); 37 g Protein; 6 g Tot Fat; 1 g Sat Fat; 2 g Mono Fat; 40 g Carb; 11 g Fiber; 9 g Sugar; 113 mg Calcium; 7 mg Iron; 642 mg Sodium; 74 mg Cholesterol

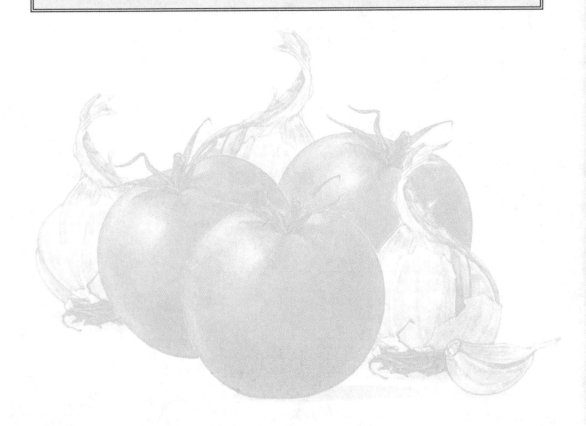

Side Dishes/ Desserts

Oftentimes, proteins are the focus of meals. However, you must not forget about the importance of side dishes and snacks. For one thing, their nutritional value can help complete a day's minimum requirements for vitamin and mineral intake. Once more, carefully chosen snacks and side dishes keep us from becoming bored with food. This is key, for it is often boredom that leads us to binge on poor food choices.

Side dishes should emphasize plenty of vegetables and include an appropriate amount of complex carbohydrates based on your daily activities.

Always keep the fat content low in your snacks and side dishes. Snacks should not be limited to food bars, but should instead feature fresh food sources, such as fruits, vegetables, or nuts. Good high protein snack choices also include cottage cheese and yogurt.

In the following section, you will find low-fat snack and side dish recipes that also feature the right balance of proteins and carbohydrates. This aids absorption of the nutrients and helps keep your metabolism up.

At the end of this section, you will also find several dessert options. No need to worry—although recipes like Chocolate and Hazelnut Pudding and Almond Chocolate Squares are certainly delicious, these are not your traditional, high-fat desserts. Instead, these healthy alternatives give you the freedom to treat yourself while still fulfilling the requirements for a healthy, fat-burning, and muscle-building diet.

Roasted Sweet Potatoes with Ginger

Yield: 2 servings

2   small sweet potatoes (about 5 ounces each)
2   teaspoons grapeseed oil
Ground ginger to taste
Ground cinnamon to taste
Salt and pepper to taste

Wash and pat dry the sweet potatoes. Prick the potatoes with a fork and microwave on high for 4 to 5 minutes. Transfer each potato to aluminum foil, close, and let stand for another 3 to 4 minutes.
  Preheat the broiler. Remove potatoes from foil, cut in half, and spread the grapeseed oil over the potato flesh. Sprinkle ginger, cinnamon, and season to taste. Broil until golden brown and serve immediately.

Per Serving (5 ounces sweet potato): 151 Cal (27% from Fat, 6% from Protein, 67% from Carb); 2 g Protein; 5 g Tot Fat; 0 g Sat Fat; 1 g Mono Fat; 26 g Carb; 4 g Fiber; 6 g Sugar; 44 mg Calcium; 1 mg Iron; 19 mg Sodium; 0 mg Cholesterol

Dandelion with Garlic

Yield: 2 servings

1   pound dandelion
2   teaspoons olive oil
1   garlic clove, minced
2   tablespoons vegetable broth (low-fat and low-sodium)
Salt and pepper to taste

Clean thoroughly the dandelion and dry with a salad spinner. Chop the dandelion. Heat the oil and garlic in a saucepan over medium heat. Add the dandelion and cook for 5 minutes mixing occasionally. Add the broth and season to taste. Continue to cook for another 5 minutes or until tender. Serve immediately.

Per Serving: 152 Cal (32% from Fat, 15% from Protein, 53% from Carb); 7 g Protein; 6 g Tot Fat; 1 g Sat Fat; 3 g Mono Fat; 23 g Carb; 8 g Fiber; 9 g Sugar; 437 mg Calcium; 7 mg Iron; 174 mg Sodium; 0 mg Cholesterol

Penne with Arugula and Tomatoes

Yield: 2 servings

1/2 cup to 2/3 cup whole wheat penne
2 teaspoons olive oil
6 ounces mushrooms, sliced
6 ounces orange bell peppers; seeded, ribs removed, and diced
2 garlic cloves, minced
2 large tomatoes, diced (about 12 ounces)

1/2 cup vegetable broth (low-fat and low-sodium)
2 bunches arugula, chopped
2 teaspoons parmesan cheese
2 tablespoons freshly minced basil
Salt and pepper to taste

Cook the pasta according to package directions.
    Heat the oil in a nonstick pan over high heat. Add the mushrooms, garlic, and cook until golden brown. Add the bell pepper, tomatoes, and sauté quickly. Add the stock and bring to boil. Reduce heat and continue to simmer for 3 minutes. Add the arugula and cook until wilted. Mix in the cooked pasta, basil, and season to taste. Sprinkle the cheese just before serving.

Per Serving (1/2 cup cooked penne): 257 Cal (23% from Fat, 14% from Protein, 63% from Carb); 9 g Protein; 7 g Tot Fat; 1 g Sat Fat; 4 g Mono Fat; 44 g Carb; 7 g Fiber; 8 g Sugar; 88 mg Calcium; 2 mg Iron; 252 mg Sodium; 2 mg Cholesterol
Per Serving (3/4 cup cooked penne): 288 Cal (21% from Fat, 13% from Protein, 66% from Carb); 10 g Protein; 7 g Tot Fat; 1 g Sat Fat; 4 g Mono Fat; 51 g Carb; 8 g Fiber; 8 g Sugar; 89 mg Calcium; 2 mg Iron; 252 mg Sodium; 2 mg Cholesterol

Asian Noodles with Peanuts

Yield: 2 servings

1 teaspoon canola oil
1 garlic clove, minced
2 teaspoons ginger, minced
2 teaspoons low-sodium soy sauce
2 teaspoons rice vinegar
3 to 4 ounces Asian noodles
6 ounces carrots, sliced diagonally (about 1 large carrot)

4 green onions, sliced diagonally
2 tablespoons peanuts
2 tablespoons Thai basil
1 tablespoon sesame oil
Pepper to taste
Dry red pepper flakes to taste

Cook the noodles according to package instructions.
    Heat the canola oil in a wok over medium heat. Add garlic, ginger, carrots and sauté 1 minute. Add green onions and sauté briefly. Add the soy sauce, rice vinegar, peanuts, basil, red pepper flakes, and bring to a boil. Add the noodles and toss to blend. Finish by adding the sesame oil, pepper to taste, and serve immediately.

Per Serving (3 ounces uncooked noodles): 315 Cal (30% from Fat, 10% from Protein, 60% from Carb); 8 g Protein; 11 g Tot Fat; 1 g Sat Fat; 5 g Mono Fat; 48 g Carb; 6 g Fiber; 5 g Sugar; 92 mg Calcium; 2 mg Iron; 1182 mg Sodium; 0 mg Cholesterol
Per Serving (4 ounces uncooked noodles): 366 Cal (26% from Fat, 10% from Protein, 64% from Carb); 10 g Protein; 11 g Tot Fat; 1 g Sat Fat; 5 g Mono Fat; 59 g Carb; 7 g Fiber; 5 g Sugar; 95 mg Calcium; 2 mg Iron; 1443 mg Sodium; 0 mg Cholesterol

Eggplant Mediterranean

Yield: 2 servings

1 pound eggplant, both ends trimmed (about 2 small eggplants)
2 tablespoons olive oil
1 teaspoon cumin
1 tablespoon paprika
1 tablespoon ground ginger
1 tablespoon garlic powder

1 teaspoon coriander
1/2 teaspoon cayenne pepper
1/4 teaspoon ground thyme
1/4 teaspoon ground oregano
Salt

Cut eggplant slices lengthwise and arrange on a baking sheet.
Mix all the spices together. On both sides of the eggplant, brush olive oil, season with salt, and sprinkle the prepared spices.

Preheat the broiler or barbecue. Broil or grill until golden brown, about 2 minutes per side.

If ground thyme and oregano are difficult to find, use regular ones and mince as small as possible.

Per Serving: 199 Cal (61% from Fat, 6% from Protein, 33% from Carb); 3 g Protein; 15 g Tot Fat; 2 g Sat Fat; 10 g Mono Fat; 18 g Carb; 9 g Fiber; 6 g Sugar; 52 mg Calcium; 3 mg Iron; 10 mg Sodium; 0 mg Cholesterol

Green Beans with Almonds

Yield: 2 servings

2 cups green beans, trimmed
2 tablespoons sliced almonds
2 teaspoons grapeseed oil
1 garlic clove, minced
Salt and pepper to taste

Place the green beans in a pan and cover with water. Add 1 teaspoon of salt and bring to a boil over high heat.
Reduce heat and simmer until crisp, about 5 to 6 minutes. Drain and set aside. Briefly heat the oil with the garlic, almonds, and add the green beans. Mix well with the beans, season to taste, and serve immediately.

Per Serving: 130 Cal (49% from Fat, 12% from Protein, 39% from Carb); 4 g Protein; 8 g Tot Fat; 1 g Sat Fat; 3 g Mono Fat; 14 g Carb; 5 g Fiber; 2 g Sugar; 81 mg Calcium; 2 mg Iron; 9 mg Sodium; 0 mg Cholesterol

Sugar Snap Peas with Garlic

Yield: 2 servings

1 tablespoon olive oil
2 cups sugar snap peas
4 garlic cloves, sliced
1 lemon
Salt and pepper to taste

Remove strings along both lengths of the sugar snap peas. Heat a wok with the olive oil over medium heat. Add the garlic and sauté quickly. Add the sugar snap peas and sauté until tender and crisp. Sprinkle a little lemon juice, season to taste and serve immediately.

Per Serving: 230 Cal (27% from Fat, 16% from Protein, 57% from Carb); 10 g Protein; 8 g Tot Fat; 1 g Sat Fat; 5 g Mono Fat; 36 g Carb; 11 g Fiber; 9 g Sugar; 121 mg Calcium; 3 mg Iron; 14 mg Sodium; 0 mg Cholesterol

Brown Rice with Mushrooms

Yield: 2 servings

2 teaspoons grapeseed oil
2/5 to 5/8 cup brown rice
1 cup to 1 ¼ cup stock or water
4 ounces onions, diced
12 ounces mushrooms, diced
1 tablespoon chives, minced
Salt and pepper to taste

Rinse the rice well and drain. Heat 1 teaspoon oil in a pan over high heat. Add the rice and sauté for a minute. Add the stock or water and bring to a boil. Cover, reduce heat, and cook until tender or about 45 minutes. Time may vary, for best results refer to package instructions.

Heat the remaining oil in a pan over high heat. Add the onion and slightly brown. Add the mushrooms and sauté until golden brown. Add the chives and season to taste. Transfer to the rice and serve immediately.

Per Serving (1/2 cup cooked brown rice): 140 Cal (22% from Fat, 14% from Protein, 64% from Carb); 5 g Protein; 4 g Tot Fat; 0 g Sat Fat; 1 g Mono Fat; 23 g Carb; 2 g Fiber; 4 g Sugar; 20 mg Calcium; 1 mg Iron; 207 mg Sodium; 1 mg Cholesterol
Per Serving (3/4 cup cooked brown rice): 184 Cal (19% from Fat, 13% from Protein, 68% from Carb); 6 g Protein; 4 g Tot Fat; 1 g Sat Fat; 1 g Mono Fat; 32 g Carb; 3 g Fiber; 4 g Sugar; 25 mg Calcium; 1 mg Iron; 259 mg Sodium; 1 mg Cholesterol

Vegetables with Tapenade

Yield: 2 servings

1 ½ ounces black olives, pitted
2   anchovy fillets, rinsed and pat dry
1 ½ teaspoon capers
1/2 small garlic clove
1   tablespoon olive oil
Lemon juice to taste
Pepper to taste
Vegetables such as carrots,
    bell peppers, cherry tomatoes,
    and mushrooms

In a food processor purée the olives, anchovies, capers, and garlic. Add pepper to taste. Slowly add the olive oil until you obtain a smooth paste. Add lemon juice to taste.

Per Serving: 104 Cal (79% from Fat, 7% from Protein, 14% from Carb); 2 g Protein; 9 g Tot Fat; 1 g Sat Fat; 7 g Mono Fat; 4 g Carb; 1 g Fiber; 0 g Sugar; 42 mg Calcium; 1 mg Iron; 397 mg Sodium; 3 mg Cholesterol (without vegetables)

Half Red Bell Pepper Stuffed with Tuna

Yield: 2 servings

6 to 8 ounces can tuna
1/2 teaspoon paprika
2   teaspoons fine herbs
1/2 teaspoon garlic powder
1   ounce onion, diced small
    (about 1/4 small onion)
1 ½ ozs carrot, diced (about half a carrot)

1   ounce celery stalk, diced small
    (about 1 celery stalk)
2   tablespoons low-fat canola mayonnaise
6   ounces red bell pepper, cut in half, seeded
    and ribs removed
Salt and pepper to taste

Mix the tuna, paprika, fine herbs, onions, carrots, celery, and mayonnaise in a bowl. Season to taste and refrigerate for 30 minutes.
Equally divide the tuna mixture between the two halves and serve immediately.

Per Serving (3 ounces tuna): 167 Cal (21% from Fat, 51% from Protein, 29% from Carb); 21 g Protein; 4 g Tot Fat; 1 g Sat Fat; 1 g Mono Fat; 12 g Carb; 3 g Fiber; 6 g Sugar; 38 mg Calcium; 1 mg Iron; 75 mg Sodium; 42 mg Cholesterol
Per Serving (4 ounces tuna): 198 Cal (19% from Fat, 57% from Protein, 24% from Carb); 28 g Protein; 4 g Tot Fat; 1 g Sat Fat; 1 g Mono Fat; 12 g Carb; 3 g Fiber; 6 g Sugar; 43 mg Calcium; 1 mg Iron; 86 mg Sodium; 54 mg Cholesterol

Radishes with Hazelnut Cream Cheese

Yield: 1 serving

10 radishes
1   tablespoon low-fat sour cream
1   teaspoon low-fat milk
1   tablespoon hazelnuts
Pinch of salt
Pinch of pepper

Crush and mince the hazelnuts with a chef knife. Mix the sour cream with the yogurt in a bowl. Add the minced hazelnuts, salt, and pepper. Serve immediately with the radishes.

Variation: Mix in a little horseradish or fine herbs.

Per Serving: 79 Cal (63% from Fat, 12% from Protein, 24% from Carb); 3 g Protein; 6 g Tot Fat; 1 g Sat Fat; 4 g Mono Fat; 5 g Carb; 2 g Fiber; 3 g Sugar; 45 mg Calcium; 1 mg Iron; 58 mg Sodium; 4 mg Cholesterol

Cottage Cheese, Raisins, and Walnuts

Yield: 1 serving

1/3 cup 2% cottage cheese, cold
1   tablespoon chopped walnuts
2   teaspoons raisins
Cinnamon to taste

Mix cottage cheese, walnut, and raisins. Sprinkle cinnamon to taste and serve immediately.

Per Serving: 136 Cal (40% from Fat, 33% from Protein, 26% from Carb); 12 g Protein; 6 g Tot Fat; 1 g Sat Fat; 1 g Mono Fat; 9 g Carb; 1 g Fiber; 5 g Sugar; 63 mg Calcium; 0 mg Iron; 307 mg Sodium; 6 mg Cholesterol

Apple and Almond Butter

Yield: 1 serving

1   small apple
    (about 4 ounces)
1   tablespoon
    almond butter

Cut the apple in half, remove core, and slice. Equally spread the almond butter among the slices.

Per Serving: 153 Cal (51% from Fat, 6% from Protein, 43% from Carb); 3 g Protein; 9 g Tot Fat; 1 g Sat Fat; 6 g Mono Fat; 18 g Carb; 2 g Fiber; 11 g Sugar; 48 mg Calcium; 1 mg Iron; 2 mg Sodium; 0 mg Cholesterol

Chocolate Pudding

Yield: 3 servings

1¼ cup low-fat milk
3   extra large egg yolks
4   tablespoons sugar
2   tablespoons cornstarch
1   teaspoon orange extract
1   teaspoon orange zest
3   tablespoons Dutch cocoa powder

Bring the milk to a boil in a saucepan. Whisk the egg yolks, sugar, cocoa, orange zest, and cornstarch in a bowl until smooth. Temper the egg mixture with a little hot milk, stirring with a whisk. Transfer the mixture to the remaining hot milk, whisking rapidly and constantly. Heat over medium heat and bring to a boil, whisking the bottom and sides of the pan to avoid scorching. The mixture will thicken in about a minute. Continue to cook and whisk until a nice shine appears, about another minute. Mix in the orange extract and divide among 3 ramekins. Place a plastic wrap over the surface of each pudding and allow cooling a bit at room temperature. Refrigerate for 2 hours and serve cold.

Per Serving: 210 Cal (32% from Fat, 15% from Protein, 53% from Carb); 9 g Protein; 8 g Tot Fat; 4 g Sat Fat; 3 g Mono Fat; 31 g Carb; 5 g Fiber; 18 g Sugar; 159 mg Calcium; 2 mg Iron; 53 mg Sodium; 213 mg Cholesterol

Pomegranate and Strawberry Parfait

Yield: 2 servings

1½ cup strawberries
2   ounces pure Acai, no sugar added
    (1 Sambazon smoothie pack)
1   teaspoon vanilla extract
1   cup low-fat yogurt
2   tablespoons pomegranate seeds

Defrost Acai.
    Mix the strawberries with vanilla extract and Acai. Marinade for 30 minutes. Spoon half the fruit mixture into four serving parfait glasses. Top with yogurt and finish with the berries. Sprinkle the pomegranate seeds and serve immediately.

Option: Add Protein Powder and/or ground flaxseeds. You may substitute cottage cheese for yogurt.

Per Serving: 138 Cal (16% from Fat, 22% from Protein, 62% from Carb); 7 g Protein; 2 g Tot Fat; 1 g Sat Fat; 1 g Mono Fat; 21 g Carb; 3 g Fiber; 16 g Sugar; 249 mg Calcium; 1 mg Iron; 87 mg Sodium; 7 mg Cholesterol

Fruit with Chocolate Sauce

Yield: 2 servings

1/2 cup strawberries
1/2 cup orange slices
1/2 cup peach slices
1   kiwi, sliced
1 ½ ounce semi-sweet chocolate, shredded
1 ½ tablespoon water

Equally divide the fruits among two plates.
Melt the chocolate with water over low heat in a double boiler. Whisk until smooth. If necessary, add a little more water. Drizzle the hot chocolate sauce over the fruits and serve immediately.

Per Serving: 179 Cal (31% from Fat, 5% from Protein, 64% from Carb); 2 g Protein; 7 g Tot Fat; 4 g Sat Fat; 2 g Mono Fat; 32 g Carb; 5 g Fiber; 25 g Sugar; 49 mg Calcium; 1 mg Iron; 5 mg Sodium; 0 mg Cholesterol

Pear and Apple Minestrone

Yield: 2 servings

5   ounces apples, brunoise (about 1 apple)
5   ounces pears, brunoise (about 1 pear)
3/4 cup jasmine green tea (or your favorite)
1 ½ teaspoon honey
1/2 teaspoon pumpkin pie spices
1   small ginger root, minced
1/2 teaspoon lemon zest
1/2 teaspoon grapeseed oil

Heat the oil in a deep saucepan over high heat. Add the apples and sauté for two minutes. Add the pears, spices, ginger, lemon zest, and sauté another minute. Add the green tea and bring to a boil. Remove from heat and transfer to a serving bowl. Cool at room temperature. Refrigerate for an hour (or best overnight) to allow flavors to develop. Serve cold.

Per Serving: 105 Cal (10% from Fat, 2% from Protein, 88% from Carb); 1 g Protein; 1 g Tot Fat; 0 g Sat Fat; 0 g Mono Fat; 25 g Carb; 3 g Fiber; 18 g Sugar; 19 mg Calcium; 1 mg Iron; 2 mg Sodium; 0 mg Cholesterol

Thin Peach Tart

Yield: 8 servings

3 ounces almond meal
2 ounces oats
3 tablespoons grapeseed oil
1 tablespoon almond extract

2 to 3 tablespoons ice cold water
2 tablespoons peach preserves
1 pound peaches (about 4 peaches)
Pinch salt

Preheat the oven to 475°F.
Place the oats in a blender and reduce to a flour consistency. Place the oat and almond flours in a bowl. Add salt, oil, almond extract, and mix until crumbly. Add one tablespoon water at a time and continue until the dough is smooth and sticks together as one ball. Lay the dough on wax paper and push down with your palm to flatten a bit. Roll out the dough to a round thin form. Turn over the dough to a cookie sheet. Brush 1 tablespoon preserves all over the pie dough surface.

Peel the peaches and cut in half. Core, quarter, and slice. Starting at the edge of the dough and working inward toward the center, arrange the slices in overlapping circles. Finish with another circle of peach slices in the center.

Bake for 15 to 20 minutes until golden brown and slightly darker around the edges. Heat the remaining preserves with a little water to thin out in the microwave. Remove the tart from the oven and brush with the preserves. Transfer the tart to a cooling rack.

Per Serving: 173 Cal (56% from Fat, 9% from Protein, 35% from Carb); 4 g Protein; 11 g Tot Fat; 1 g Sat Fat; 1 g Mono Fat; 16 g Carb; 3 g Fiber; 9 g Sugar; 31 mg Calcium; 0 mg Iron; 6 mg Sodium; 0 mg Cholesterol

High Fiber Salad

Yield: 8 servings

2 oranges, skin removed and sliced
1 granny smith apple, skin removed and diced
1 Anjou pear, skin removed and diced
1/2 cup grapes (combination of white and red)
1 cup strawberries
1/2 cup blueberries
1/2 cup raspberries
1/2 cup blackberries
1 mango, diced
1/2 pineapple, wedged
Juice of 1 orange (or lime, lemon)

Place the fruits in a bowl. Add the orange juice and mix well. Refrigerate until use.

This is a great healthy fruit salad for a party. You may add fresh minced herbs such as rosemary, basil, or mint.

Per Serving: 127 Cal (3% from Fat, 4% from Protein, 93% from Carb); 2 g Protein; 0 g Tot Fat; 0 g Sat Fat; 0 g Mono Fat; 33g Carb; 5 g Fiber; 24 g Sugar; 46 mg Calcium; 0 mg Iron; 3 mg Sodium; 0 mg Cholesterol

Acai and Soy Milk Popsicle

Yield: 4 popsicles

    3.5 ounces Pure Acai, no sugar added
      (Sambazon smoothie pack)
    4 ounces berries
    4 ounces banana (about a small banana)
    4 ounces soy milk

Place all the fruits and soy milk in a blender. Purée on high speed. Divide equally among 4 popsicle molds and freeze.

Per Serving: 69 Cal (27% from Fat, 10% from Protein, 63% from Carb); 2 g Protein; 2 g Tot Fat; 0 g Sat Fat; 0 g Mono Fat; 12 g Carb; 3 g Fiber; 5 g Sugar; 10 mg Calcium; 0 mg Iron; 6 mg Sodium; 0 mg Cholesterol

Strawberries and Spinach Smoothie

Yield: 2 servings

    2 cups strawberries
    1 bunch fresh spinach
    1 banana
    1 tablespoon flaxseeds
    Aged balsamic vinegar to taste (optional)
    Ice cubs

Place strawberries, spinach, and banana into a blender. Puree and mix in the aged balsamic vinegar (optional). Serve immediately.

Option: Add Protein Powder which adds 100 calories

Per Serving: 178 Cal (13% from Fat, 15% from Protein, 72% from Carb); 8 g Protein; 3 g Tot Fat; 0 g Sat Fat; 0 g Mono Fat; 37 g Carb; 10 g Fiber; 17 g Sugar; 206 mg Calcium; 6 mg Iron; 138 mg Sodium; 0 mg Cholesterol

Flourless Walnut Cake with Chocolate Drizzles

Yield: 12 servings

10 ounces walnuts
3 eggs
3 ounces light brown sugar
2 ounces unsalted butter, melted and cooled
1/2 teaspoon vanilla extract

3 tablespoons Dutch cacao powder
5 to 6 tablespoons evaporated 2% milk
2 tablespoons honey
Pinch salt

Preheat the oven to 355 F. Grease an 8 inch diameter cake pan and place wax paper on the bottom of it.
In a food processor, chop down the walnuts. You need to end up with a meal consistency but with still lots of small chopped nuts pieces in it in order to maintain the texture of the cake.

Separate the egg whites from the yolks. Beat the yolks with the sugar until it becomes a light pale color. Add the vanilla, salt, melted butter, and mix until well incorporated. Start to whip the egg whites, adding a teaspoon of sugar half way through. Once the egg whites are firm, fold a third of it into the prepared mixture. Add remaining egg whites while folding carefully not to break them. Transfer to the cake pan and bake for 40 minutes or until a cake pick inserted in the center comes out dry. Be aware that the cake will not rise much—that is normal. Cool over a rack before unmolding. Remove wax paper and cut into 12 slices.

Mix the cacao and evaporated milk. Add the honey and warm up in the microwave for 15 to 20 seconds. Mix again before use. Plate each cake slice, drizzle 1 tablespoon chocolate sauce, and serve immediately.

Many twists can be given to this basic recipe. Keep in mind it will change calories.

- Melt 1 teaspoon almond butter into the chocolate sauce
- Add 1 apple, diced into the cake mixture
- Add cinnamon into the cake mixture
- Substitute the vanilla with rum or walnut liquor
- Substitute butter with grapeseed oil. Be aware it will change the cake texture and flavor.

Per Serving: 254 Cal (70% from Fat, 9% from Protein, 21% from Carb); 6 g Protein; 21 g Tot Fat; 4 g Sat Fat; 4 g Mono Fat; 14 g Carb; 2 g Fiber; 10 g Sugar; 60 mg Calcium; 1 mg Iron; 30 mg Sodium; 72 mg Cholesterol

Recipes inspired from:

THE SAINT-TROPEZ DIET
—Apostolos Pappas, Marie-Annick Courtier

THE PARK AVENUE DIET
—Dr. Stuart Fisher, Marie-Annick Courtier

THE PROFESSIONAL CHEF
—Culinary Institute of America

THE FLAVORS OF BON APPETIT 1998

FRENCH CLASSICS
—Richard Grausman

Workout Journal

E

THE **BODY**
SCULPTING
BIBLE
FOR**WOMEN**

BREAK-IN ROUTINE #1

Daily Workout Journal — Week ⬤ Day ⬤

	Exercise Main (Alternate)	Rest	Set 1 Reps	Weight	Set 2 Reps	Weight	Set 3 Reps	Weight	Set 4 Reps	Weight	Set 5 Reps	Weight	
Group 1													**Group 1**
Group 2													**Group 2**
Group 3													**Group 3**
Group 4													**Group 4**
Abs													**Abs**

Cardio

Cardio Activity:

Average Heart Rate:

Duration:

Notes:

Notes

BREAK-IN ROUTINE #2

Daily Workout Journal

Week ⬤ Day ⬤

	Exercise Main (Alternate)	Rest	Set 1 Reps / Weight	Set 2 Reps / Weight	Set 3 Reps / Weight	Set 4 Reps / Weight	Set 5 Reps / Weight	
Group 1								Group 1
Group 2								Group 2
Group 3								Group 3
Group 4								Group 4
Abs								Abs
Cardio	Cardio Activity: Average Heart Rate: Duration:		Notes:					Notes

14-DAY BODY SCULPTING WORKOUT #1

Daily Workout Journal

Week ◯ Day ◯

	Exercise Main (Alternate)	Rest	Set 1 Reps	Set 1 Weight	Set 2 Reps	Set 2 Weight	Set 3 Reps	Set 3 Weight	Set 4 Reps	Set 4 Weight	Set 5 Reps	Set 5 Weight	
Group 1													Group 1
Group 2													Group 2
Group 3													Group 3
Group 4													Group 4
Abs													Abs

Cardio

Cardio Activity:

Average Heart Rate:

Duration:

Notes:

Notes

14-DAY BODY SCULPTING WORKOUT #2

Daily Workout Journal   Week ◯ Day ◯

Exercise Main (Alternate)	Rest	Set 1 Reps Weight	Set 2 Reps Weight	Set 3 Reps Weight	Set 4 Reps Weight	Set 5 Reps Weight
Group 1						
Group 2						
Group 3						
Group 4						
Abs						

Cardio

Cardio Activity: Notes:

Average Heart Rate:

Duration:

Notes

14-DAY BODY SCULPTING WORKOUT #3

Daily Workout Journal   Week ⬤ Day ⬤

Exercise Main (Alternate)	Rest	Set 1 Reps	Set 1 Weight	Set 2 Reps	Set 2 Weight	Set 3 Reps	Set 3 Weight	Set 4 Reps	Set 4 Weight	Set 5 Reps	Set 5 Weight
Group 1											
Group 2											
Group 3											
Group 4											
Abs											

Cardio

Cardio Activity:

Average Heart Rate:

Duration:

Notes:

14-DAY RAPID BODY SCULPTING WORKOUT #1

Daily Workout Journal Week ◯ Day ◯

	Exercise Main (Alternate)	Rest	Set 1 Reps	Set 1 Weight	Set 2 Reps	Set 2 Weight	Set 3 Reps	Set 3 Weight	Set 4 Reps	Set 4 Weight	Set 5 Reps	Set 5 Weight	
Group 1													**Group 1**
Group 2													**Group 2**
Group 3													**Group 3**
Group 4													**Group 4**
Abs													**Abs**

Cardio	Cardio Activity:	Notes:	**Notes**
	Average Heart Rate:		
	Duration:		

14-DAY RAPID BODY SCULPTING WORKOUT #2

Daily Workout Journal   Week ⬤   Day ⬤

	Exercise Main (Alternate)	Rest	Set 1 Reps · Weight	Set 2 Reps · Weight	Set 3 Reps · Weight	Set 4 Reps · Weight	Set 5 Reps · Weight
Group 1							
Group 2							
Group 3							
Group 4							
Abs							

Cardio	Cardio Activity:	Notes:	**Notes**
	Average Heart Rate:		
	Duration:		

14-DAY ADVANCED BODY SCULPTING WORKOUT #1

Daily Workout Journal

Week ⬤ Day ⬤

Exercise Main (Alternate)	Rest	Set 1 Reps	Weight	Set 2 Reps	Weight	Set 3 Reps	Weight	Set 4 Reps	Weight	Set 5 Reps	Weight
Group 1											
Group 2											
Group 3											
Group 4											
Abs											

Cardio

Cardio Activity:

Average Heart Rate:

Duration:

Notes

Notes:

14-DAY ADVANCED BODY SCULPTING WORKOUT #2

Daily Workout Journal

Week ◯ Day ◯

Exercise Main (Alternate)	Rest	Set 1 Reps	Weight	Set 2 Reps	Weight	Set 3 Reps	Weight	Set 4 Reps	Weight	Set 5 Reps	Weight	
Group 1												**Group 1**
Group 2												**Group 2**
Group 3												**Group 3**
Group 4												**Group 4**
Abs												**Abs**

Cardio

Cardio Activity: Notes:

Average Heart Rate:

Duration:

Notes

14-DAY BODY SCULPTING DEFINITION WORKOUT

Daily Workout Journal   Week ◯ Day ◯

	Exercise Main (Alternate)	Rest	Set 1 Reps · Weight	Set 2 Reps · Weight	Set 3 Reps · Weight	Set 4 Reps · Weight	Set 5 Reps · Weight	
Group 1								Group 1
Group 2								Group 2
Group 3								Group 3
Group 4								Group 4
Abs								Abs

Cardio	Cardio Activity:	Notes:	Notes
	Average Heart Rate:		
	Duration:		

14-DAY BODYWEIGHT BODY SCULPTING WORKOUT

Daily Workout Journal   Week ⬤   Day ⬤

	Exercise Main (Alternate)	Rest	Set 1 Reps / Weight	Set 2 Reps / Weight	Set 3 Reps / Weight	Set 4 Reps / Weight	Set 5 Reps / Weight	
Group 1								**Group 1**
Group 2								**Group 2**
Group 3								**Group 3**
Group 4								**Group 4**
Abs								**Abs**

Cardio	Cardio Activity:	Notes:	**Notes**
	Average Heart Rate:		
	Duration:		

Appendix F
Nutrition Journal

F

THE **BODY**
SCULPTING
BIBLE
FOR **WOMEN**

Daily Nutrition Journal
Week ◯ Day ◯

	Food	Serving Size	Calories	Carbs (grams)	Protein (grams)	Fat (grams)	
Meal 1							Meal 1
Meal 2							Meal 2
Meal 3							Meal 3
Meal 4							Meal 4
Meal 5							Meal 5
	Total						

Daily Nutrition Journal

Week ⬤ Day ⬤

	Food	Serving Size	Calories	Carbs (grams)	Protein (grams)	Fat (grams)
Meal 1						
Meal 2						
Meal 3						
Meal 4						
Meal 5						
	Total					

Daily Nutrition Journal

Week ◯ Day ◯

	Food	Serving Size	Calories	Carbs (grams)	Protein (grams)	Fat (grams)
Meal 1						
Meal 2						
Meal 3						
Meal 4						
Meal 5						
Total						

Daily Nutrition Journal

Week ⬤ Day ⬤

	Food	Serving Size	Calories	Carbs (grams)	Protein (grams)	Fat (grams)
Meal 1						
Meal 2						
Meal 3						
Meal 4						
Meal 5						
	Total					

Daily Nutrition Journal   Week ⬤ Day ⬤

	Food	Serving Size	Calories	Carbs (grams)	Protein (grams)	Fat (grams)
Meal 1						
Meal 2						
Meal 3						
Meal 4						
Meal 5						
Total						

Daily Nutrition Journal

Week ⬤ Day ⬤

	Food	Serving Size	Calories	Carbs (grams)	Protein (grams)	Fat (grams)
Meal 1						
Meal 2						
Meal 3						
Meal 4						
Meal 5						
Total						

Daily Nutrition Journal

Week ● Day ●

	Food	Serving Size	Calories	Carbs (grams)	Protein (grams)	Fat (grams)
Meal 1						
Meal 2						
Meal 3						
Meal 4						
Meal 5						
Total						

Tracking Your Progress

THE BODY SCULPTING BIBLE FOR WOMEN

G

The only way to know if your program is working is to track your progress. A simple way to do this is by using the following formulas excerpted from the book Hardcore Bodybuilding: A Scientific Approach, written by strength training authority Frederick C. Hatfield, Ph.D. Dr. Hatfield, better known as Dr. Squat, is the co-founding Director of Sports and Fitness Sciences for the prestigious International Sports Sciences Association (ISSA). As a three-time winner of the World Championship of Powerlifting, Dr. Hatfield not only is well versed on weight training theory, but on its application as well.

FOR WOMEN:

Before you use the formulas, there are five measurements required:

Measurement 1:   Body weight.
Measurement 2:   Wrist Circumference (measured at the widest point).
Measurement 3:   Waist Circumference (measured at your umbilicus).
Measurement 4:   Hip Circumference (measured at the widest point).
Measurement 5:   Forearm Circumference (measured at the widest point).

PROCEDURE:

#1-   Multiply your body weight by 0.732. Body weight x 0.732 = Result 1.

#2-   Add the result above to 8.987. ❰ Result 1 + 8.987 = Result 2.

#3-   Divide your wrist circumference by 3.14. ❰ Wrist divided by 3.14 = Result 3.

#4-   Multiply your waist measurement by 0.157. ❰ Waist x 0.157 = Result 4.

#5-   Multiply your hip measurement by 0.249. ❰ Hip x 0.249 = Result 5.

#6-   Multiply your forearm measurement by 0.434. ❰ Forearm x 0.434 = Result 6.

#7-   Add results 2 and 3. ❰ Result 2 + Result 3 = Result 7.

#8-   Subtract Result 4 from Result 7. ❰ Result 7 - Result 4 = Result 8.

#9-   Subtract Result 5 from Result 8. ❰ Result 8 - Result 5 = Result 9.

#10-   Add Result 6 and Result 9. The result is your Lean Body Mass (your fat-free weight) ❰ Result 6 + Result 9 = Lean Body Mass.

#11-   Subtract your Lean Body Mass from your body weight. Once you get the result, multiply that number by 100. Once you get this result, divide it by your Body weight. ❰ [(Body weight-Lean Body Mass) x 100] divided by your body weight.

EXAMPLE:

A woman that weighs 125 and has a wrist measurement of 6.0, a waist measurement of 24, a hip measurement of 38, and a forearm measurement of 9.5 would calculate her body fat percentage in the following manner.

Step 1:   125 x 0.732 = 91.5.

Step 2:   91.5 + 8.987 = 100.487.

Step 3:   6 divided by 3.14 = 1.91.

Step 4:   24 x 0.157 = 3.768.

Step 5:   38 x 0.249 = 9.462.

Step 6:   9.5 x 0.434 = 4.123.

Step 7:   100.487 + 1.91 = 102.397.

Step 8:   102.397 - 3.768 = 98.629.

Step 9:   98.629 - 9.462 = 89.167.

Step 10:   4.123 + 89.167 = 93.29 (Lean Body Weight: Fat-Free Weight).

Step 11:   [(125-93.29) x 100] divided by 125 = (31.37 x 100) divided by 125 = 3171 divided by 125 = 25.368 (Body Fat Percentage).

Notes:

The formulas above are approximations. The goal is to have a point of reference from which to work. I recommend that you measure your body fat every three weeks. If you see a pattern of gaining muscle and losing fat, then you know your program is on track. If not, examine which part of your program is not optimal. Assuming that you are following the recommended training routines, the only things that could be going wrong are either you are not getting enough rest at night, or more likely, are not following the nutrition plan properly.

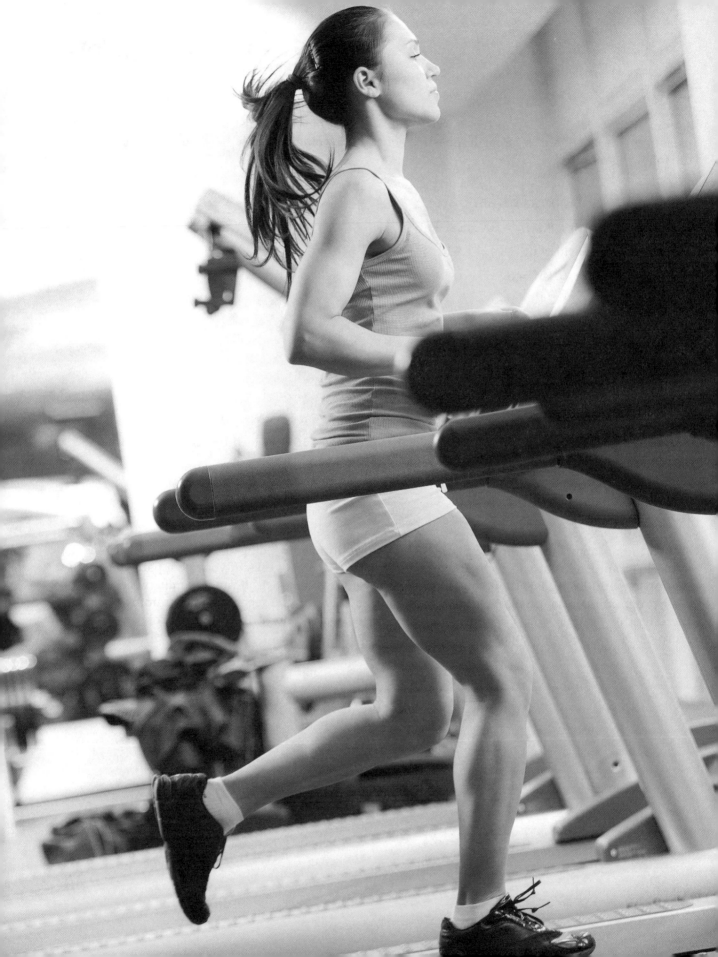

Appendix H
Grocery Shopping List

H

THE **BODY SCULPTING BIBLE** FOR **WOMEN**

Note: Eat a meal prior to going grocery shopping to ensure that you don't buy junk foods. Another strategy is to do your grocery shopping on Sundays, when you are allowed to eat whatever you want for one meal.

Obviously, you do not need to purchase all of the items on this grocery list. We provide it as a reminder of the types of foods that your shopping list should include.

CARBOHYDRATES

- Brown rice
- Chickpeas
- Cream of rice
- Yams (sweet potatoes)
- Whole wheat bread
- Plain oatmeal (old fashion, not instant)
- Corn
- Baking potato
- Pita bread
- Lentils
- Grits
- Fruits
- Fresh green vegetables

PROTEINS

- Chicken breasts (avoid deli meats; they are high in sodium and low in protein)
- Turkey breasts (avoid deli meats; they are high in sodium and low in protein)
- Water-packed Tuna
- White fish
- Eggs
- Halibut
- Cod
- Round steak
- Top sirloin

FATS

- Flaxseed Oil

SUPPLEMENTS

- Vitamin and mineral formula
- Vitamin C
- Chromium picolinate
- Fish oil capsules (if you don't use flaxseed oil)
- Meal replacement powders
- Whey protein powders
- Protein bars
- Creatine
- Glutamine

DAIRY

- Skim Milk

MISCELLANEOUS ITEMS

- Garlic powder (for flavoring)
- Onion powder (for flavoring)
- Balsamic vinegar
- Crystal light
- Any sugar-free and salt-free seasoning

(Photocopy these pages for your own personal use)

Appendix I
Body Sculpting Under Special Circumstances

THE **BODY**
SCULPTING
BIBLE
FOR **WOMEN**

BODY SCULPTING DURING PREGNANCY

Much research in this area has determined that remaining active during pregnancy offers several benefits to the mother and baby. The key to reaping such benefits is to adjust your exercise program in order to make it safe for you and your baby during this period. Keep in mind that the goal of **exercising during pregnancy is to maintain your present level of fitness, not to improve it.**

Some of the benefits that exercise offers to expecting mothers are:

- Speedier recovery after delivery.

- Increased sense of well-being and self esteem during and after pregnancy.

- Fewer leg cramps.

- Larger placenta, which in turn provides an increased nutrient base for the baby.

- Decreased risk of excessive weight gain caused by an increase of fat storage.

- Stronger lower back, which in turn reduces the risk of lower back pains.

- Boost in energy levels.

- Decreased likelihood of varicose veins.

- Reduced chances of having a Caesarean birth.

- Higher chances of achieving labor either a few days earlier or on time.

- Preparation for the stresses imposed by labor and delivery.

The amount of exercise that mothers-to-be will be able to tolerate during these nine months is directly related to how active they were before becoming pregnant. If a woman has never exercised before in her life, pregnancy is not the time to start a full-blown weight training and intense aerobics program. Starting a weight-training program is very traumatic on the body. A more sensible approach for someone who has never exercised before is to start a mild daily 20 to 30 minute aerobics program consisting of walking at a normal pace. Why walking? Because walking is one of the most natural and safest forms of exercise. During pregnancy, it is crucial to choose exercises that do not result in a loss of balance, since a fall could prove fatal for both the mother and the baby. Therefore, aerobic activities such as aerobic dance, bench step classes, kickboxing aerobics, and roller blading are all out of the question.

There are certain precautions you will need to incorporate in your walking program in order to make it safe. Remember that the goal during this period is to maintain, not to improve, so your workout intensity should be mild to moderate. In other words, you should walk at a normal pace and should not attempt to push yourself. Pushing yourself can create undue stress upon your body and will increase your chances of reaching two conditions that should be avoided at all times during pregnancy. They are:

Your heart rate should never exceed 140 beats per minute. Be especially careful to monitor your heart rate during exercise. This can easily be done by counting the amount of times your heart beats in 10 seconds while you are performing the activity and then multiplying that number by 6. This will give you the amount of beats per minute. To avoid raising your heart rate too high, walk at a normal pace.

Your body temperature should never exceed 100 degrees Fahrenheit (or 38 degrees Celsius). Walk at a normal pace and choose a time and place where it is neither hot nor humid. Walking either early in the morning or in the late afternoon is best. Also, avoid wearing clothing that is too warm. If you'd rather walk indoors, do not use a motorized treadmill since it is easy to trip and fall while using this equipment. Instead, use the non-motorized models where you are the one that sets the pace. Other good forms of indoor exercises for expectant mothers are swimming and water walking.

What if you have been active prior to your pregnancy? Then you may continue your activities *as long as they are not activities that could result in a loss of balance and as long as you remember to lower your intensity levels to prevent an increased body temperature and heart rate.* Again, we cannot overemphasize that the goal during this period is maintenance and not improvement. Therefore, don't push yourself. Women who are involved in weight training should follow a program with the following modifications:

- Increase your rest periods in between sets to two minutes in order to maintain a normal body temperature and a low pulse (below 140 beats).

- Perform only 3 sets per exercise.

- In order to stay away from reaching muscular failure choose a weight that you can perform for 12-15 repetitions and perform 8-10 repetitions per set instead.

- Eliminate exercises where you have to lay down flat on your back (such as flat dumbbell bench press) since this position can decrease blood flow to the uterus and therefore to the baby.

- Eliminate exercises that may cause a loss of balance such as lunges and squats. Instead, substitute exercises like seated leg curls and leg exten-

sions. If you have access to machines, this is the perfect time to use them.

Remember we previously said we recommend free weights since our body is designed to operate on a three-dimensional universe and machines lock us in a two dimensional one? During pregnancy, being locked in a two-dimensional universe is a good thing since it makes the exercises safer and eliminates the possibility of losing balance. Also, by using machines, secondary stabilizer muscles, such as abdominal and pelvic muscles, are not activated. This is good because we don't want to create any undue stress in these areas during pregnancy. Machines also greatly decrease a chance of joint injuries.

During pregnancy, a loosening of the joints occurs—allowing ligaments and tendons to stretch in preparation for delivery. Because of this, there is a higher risk of incurring a soft tissue injury if free weights are used. If you choose to continue using free weights during this period, remember to pay close attention to your exercise form and to choose your exercises carefully.

- Eliminate the abdominal exercise portion of the 14-Day Body Sculpting Workout. You must avoid any exercise that may risk even mild abdominal trauma. In addition, avoid exercises where you have to lay down flat on your stomach. For instance, do standing or seated leg curls rather than lying leg curls.

- Don't hold your breath while exercising; otherwise you can cut the oxygen supply to your baby.

Taking all of these points into consideration, we have created a new weight training program for use during pregnancy.

Special Instructions: Use modified compound supersets. Perform the first exercise, rest for the prescribed rest period, perform the second exercise, rest the prescribed rest period and then go back to the first exercise. Continue in this manner until you have performed all of the prescribed number of sets. Then continue with the next modified compound superset.

DAY 1

MODIFIED COMPOUND SUPERSET # 1

BACK-Wide-Grip Pull-downs to Front

Reps: 8-10
Sets: 3
Rest: 2 minutes

CHEST-Seated Chest Press Machine

Reps: 8-10
Sets: 3
Rest: 2 minutes

MODIFIED COMPOUND SUPERSET # 2

BACK-Close-Grip (Palms facing you) Pull-downs

Reps: 8-10
Sets: 3
Rest: 2 minutes

CHEST-Pec Deck Machine

Reps: 8-10
Sets: 3
Rest: 2 minutes

MODIFIED COMPOUND SUPERSET # 3

BICEPS-Seated Dumbbell Curls

Reps: 8-10
Sets: 3
Rest: 2 minutes

TRICEPS-Triceps Pushdowns

Reps: 8-10
Sets: 3
Rest: 2 minutes

MODIFIED COMPOUND SUPERSET # 4

BICEPS-Seated Incline Curls

Reps: 8-10
Sets: 3
Rest: 2 minutes

TRICEPS-One-Arm Cable Extensions

Reps: 8-10
Sets: 3
Rest: 2 minutes

DAY 2

MODIFIED COMPOUND SUPERSET # 1

THIGHS-Leg Extensions

Reps: 8-10
Sets: 3
Rest: 2 minutes

HAMSTRINGS-Seated Leg Curls

Reps: 8-10
Sets: 3
Rest: 2 minutes

MODIFIED COMPOUND SUPERSET # 2

HAMSTRINGS-Standing Leg Curls

Reps: 8-10
Sets: 3

Rest: 2 minutes

THIGHS-One Legged Leg Extensions

Reps: 8-10
Sets: 3
Rest: 2 minutes

MODIFIED COMPOUND SUPERSET # 3

CALVES (LOWER/UPPER)-Seated Press Machine

Reps: 8-10
Sets: 3
Rest: 2 minutes

SHOULDERS-Lateral Raises

Reps: 8-10
Sets: 3
Rest: 2 minutes

MODIFIED COMPOUND SUPERSET # 4

SHOULDERS-Overhead Shoulder Press Machine

Reps: 8-10
Sets: 3
Rest: 2 minutes

CALVES-Seated Calf Raise Machine

Reps: 8-10
Sets: 3
Rest: 2 minutes

If you experience any type of abnormal conditions such as bleeding, sharp abdominal pain, loss of breath, exhaustion, or any other symptom that does not feel normal,

If for any reason your doctor recommends complete bed rest, continue your healthy eating and do not attempt to engage in any type of physical activity.

> ## STOP EXERCISING AND CONTACT YOUR DOCTOR IMMEDIATELY!

For more information on training during pregnancy, contact the American College of Obstetricians & Gynecologists (ACOG) at (202) 484-3321.

NUTRITION DURING PREGNANCY

Nutrition becomes even more important than ever before during these nine months. Your health, and that of your baby, depends on it. Do you know that the following conditions are mostly caused by a lack of good nutrition during pregnancy?

- Anemia (which is caused by lack of protein and vitamins in the diet).

- Miscarriage.

- Babies born with brain damage, low intelligence, below average birth weight, and low immune systems.

- The afterbirth can break loose in the uterus before labor begins, a condition that causes internal bleeding in the mother and can cause the baby to die (50 percent of births in this manner result in death).

- Metabolic Toxemia (caused by lack of protein and vitamins) which can cause death to both the mother and the baby.

Therefore, continue to follow the nutrition guidelines from Chapter 6. In addition, keep the following points in mind:

- **It is more important than ever to remain hydrated throughout the day.** Drink plenty of water, especially before, during and after exercise. Remember that water not only helps flush bad toxins out of the body, but the body also uses it as a coolant to keep body temperature down.

- **This is no time to be preoccupied with losing weight.** Attempting to go on a strict and restricted diet during this period will ensure that your baby does not get all of the necessary nutrients that he/she needs in order to be born strong and healthy. In order to avoid excessive weight gain and properly nourish your baby, take the amount of calories that you are currently taking in and add an additional 300 calories per day (remember to follow the ratios recommended in Chapter 6). If after two weeks you see that you are losing weight, add an additional 300 calories. Remember, don't panic if you start gaining more weight than anticipated. This is a normal part of the pregnancy process. As long as you are eating good foods, there is nothing to worry about. Besides, by remaining active during this period, as soon as you have the baby, you will get back to normal very quickly.

- **Absolutely no diet pills during this period, even if they claim to be "all natural."** Most natural diet pills are made up of caffeine (in its standardized herbal form Guaranna) and ephedrine (in its standardized herbal form MaHuang). Both of these substances, which are far from being "natural", not only suppress your appetite and give you an unnatural energy boost as they stimulate your nervous system, but they also increase your resting heart rate and

body temperature—the two things that we are trying to avoid at all costs. In addition, let's remember that whatever you ingest is ingested as well by the baby. It would be impossible to determine what kind of effects these substances would have in the development of your baby, especially in the first trimester when the heart, brain and nervous system are just beginning to develop. So please, no diet pills, even if they claim to be "all natural." The risks are not worth it.

- **Another type of drug to be aware of are diuretics or water pills.** These pills dehydrate you and as a result your body temperature will rise (one of the things that you need to avoid). Unfortunately, in an effort to reduce the normal swelling that occurs during pregnancy due to water retention, some people recommend these drugs. They are dangerous and harmful to yourself and to your baby. The following are some of the side effects that these drugs produce:

  Diarrhea.

  Dizziness.

  Nausea and vomiting.

  Headache.

Even while eating a healthy diet, swelling is a natural part of pregnancy. If the swelling in your feet is bothering you too much, lie down on the sofa and raise your feet above your head. You can repeat this procedure several times a day. It should help to reduce the swelling. But no matter who recommends diuretics, **Don't use them!**

FITASTIC AT AND AFTER 40

Placing A Proactive Pause On Menopause!

This section is based on our response to numerous questions that women have asked us about our stance on hormone replacement. We've all heard the jokes about hitting age 40 and being "over the hill". The truth is, this is an approximate age when both men and women begin to lose lean muscle. In fact, women over 35 can begin losing about ½ pound of muscle and over 3% bone density per year. Aside from losing that great-looking lean muscle tissue, when you lose muscle, your resting metabolism also becomes affected and the result means burning fewer calories, naturally. A sedentary lifestyle with minimal physical activity can quickly turn into a vicious slope of deficiencies. The sedentary female will also lose bone density, which can lead to conditions like osteoporosis.

In our men's edition of the *Body Sculpting Bible*, we also talk about changes that men face when they hit the 40-year mark (Ladies, this is something to consider for the men in your lives!). You ladies know all too well that the typical mind-set of a female is different compared to a male when it comes to fitness training and physique transformation. Men tend to let ego guide them and this usually translates to lifting as heavy as we can, by any means necessary—many men heave-ho, jerk, catapult and use inertia to simply prove that they can command the lift. This often leads to little or no worthy result and can quickly lead to a pretty ugly injury in the connective tissues. Women tend to be a little tamer when it comes to weight training and seem to be more focused on the quality of exercise performed over the quantity of weight that they lift.

Many changes during the years leading up to menopause are brought on by changing levels of hormones produced by the ovaries, mainly estrogen. Estrogen is a female marker hormone that promotes the growth and health of many tissues throughout the whole body. In addition, the ovaries produce progesterone and testosterone.

Although testosterone is the predominant male marker hormone, it has a key role in the female body as it is responsible for estrogen production and helps to maintain bone density and muscle mass. Fluctuations in these key hormones during menopause can lead to the followings adverse conditions:

- Heart and blood vessel (cardiovascular) disease
- Osteoporosis
- Urinary incontinence
- Loss of sexual function
- Colon cancer
- Premature ovary failure
- Parkinson's disease
- Type 2 diabetes
- Physical and mental exhaustion
- Depression and emotional chaos
- Weight (body fat) gain

THE WEIGHT LOSS SCENARIO

Trying to lose weight is an uphill battle for many women during menopause. Calorie controlled diets worked pre-menopause and this was a great strategy for losing those extra pounds of body fat. However, for some women during menopause this is no longer the case, and continuing to follow these low or restricted calorie diets, more often than not will lead to failure.

All is most definitely *not* lost in the battle of the bulge, and by following the simple diet, exercise, and supplement guidelines set out in this section, you will re-set your body's fat burning mechanisms and start to drop that unflattering body fat, once and for all.

THE HORMONES

Estrogen and progesterone are lower down the fat-burning continuum when compared to insulin, cortisol, the thyroid hormones, and the catecholamines. Regardless of being lower down the pecking order, they still have their part to play in fat burning, especially during menopause.

Estrogen is an insulin sensitive hormone and helps to regulate the adverse effect of insulin. Progesterone blocks the impact of estrogen on insulin, but works together to control the adverse effects of cortisol. You may be thinking, "why is this important?"

Well, insulin and cortisol are a bad concoction for burning body fat and are the main culprits for unwanted fat distribution around the middle of the body. Hence the name "middle-aged spread!"

When insulin and cortisol are both present in high amounts, they are a catalyst for storing fat and preventing muscle growth, especially when your calorie intake is high. In addition, when your calorie intake is too low, the fat burning potential is halted, and a major consequence of this disruption is that skeletal muscle enters into a catabolic state.

Due to the muscle being in a catabolic state, its building potential is vastly hindered. This is directly related to a decrease in the resting metabolic rate and an overall reduction in energy expenditure.

Just remember that muscle is more metabolically active than fat and this again is another reason why fat is gained during menopause; especially in women who are sedentary and/or performing the wrong types of exercises. This will be discussed later on in this section.

THE SOLUTION

In a nutshell, you are more carbohydrate sensitive and stress sensitive during menopause. This means that the amount of carbs you ate when you were younger are now too much for your body to handle. The consequence of this carbohydrate sensitivity is an unwanted increase to your waistline and a surge in overall body fat.

Additionally, the stressful lifestyle and lack of sleep that you used to tolerate earlier on in your life is now a huge catalyst for adding inches to your belly and waist.

Simply limiting the calories you eat is not necessarily the best strategy for combatting the girth of your waistline during menopause; doing so will often only lead to failure. The best approach is to have a broader knowledge of nutrition and exercise and to understand how these two important variables impact the fat burning hormones within your body. Therefore, the following approach to these key hormones is definitely more robust in terms of improving the body's fat burning potential, and is not just a pigeonholed approach like counting calories.

NUTRITIONAL KNOWLEDGE

Not surprisingly, the main culprit in your weight gain is more likely to be refined sugars, as these cause your insulin levels to spike drastically. However, there are foods that are still a major part of many people's staple diets, which also play a role in causing insulin levels to spike. These include whole grain breads, fruits that are high in sugars, dairy products, and starchy vegetables. The influence of these foods that were initially part of your diet and kept you lean during your younger days are now counteracting your weight loss goals.

A key solution to this issue is to switch to foods that are higher in proteins, non-starchy carbs, and low sugar fruits; this will help with better insulin control and will increase your fat burning potential. The following is some simple advice to help you more effectively control the insulin levels within your body:

- Cut back on starchy carbs, dairy, and grains. Replace with non-starchy carbs such as leafy green vegetables and rainbow-colored vegetables. These foods are high in vital micronutrients and are a healthier approach toward optimal health. These whole foods are also better than simply relying on over-the-counter supplements.

- Increase your consumption of lean proteins and fatty fish as a substitute for your carb intake. Fatty fish such as herring, mackerel, and tuna are high in omega-3s which are an essential part of the fat molecules within the body that help to mop up triglycerides and have an anti-inflammatory effect. Basically, they keep the body a well-oiled machine!

- Non-starchy vegetables and proteins take longer to digest, which is caused by a reduction in HCL. Also, the pancreas enzymes that are needed to break down these food types is slowed down with age. A shot of vinegar and a leafy green salad will help with this issue.

KNOWLEDGE OF EXERCISE

Exercise should also be approached in a different manner and again it is all about hormonal control. The hormone cortisol is manufactured during exercise sessions and can last for a long time. Overworking with long sessions of high intensity training and drawn-out cardio sessions can skyrocket your cortisol. However, periodized and cycled training—like we've developed in our 14-Day Body Sculpting plans—are meant to counter the cortisol effect. Also, short bursts of high intensity exercise such as Tabata training has been proven to greatly enhance testosterone and human growth hormone (HGH) levels.

These two hormones improve the body's fat burning and muscle building potential by working with cortisol. Cortisol is fickle as it can either help to store fat or burn fat. However, this is dependent on which other hormones it is paired off with. Bearing this in mind, exercise sessions that last longer in duration will increase cortisol levels and reduce HGH levels. Therefore, the major consequence to the exhausted training sessions is that cortisol is given free reign to store more body fat. This increase in cortisol and weight gain is further exacerbated by menopause due to your physiology being more vulnerable to the adverse impact of cortisol.

Exercise made up of shorter sessions and with higher intensity is more beneficial in terms of cortisol control when compared to longer exercise sessions with moderate intensity. The following are some additional recommendations for tackling menopausal weight gain and helping to manage stress levels:

- Take a leisurely walk for one hour per day in a relaxed setting, as this lowers cortisol levels.

- Perform compound weight training exercises for a maximum of 45 minutes per session, three times per week.

- Incorporate some rest-based living into

your daily routines, which should be both restorative and relaxing in nature. These should include sleeping, napping, massage, the Zone-Tone, meditation, breathing exercises, sauna, Tai Chi, and restorative yoga.

THE USE OF SUPPLEMENTS

Bioidentical hormone replacement therapy (BHRT) has changed the manner in which women age. This natural replacement therapy has proven to help women during menopause to improve the quality and length of their lives. The remedy is very simple in that it helps to battle the effects of menopause and its associated conditions by using hormone pellets that are injected under the skin. These pellets replace low estrogen and testosterone hormones that have been reduced and it creates an optimized hormonal balance within the female body.

PELLETS COMPARED TO OTHER BHRT MODALITIES

Pellets work best because they offer the only true balancing method of your hormone levels. Since the all-natural pellets are placed in your sub-cutaneous fat and hormones are delivered through cardiac output (blood flow), this ideal delivery system gives the body the chance to optimally regulate hormone delivery, naturally and not manually.

This is a big deal! Also, because the pellets remain in the body, it gives the body a chance to optimally stabilize your hormone level, resulting in the optimized health of your heart, brain, bones, and breasts. No other hormone delivery can accomplish this; every other delivery modality is dependent on the manual deliverer. This results in a destabilized hormone

environment and is precisely what causes something that professionals refer to as the hormonal roller-coaster effect, when hormone levels are all over the place.

The solution for optimized health truly does reside in these tiny powerful pellets. This is evidence-based medicine at its finest and there exists the clinical study literature to back it all up.

If you're ready to start feeling your best and take a proactive approach in achieving your best state of health, please reach out to us and we will guide you in the right direction.

ESTROGEN PELLET THERAPY

Estrogen is undoubtedly the most important hormone for women. The longer a woman is without the protection of this vital hormone, the more prone she will be to the deficiencies discussed at the beginning of this section. There are estrogen receptors at the various regions within the brain and body. This is the main reason why an imbalance in estrogen can lead to skin issues, bone shrinkage, moodiness, and cognitive decline.

Bioidentical hormone replacement pellet therapy helps by replicating the serotonin available within the brain cells and this markedly helps to stabilize mood, which is often affected with menses and when estrogen levels are high.

TESTOSTERONE PELLET THERAPY

This is similar to the above in terms of administration, but it helps with the following:

- Balances with estrogen to produce serotonin

- Helps with emotional stability

- Reduces anxiety and bouts of depression

- Helps with mental clarity
- Helps with sleep issues
- Helps to combat muscle atrophy
- Reduces pain in the muscle and joints
- Improves muscle tone
- Helps to fight weight gain

When it comes to the superficial benefits associated with bioidentical hormone replacement pellet therapy, most women get very excited about having more energy, a boost in libido, less moodiness, less body fat, and an overall increased sense of well-being. What you don't hear them talk about, and realize that they should be shouting from the rooftops, is how bioidentical estrogen and testosterone pellet therapy, together, ultimately protects and enhances the female heart, bones, brain, and breast. What more could you ask for?

For more information on bioidentical hormone replacement therapy and pellets, please visit us at www.BodySculptingBibles.com and we will give you our opinions on your best course of action.

BODY SCULPTING FOR SENIOR WOMEN

During the past several years, many studies have been conducted that point to the many benefits and safety of weight training exercise for aging adults. Among these benefits are the usual benefits of reduced cholesterol, reduced blood pressure, reduced resting pulse rate, increased levels of muscle mass, increased levels of bone density and decreased levels of body fat. In addition to those benefits, weight training for seniors offers the following:

- Improved digestion.
- Improved blood glucose levels.

- Reduced discomfort caused by arthritis.
- Reduced lower back pain.
- Increased mobility (due to an increase in muscle strength).
- Reduced possibility of a fall due to loss of balance caused by loose joints and weak leg muscles.

In order for seniors to get all of the benefits strength training has to offer the following guidelines must be followed:

- **First and foremost, consult with your doctor and/or physical therapist before you start any exercise program.** Depending on your present condition, you may or may not need someone to supervise you during your weight training session. If you have been physically active all your life, you should have no problems going into a weight training routine. If you have never been very physically active and you suffer from ailments like loss of balance, then supervision may be required.

- **Educate yourself on how to perform the exercises correctly!** Read the exercise description section of this book as many times as necessary. Study the illustrations and practice the movement mentally. It is crucial that exercise form is followed in order to avoid injury.

- **Ensure that you follow the nutritional guidelines of our Nutrition Chapter.** Many senior citizens in this country are malnourished, as their appetites have decreased over the years. Also, certain medications cause a loss of appetite. Force yourself to follow our nutrition guidelines and we guarantee that you won't be malnourished. Remember that in order to get the maximum effect from training, the diet has to be in order. Being malnourished leads to a loss of muscle mass (the body is using such mass as fuel) and a resulting loss of strength and bone density (which leads to brittle bones).

As far as the exercise program, you have two choices. If you have always been physically active and you are in good health, go ahead and start with our Break-In Routine and progress to the 14-Day Body Sculpting Workout. If on the other hand, you suffer from ailments like loss of balance and have perhaps limited mobility, use the following program that utilizes machines:

- Leg Extensions
- Seated Leg Curls
- Leg Press
- Calf Press
- Lower Back Machine
- Abdominal Machine
- Pulldown to Front
- Close-Grip Pulldown
- Overhead Press Machine
- Rear-Delt Machine
- Biceps Curl Machine
- Triceps Extension Machine

HOW TO PROGRESS:

Follow the same structure of the 14-Day Body Sculpting Workout:
- Use weights on Monday/Wednesday/Friday alternating between Day 1 and 2.
- Do cardio on Tuesday/Thursday/Saturday.

- Sundays are for complete rest.

Weeks 1-2 perform 2 sets of 15-18 repetitions per exercise. Take 2 seconds to lift the weight and 4 to lower it. Rest 1 minute in between sets. No weight training techniques such as modified compound supersets are to be utilized. Perform one set after the other in straight set fashion.

Weeks 3-4 increase to 3 sets of 12-15 repetitions. Take 2 seconds to lift the weight and 4 to lower it. Rest 1 minute in between sets. No weight training techniques such as modified compound supersets are to be utilized. Perform one set after the other in straight set fashion.

Weeks 5-6 go up to 4 sets of 10-12 repetitions. Take 2 seconds to lift the weight and 4 to lower it. Rest 1 minute in between sets. No weight training techniques such as modified compound supersets are to be utilized. Perform one set after the other in straight set fashion.

On cardio days, build up to 25 minutes of continuous aerobic exercise performed at 70-75 percent of your maximum heart rate. Start with 5 minutes of aerobics 3 times a week, and add 2 minutes every week to the original 5 minutes. At the end of 10 weeks you should be able to do 25 minutes of continuous aerobic exercise with no problems. Use Sundays as your complete rest day from diet and exercise. If after a while using this routine you feel that you are in shape for the 14-Day Body Sculpting Routine, then by all means do so by using the exercises listed above. If you feel that you are ready to incorporate some free weight exercises as well, then go for it!

YOUNGSTERS AND WEIGHT TRAINING

At what age a teenage girl can start working out with weights has always been a topic of debate. Some people say that weights should not be touched until after all growing is done or else the growth platelets could be affected and and stunt growth. Others say it is okay to start lifting weight at an early age. We have arrived at the following conclusions based on the latest research on this subject.

We believe that youngsters (anybody **less than 12 years old**) are better off doing exercises with just their body weight. The following exercises should compose a youngster's program:

- Running
- Dips
- Push-ups
- Pull-ups
- Chin-ups
- Squats with no weights
- Lunges with no weights
- Calf raises with no weight
- Crunches
- Leg raises

Depending on the age and motivation of the person, anywhere between 2-5 sets of each exercise for the maximum amount of reps possible is sufficient. There should be 30 seconds of rest in between exercises and they should be performed 3 times a week.

An additional 15-20 minutes of running on the rest day is enough exercise for anyone who wishes to start an exercise program before the age of 13.

13-year-olds can start working out with weights as long as they're using weights light enough to allow 20-30 reps per set. They should basically follow the same program described above with the same set, repetition and rest scheme, plus adding the following dumbbell exercises: dumbbell curls, dumbbell overhead triceps extensions, and lateral raises. In addition, dumbbells can also be used to perform lunges, squats and calf raises. The complete program will look like the following:

- Running
- Dips
- Push-ups
- Pull-ups
- Chin-ups
- Lateral raises
- Dumbbell curls
- Dumbbell overhead triceps extensions
- Dumbbell squats
- Dumbbell lunges
- Dumbbell calf raises
- Crunches
- Leg raises

Continue this program for the next three years.

15-year-olds can start increasing the weight but should stay within 13-20 reps. For the next two years they should concentrate on perfecting their exercise technique. They must make sure to only increase the weight when they can do over 20 repetitions easily. They should not go to absolute muscular failure or use any fancy weight training techniques, since there is still some bone growth and development occurring in their bodies. Remember, strenuous and heavy weighted exercise can interfere with the growth process, so keep it simple!

At this age it is okay to use the 14-Day Body Sculpting routines from this book as long as the 13-20 repetition rule is kept (Weeks 1-2: 18-20 reps are used, weeks 3-4: 16-18, weeks 5-6: 13-15).

After 18, you can start using heavier weights with no problems; by then all of the growth platelets, bone and joint structure should be fully developed.

FITNESS WHILE TRAVELING

We always use traveling as an excuse to not get in shape. Getting in shape while traveling is more challenging, but it is certainly possible. Provided that you are determined, the key is planning and preparation.

Before you go on your next trip, find out if the hotel that you are going to stay in has a fitness facility or at least a set of dumbbells. If not, then find out where the closest fitness facility is and plan to work out there. If, by some twist of fate, there are no fitness facilities in the area (hard to believe), then try to do the youngsters weight training routine which consists of dips, push-ups, pull-ups, chin-ups, squats with no weights, lunges with no weights, calf raises with no weight, crunches and leg raises performed 3 times a week for 5 sets with 30 seconds of rest in between sets of as many reps as possible. Run for 20-30 minutes first thing in the morning on rest days. All you need for this routine is a park with a chin-up bar and parallel bars. If there is no park within the area, then you can still do push-ups, pull-ups, chin-ups, squats with no weights, lunges with no weights, calf raises with no weight, crunches and leg raises. All you need to carry is a portable chin-up bar that you can place in the hotel room. Once you get back home, you can start doing the 14-Day Body Sculpting Workout as laid out with the only exception being that you should start it on Week 3, since you have already done high repetition, light weight work.

With diet, you will need to get creative. Follow the rules from the section on eating out. Also, carry with you protein bars so that you are prepared with all of the required meals for the day. Missing meals too often guarantees failure with this program.

As you can see, even though it will take more effort to get in shape if you travel, it is not impossible. If you are determined enough to change your body, then nothing is impossible!

TRAINING WHILE YOU ARE SICK

Nothing can bring progress to a halt more than when you are sick. We are often asked the question, should I train while I am sick? The answer to that question really depends on what you mean by sick. Is it a cold? The flu? Allergies? Most people confuse the common cold for the flu. However, these are different types of illnesses. The flu is caused by viruses known as Influenza A or Influenza B, while the common cold is caused by viruses called coronaviruses and rhinoviruses. There are over 200 different types of coronaviruses and rhinoviruses. If one of them hits you, your immune system builds a lifelong immunity to it (therefore, the same virus will never hit you twice). However, you have the rest of the viruses that have not yet affected you to worry about; and there are enough to last a lifetime.

The flu, as you may have already found out by experience, is much more severe as it is usually accompanied by an array of body aches and fever. Therefore, your body's immune system is taxed much more by the flu than by the common cold. At this time, training would not only be detrimental to muscle growth, but it would also be very detrimental to your health as well. Remember that while training can help us gain muscle, lose fat, feel good and energetic, it is still a catabolic activity. The body needs to be in good health in order to go from the catabolic state caused by the exercise to an anabolic state of recuperation and muscle growth. So if you have the flu, your body is already fighting a catabolic state caused by the Influenza virus. In this case, weight training would only add more catabolism, which in turn would negatively affect the efficacy of the immune system against the virus, causing you to get sicker. Therefore, absolutely no training if you have the flu. Instead, concentrate on very good nutrition and on drinking large amounts of fluids (water and electrolyte replacement drinks like Gatorade in order to prevent dehydration). Once the flu completely runs its course, you can slowly start up the 14-Day Body Sculpting Workout on week 1 starting with light weights. Don't push yourself too hard during this first week. The next week you'll repeat week 1 again, but pushing yourself closer to muscular failure. By the second week of the program you should be back on track.

If it is the common cold that is hitting you and the particular virus is mild (you know that it is mild when your symptoms are just a runny nose and slight coughing), you may get away with training as long as you stop the sets short of reaching muscular failure and you decrease the weight poundages by 25 percent (divide the weights that you usually use by 4 and that will give you the amount of weight that you need to take off the bar) in order to prevent you from pushing too hard. Again, if the cold virus is causing you to feel run down, achy, with a sore throat and headaches, it would be best to stop training all together, until the symptoms subside. If this is the case, follow the exercise program start-up recommendations described above for after the flu. Remember that we do not want to make it any harder for the immune system to fight the virus by introducing more catabolic activity, so intense training is out during that time.

If your ailment is something other than the common cold or the flu, consult your doctor.

Now that we have seen how a flu or a cold can throw a wrench into your progress, let's see how we can prevent them from affecting us during the flu season or during any other season for that matter.

While it is still unknown why the cold and flu season generally comes during the winter months, it is known that you have to let the virus into your system in order for it to affect you. Therefore, it is only logical that we implement a two-fold prevention approach:

Prevent the virus from infiltrating your system. Keeping in mind that cold viruses spread by human contact, that they get into your system through the mouth, eyes and nose, and that they can remain active for up to three hours, you can accomplish this by doing the following:

- Keep your hands away from your face
- Wash your hands with anti bacterial soap frequently throughout the day (especially as soon as you finish your workout at the gym).

Maintain immune system operation at peak efficiency levels at all times. Remembering that excessive exercise, a bad diet, and losing sleep are all catabolic activities, do the following:

- Avoid overtraining by using the principles advocated in this book.
- Maintain a balanced diet as described in the nutrition chapter and avoid processed foods that contain high levels of saturated fats, refined flours or sugar since these types of foods lower the immune system function.
- Get a healthy dose of sleep a day (anywhere from 7 to 9 hours depending on your individual requirements).

So remember, stay healthy by following the tips above, and if you get sick, then "don't beat a tired horse" as former Mr. Olympia Lee Haney used to say. Rest until you get better! If you don't you will end up more seriously ill and this will take you out of the gym for a longer period of time.

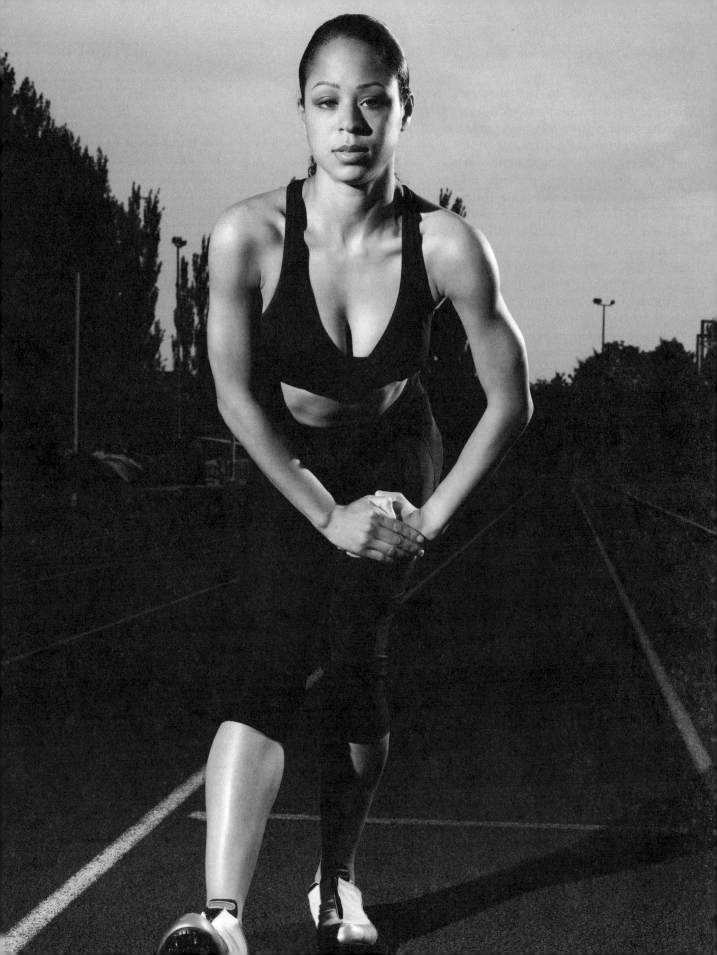

Appendix J
Anatomy Charts

THE **BODY**
SCULPTING
BIBLE
FOR**WOMEN**

J

FEMALE MUSCULAR AND SKELETAL ANATOMY

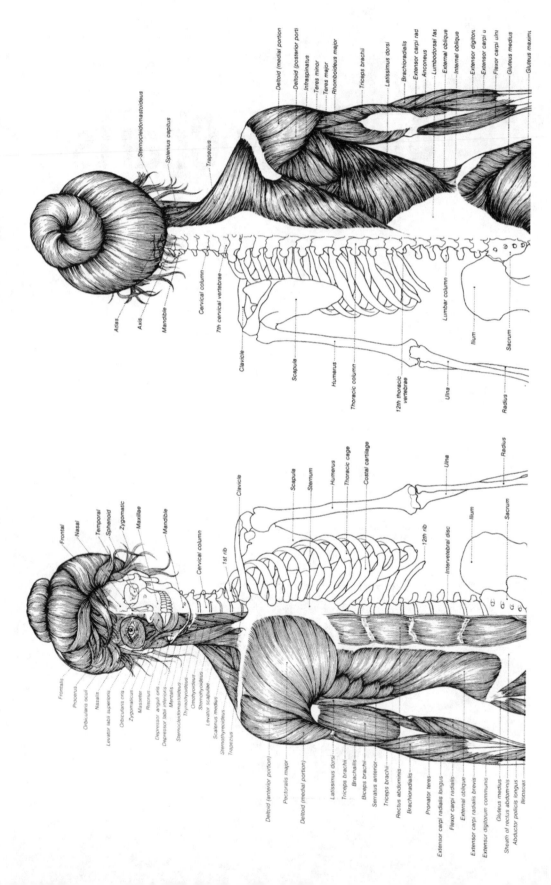

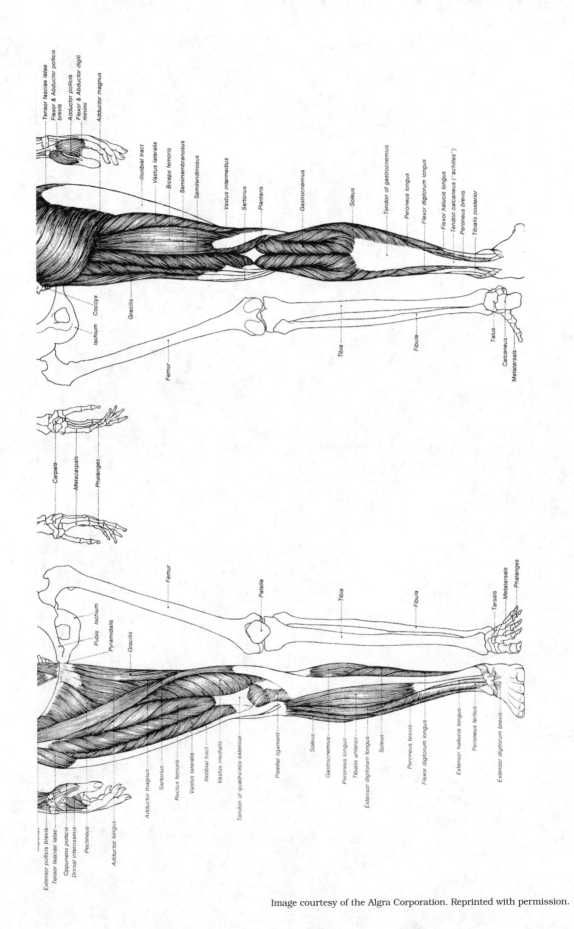

Image courtesy of the Algra Corporation. Reprinted with permission.

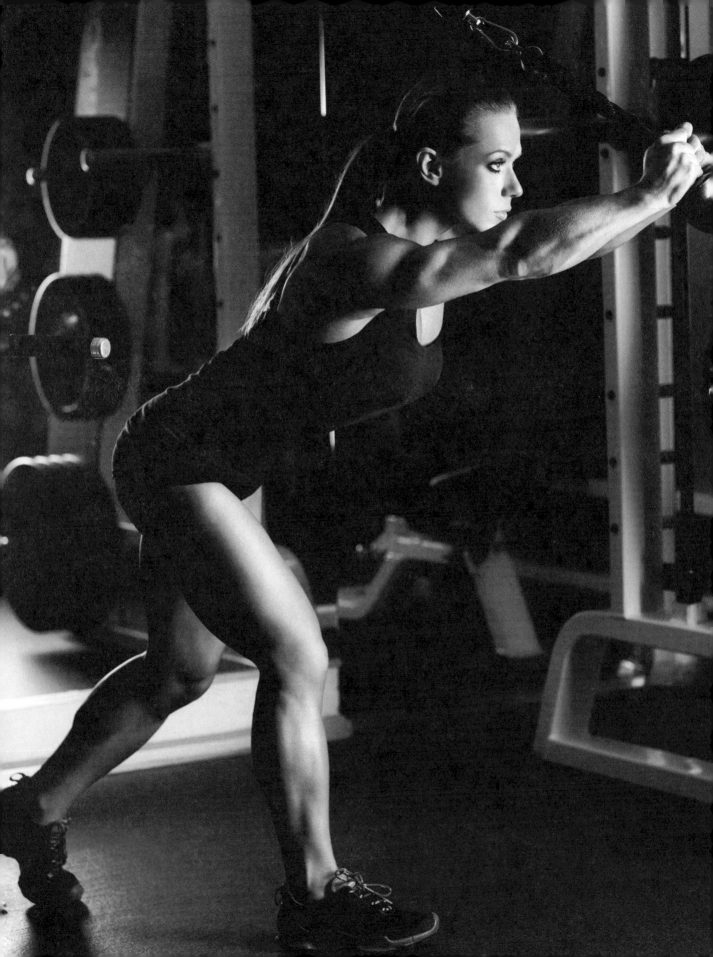

The Zone-Tone

K

THE**BODY**
SCULPTING
BIBLE
FOR**WOMEN**

THE EVOLUTION OF THE ZONE-TONE BREAKTHROUGH SYSTEM

When the *Body Sculpting Bible* books were first printed almost sixteen years ago, it was a time when mind-based practices like meditation, quantum physics, and the mind/muscle connection had not yet been accepted by the mainstream. At first we had received both praise for our work and also concern by some who thought we might be "losing it"!

That has now all changed drastically. Today, these practices are much more commonplace—so much so, that it's now actually odd if you're not tapping your brain to bring about your greatest fitness results possible. We live in a time when stress is at an all-time high and because of it, we need the power of the mind to help us cope and conquer in everything we do. If you're someone who's neglected to tap the powers of the mind, paying close attention to this updated section may very well prove to become your greatest fitness asset.

In its early stages, Zone-Tone was pretty much just a technique that we used to zero in and achieve better results from our workouts, simply by laser focusing on each muscle group before and during exercise action/exertion. But now, it's evolved into a stand-alone, complete training system that is enhancing fitness as a whole in extraordinary ways. It's not just a philosophy or a single tool—it's an entire system of robust tools, tips, tactics, and a results-driven mindset.

Most people are losing out on the benefits of involving their mind in their workout. Lots of bodybuilders, athletes, and beginning exercisers are wasting their time by simply training without thinking about what they're doing. Their focus is totally on the physical while ignoring the mental aspects. I suppose that's fine if you're content with average results. But who wants to be average? You're in it to win it.

That is, you're after the body of your dreams—not the body of an average Joe or Jane. This section will help you get there. By developing and optimizing your mind-to-muscle connection, you'll compound your efforts exponentially. You'll not only achieve the body you dream about, you'll achieve it faster than you ever thought possible.

HOW DO WE USE THE ZONE-TONE METHOD?

Like all new things, Zone-Tone might seem difficult to master at first. It's not! When you follow the simple, detailed instructions we've laid out in this book, you'll pick up on the tools, tips, and techniques quickly. You'll be effectively using Zone-Tone in your workout—and your life—in no time at all. The proof is in the pudding, as they say. We have successfully taught millions of people how to use the Zone-Tone technique. We're about to do the same for you!

You achieve a successful mind-to-muscle connection when you effectively communicate with a specific muscle before you begin the exercise. Basically, you're preparing it for the upcoming set. By maintaining this connection throughout the duration of the exercise, one set will be much more effective than you'd even imagine. In fact, some people have reported getting better results from fewer sets using Zone-Tone than they had doing multiple sets without it. Unless you've recently won the lottery, I'm guessing that's the best news you've heard in a long time. When you implement the Zone-Tone principles into your training, you can create superbly toned and defined muscles in far less time than it would otherwise take. We guarantee that by combining these concepts you will achieve an unbelievable physical transformation in a minimal amount of time.

An important function of mental practice is

being able to adapt these skills to special circumstances. For example, a master violinist would use mental preparation to memorize and rehearse a piece right before an important concert. Another use would be considered organizational. For instance, a figure skater could use mental preparation to ingrain a complex sequence of stunts and dance movements in his/her mind as easily as you can remember your phone number. Yet another use of mental preparation is motivational. Roger Clemens could have used mental preparation to picture the pay-off of a goal-focusing technique—perhaps to throw a shut-out during the World Series—seeing it in his mind's eye long before it ever happened.

There's at least one other use for mental preparation prior to a specific event. We'll call it "activational". Some power lifters engage in mental preparation that involves almost theatrical activities. The outcome is to generate the maximum level of excitement prior to executing a competitive lift. Similarly, an athlete might use mental preparation to achieve a high level of arousal right before a specific competitive task.

Certain athletic feats, such as the high jump, center on neuromuscular facilitation. In these cases, it's fairly common to see an Olympic jumper mentally practice their jump prior to an attempt. You'll see them going through the head, arm, and leg movements of the jump on a minor scale. The movements will precisely follow the rhythms and sequences of an ideal jump.

The examples above constitute a different use of mental preparation than we would use for mastering a specific skill. When preparing for a specific event, the mental focus is brief and narrowed, like a laser, on a precise performance. When learning a new skill, on the other hand, mental practice is long-term. The goal is to bring about a permanent change in behavior. Gradually, over a prolonged period of time, you not only master the skill, but come to feel like it's second nature. As you can see, this temporal factor is an important way to distinguish performance-preparation imagery from skill-learning imagery.

The performance preparation is applied to tasks that have become fully automated, like the "second nature" we referred to above. In this case, you'd focus on the event as a whole, rather than breaking it down into smaller tasks. Let's look at an example.

Before a tournament, a great golfer like Tiger Woods should focus on the vision of hitting a 400-yard drive. What he should not do is individually picture taking the perfect stance and grip, executing an ideal swing, etc. In fact, in performance preparation procedures, breaking down the smaller tasks can actually be destructive to your performance. Executing the perfect swing comes almost automatically for Tiger. The energy and focus needed for mental energy can be spent elsewhere. There's no need to "waste" that time on envisioning something he'll have no problem doing.

Now, take a look at that. Why won't he have any trouble executing the perfect swing? It's a technical matter. Anyone who's had golf lessons knows how complicated the perfect swing is, no matter how effortless it looks. To get it, though, it's a process of practice, learning, development, and polishing. What's the payoff for all that hard work? Perfection.

ZONE-TONE TIMING

Mental preparation begins before you ever set foot in the gym. The idea here is to get yourself into the right mindset to succeed. You have to go into the gym focused in order to maintain your focus throughout your workout. The journey of a thousand miles begins with a single step, as they say. Mastering the mind-to-muscle connection works the same way. Start with the basics. Once you've got the basics down, you'll be able to expand on them and maybe even create some mental exercises of your own.

The most basic of basics is the need to focus on details. When we want to "get ahead" we're so focused on the goal at the end of the road that we miss out on the journey. Blame it on our cavemen ancestors, when we were clubbing each other over the head for the best caves. The "survival of the fittest" mentality is still a part of human nature. As a result, we humans are competitive creatures. Think about it. How often have you measured success in terms of doing better than someone else, whether it's running faster, making more money, driving a cooler car? The problem with this kind of thinking is that your focus is directed outward. Instead, you should direct it inward. Like we said, you can become obsessed with the end result and lose sight of the precious details wherein the power of your mind lies. Instead of missing the forest for the trees, you're missing the trees for the forest.

A competitive streak isn't a bad thing. However, the goal should be to compete with yourself. Winning your last ball game brings on only a temporary satisfaction. One failure later, you've completely forgotten the feeling of success. As athletes (if you're exercising, you're an athlete!), we need to get inside of ourselves. The other players are part of the game, but they're not part of your drive.

AFFIRMATIONS

Repeating a mantra (also known as an affirmation) is one way to achieve the right mindset. A mantra is a few words (it can be one word, several words, or even a whole sentence) that are meaningful to you. One of the most famous sports mantras of all time is Muhammad Ali's "I am the greatest." I think we can all agree that it worked!

Here are a few tips on getting the most from your affirmations. If you practice doing affirmations correctly, you'll see great results. If you do them half-heartedly, or with poor form, just like bicep curls gone awry, you're wasting your time.

- Select a mantra that's positive. Phrase it as a declarative statement, and keep it in the present tense. For example, say "I move faster than a speeding bullet" instead of, "I will move faster than a speeding bullet." The difference is subtle, but the mental effect is huge. Phrasing it this way makes it an "affirmation." An affirmation is defined as "a statement asserting the existence or the truth of something." The sentence "I move faster than a speeding bullet" is the plain and simple truth to your mind, not just a possibility or a goal.

- Phrase them in a positive way. So, instead of saying, "I won't smoke anymore," say, "I enjoy breathing fresh, clean air and having healthy lungs."

- Use "I desire" rather than "I want." The word "want" actually means that you lack. That's not quite what you want to communicate, is it? "I want sculpted abs"? No! "I have the sculpted abs I desire."

- First person or second person? ("I am" vs. "you are".) That's your call. See which works better for you.

- Say your affirmations out loud. It's far more effective when it's your own voice speaking, your own ears hearing your voice, and your own brain processing what you've said. If you feel silly, get over it. Stand in front of a mirror, look your-self in the eye, and speak clearly and loudly.

- Use driving time for affirmations. Stuck in traffic? That's the ideal time to work on your affirmations. With half the dri-vers around you using BlueTooth or speaker phone, you won't even attract attention as you speak. Better yet, if you don't already have one, purchase an ear-piece and simply wear it when speaking your affirmations. No one will even glance at you!

- How often should you do your affirma-tions? Several times daily—ideally, about ten times a day. You'll be amazed to see how much more natural they feel after you've done them several times. Some affirmations may seem like such a stretch that you can barely say them with a straight face at first. Once you're in the habit of saying them frequently, you'll be surprised to find that they "fit"

a whole lot better.

Memorize a mantra that you can repeat right before a competition, game, or any other big event—it doesn't even have to be related to sports. Doing so focuses your mind solely on the positive. It leaves no room for any negative thoughts to creep in.

Here are some other examples of great affir-mations that will really help you get your head in the right place:

1. I love taking great care of myself.

2. I let all stress and negative feelings sim-ply melt away.

3. All the muscles in my body feel so pow-erful.

4. Day by day, in every way, I am getting better and better.

5. My body is physically improving while I rest.

6. I love physical exercise and recreation.

7. I feel so strong and fit.

8. I am in better shape with every passing second.

9. I love eating healthy food.

10. My endurance is super-charged.

11. I am achieving all of my athletic goals.

12. I train harder than anyone else.

13. I am constantly improving.

14. I am in the best shape of my life.

15. My body is dramatically changing right now.

16. I have great workouts.

17. I am always in control.

18. I am mentally tough.

19. I feel better than ever.

20. My muscles are fully recovered.

21. I feel so strong.

22. I am fast.

23. I am determined.

24. I feel great.

25. I am fully energized.

26. I can handle it.

27. I feel thinner and stronger today.

28. I'm burning body fat right this second.

29. My body feels light.

30. I'm making great progress.

31. Shedding extra weight is easy.

32. I feel so slim that I'll be buying new clothes soon.

33. I'm in the best shape of my life.

34. I get better every time I train.

35. Being active is fun.

36. My body changes with each workout.

37. I am more focused than anyone.

38. I get better and better every day.

39. I'm very relaxed.

40. I'm focused.

41. I learn from my mistakes, and get even better.

42. I do everything full-out.

43. I get better by watching others succeed, too.

44. My body knows exactly what to do.

45. This weight is so light.

46. I run like the wind.

47. My muscles are getting stronger right now.

48. I can jump like there's no gravity.

49. I am the master of my body.

50. I do everything with a joyful heart.

The trick is this—every time you repeat your affirmations, you've got to really feel it and believe it. Say them with complete confidence, knowing that you're really making it happen now. If you're not doing them full-out, you're wasting your breath. And then, after you've stated this new truth about yourself, get into action!

One way to brace yourself for potential distractions and interruptions is by using the on-site psych plan. The premise is simple: prepare for any reasonable interference so that you're ready to deal with them as quickly and efficiently as possible. Doing so helps put you in a positive frame of mind. You're free to focus on the event ahead, with no need to fret over possible distractions.

Start by walking through every step between arriving at the site of the event and the actual start of your performance. Make a list of each of those steps, both mental and physical. For example, you would include "visualizing a successful performance" (mental) as well as "suiting up" (physical).

Next to each item on your list, write down what you will you do if something goes wrong. For instance, next to "suiting up" you could jot down a plan for what to do if you can't find your shoes. With the visualizations, write out how you'll handle it if your friend wants to chat while you're trying to concentrate (I'm sure you've experienced this!). The last step is to write out a Plan B. That is, what will you do if your first plan of action fails?

Knowing that you have a game plan for overcoming any potential obstacle will greatly reduce your anxiety. You'll feel even better knowing that you're prepared if any part of your game plan doesn't work out.

There are lots of ways to prepare in advance. For example, you might have an upcoming event in mind. The idea of winning that event will get your energy levels high. This is one of the first places that visualization comes in. It's not enough to say, "I want to win the powerlifting contest next month." Instead, see, hear, smell, and feel (heck, even taste!) what winning will be like.

Here's an example of how you might visualize the experience of winning the lifting contest:

Imagine waking up on the morning of the competition. Hear your alarm going off, that awful "beep, beep, beep" blaring in your ear. Now you get out of bed. Walk into your kitchen. Have a bite to eat. Imagine eating or drinking whatever it is that you would normally consume on the morning of a competition. Smell the coffee brewing and hear the "glurg glurg" of the coffee maker. After you eat, you hop in the shower. Feel the hot water soothing your muscles. Smell the shampoo and the bar of soap. Feel the terry cloth towel when you step out to dry off.

You head back to your bedroom to get dressed. You walk over to the closet and take out your clothes for the competition. Hear the plastic hangers clink as you flip through your clothes. Really visualize the color of your clothes in your mind's eye. Feel the texture of the fabric.

Now you're in your car driving to the competition. What do you see and hear along the way? What buildings, stores, or neighborhoods do you pass? Are you listening to the radio? What kind of music?

After you've arrived, visualize yourself walking through the front doors. You see and greet fellow contestants. You feel some butterflies in your stomach, a mixture of nerves, excitement, and adrenaline. Mentally walk through your preparation routine. Put on your gloves, feel the leather. Feel the cinching of your waist as you tighten your belt.

Next you'll sit on a chair or in the stands watching the other competitors. Smell the gym, that unmistakable mixture of sweat, metal, and rubber. There are lots of sounds for you to take in: the clank of the weights, the shouts of encouragement, the grunts of exertion from your fellow competitors.

You're up next. See yourself walking over to the weights. Take a deep breath. Feel the bar in your hands, the smooth, round metal. Really imagine the contraction of every muscle as you lift the weight. You can hear the judges repeating "Lift. Good lift." Here's the really important part: imagine yourself succeeding. It's a good, clean lift. You've executed perfect form. Everyone around you is impressed with your spot-on technique. Whatever your goal weight is, you successfully lifted it. Put the weight down. Hear the thud. Feel your muscles ache. You're short of breath. But it feels great. It's the exhaustion of success. You notice the sweat dripping from your face. When the cool air hits it, you feel refreshed. It's been a perfect day. You performed to the very best of your abilities.

As you can see, this scenario is incredibly detailed. The more details you include, the more real the visualization will seem. When you see yourself succeeding, it's like you're predicting the future. Your brain says, "This is how our day is going to go." It's not a "maybe" or "gee, that'd be nice." It's a fact. Your mind and your body will conform to that fact, making sure that your ideal day happens. Even when glitches in your plan pop up, you're prepared for them. Your brain refuses to let a bump in the road interfere with the day it's got planned. The unexpected (and the unappreciated) is bound to come up. Mental preparation doesn't eliminate rocky spots. It equips you to overcome them. When you've visualized a successful day, you're not going to be derailed. Subconsciously, your mind does what it takes to keep you from being derailed.

4 WAYS TO BECOME UNSTOPPABLE

There are four beliefs that can get you focused and pumped up in any situation. Feeling great about yourself and your settings will give you unstoppable energy.

1. All that matters is the here and now. If you're about to do barbell squats, for example, tell yourself, "I'm only performing this one set." It's as if this one set of squats is all that exists in the whole

world at this moment—no sets were performed before it, and there will be no sets after it. Banish thoughts of past or future performances from your mind.

2. I am unstoppable today. Tell yourself you are a lean, mean, fitness machine. Absolutely nothing and no one can affect you today. There's an invisible force field around you repelling any would-be distractions.

3. These conditions are ideal! Regardless if its bright and sunny or gray and rainy, tell yourself that the conditions are perfect for having an amazing workout.

4. I have no limits, not even the sky! Today you are capable of achieving absolutely anything. There are no limits on what your mind and body can do when they work together.

INSTANT ENERGY

Your eyes are glued to the clock, and the numbers actually seem to be moving backwards. When will this workday finally end? You can't concentrate, and overall, you feel like a slug. Next time this happens to you, try one of these tricks for beating the midday slump and putting some pep back in your step:

- Work those muscles. Being physically active gives you instant energy. Get up and take a brisk walk, preferably outdoors.

- For a quick fix, nix the caffeine. Caffeine can leave you jittery and dehydrated. Opt for a sports drink with added electrolytes instead.

- Have a healthy breakfast feast. You've got to fuel up your body before you can face the day and breakfast is the best meal for eating mean and staying lean. You wouldn't drive to work with no gas in your car, would you?

- Put your hands in the air and step away from the vending machine. Opt for an apple over a chocolate bar when you need an energy boost. Sugary foods will cause you to crash, and you'll wind up feeling more tired than before you ate. Even better, drink some cold water with that apple and in less than ten minutes you will feel satisfied! Allow that time for your brain to receive the message from your stomach.

- Take time for a tea party. Drinking the right tea on a regular basis can increase your stamina. Buy natural herbal teas or boil your own using dried herbs.

- Take supplements. Energy is the product of chemical reactions taking place in our body. Vitamins and minerals trigger these reactions. Use supplements to make up for any nutrient deficiencies in your diet and feel your energy soar! (Check out our Resources page in the back of the book for great deals on superb products.)

- Grab an energy bar. Energy bars are specifically formulated to give you a short-term energy boost. Just make sure you don't choose one that contains more fat and sugar than a candy bar. We love bars like Kind Bars and products that contain healthy and limited ingredients. Even bar brands like Quest Bars are decent and happen to be delicious supplemental food/snack options.

- Drink plenty of water. You need lots of water to stay hydrated. Proper hydration curbs your desire for snacks and keeps you alert. Again, try to make it cool water, as this will further help combat hunger. Also, your body will actually begin working at warming up that water, which means more calories burned. Not a ton, but those calories burned can add up.

- Pack a lunch and eat it. If you skip this important meal, you're guaranteeing a mid-afternoon slump. Eating a nutritious lunch doesn't have to take more than 15 minutes.

- Snack often. You're better off eating several small meals than three big ones. Loading up in one sitting diverts blood from your brain to your digestive system, leaving you sluggish and tired.

- Take some deep breaths. Every time you take a breath, your cells' oxygen levels are replenished. Your cells need oxygen to perform their essential tasks. Here's the right way to breathe: sit comfortably, clear your mind, and breathe in through your nose and out through your mouth. Also, tap that mind power; imagine in your mind's eye, breathing in clean and refreshing white energy and exhaling dark and toxic smog-like energy.

- Get comfortable. Sitting in an uncomfortable position can actually stress out your body and drain your energy. Practice your good posture, just as mother said! Sitting upright helps your spine relax and allows you to breathe properly.

- Laughter is the best medicine. For an instant energy boost, find someone or something that makes you laugh. Laughter kicks depression and lethargy in the butt!

- Washing your face in cool water can refresh your body and mind. Splash a bit of cold water on your face or even just wash your hands.

- Take a quick break. Standing up and stretching can get the blood flowing and restore your energy. Plus, it will loosen up your muscles.

- Get some sunshine. Fluorescent lighting is an energy vampire. Our brains need the color spectrum of natural daylight. Plus, sunshine helps us produce vitamin D. Vitamin D supplements are also awesome nutritional supplements to consider taking.

- Give your nose a treat. Breathing in a fresh citrus scent is a tried-and-true method for fighting off drowsiness.

- Switch to a different task. Feel stuck in a rut? Hit a dead end with your current project? Switch to a different task to stimulate your brain.

- Say hey to a co-worker. Chat with a co-worker over the water fountain or opt for a face-to-face over sending an e-mail. Feelings of friendship and camaraderie make the workplace more pleasant.

- Find the good in the bad. Next time you're dreading a task, try this: don't focus on the misery of trudging through the task. Instead, think about how good you'll feel when it's done.

- Keep it cool. Cooler temperatures keep you more alert than warm ones. Warmth reminds our bodies of nestling up in bed for a good sleep. Even if you aren't master of the thermostat, you can still wear lighter clothes.

- Focus on fun. What are your plans after work? Cooking a delicious dinner or taking a walk with your dog? Whatever pleasant activity you have planned, focus on it and know that there's a light at the end of the workday tunnel.

- Get plenty of sleep. Avoid burning the midnight oil. Sleep is fuel for our bodies. Starting out the day well-rested is key to feeling productive.

SCIENTISTS SAY...

Studies reported in reputable scientific journals have shown that by participating in physical activities you can improve your mind, your job performance, and your overall health. Imagine, then, how many more benefits you can achieve by pairing activity with imagery.

Brain scans show that people who visualize that they are exercising stimulate the same parts of the brain as if they were really exercising. A 2004 study published in *World Disease Weekly* reported that guided imagery briefly— but measurably—reduces one's anxiety as well as the physical symptoms of anxiety. It also improves your memory.

How does all of this work? Your brain has various physiological systems that can positively affect our central and sympathetic nervous systems. Ultimately, exercise enhances the workings of these systems, which together control all your bodily processes. When you lead a sedentary lifestyle, your physiological stress system is out of practice so to speak. It's kind of a "use it or lose it" concept.

Gradually the system becomes less and less able to respond to stress. We can think of DNA as the genetic blueprint of our bodies. That little double-helix determines many of our physical and mental characteristics. If your DNA says you've got blue eyes, you've got blue eyes. Ever since science has understood the nature of DNA, we've thought of it as the 800-pound gorilla—you just can't argue with it. But what

if our emotions and state of mind could actually change our DNA? That's what a study conducted in the mid-nineties suggests.

Basically, these global blood studies found that life events, such as illness or emotional trauma, change our belief system and that change is mirrored in our DNA. This claim sounds incredibly far-fetched at first. But it starts with the basic premise most of us can agree on. For every thought or emotion we experience, a chemical reaction in our body creates a physical manifestation of those feelings. The studies I mentioned above suggest that happy feelings make for happy DNA.

Some scientists believe that this phenomenon is evident in changes in the DNA of children born HIV-positive. The children were unaware of the terminal illness lying dormant inside them. They were simply joyful, carefree kids leading happy lives. It was discovered that the DNA began to mirror the innocence and happiness of the child, and the HIV had no place for expression. By the time the children reached school age, they tested negative for HIV.

I can hardly think of more striking evidence for the power of our minds than the possibility of altering our DNA. But this next study may come close!

The Buck Institute for Age Research in Novato, California did a study comparing the strength and physiological makeup of two groups—one made up of people age 20-35, and the other of people age 65 and up. Part of the over 65 group participated in a strength training program for six months. Of course, you'd expect to see strength gains, that's no huge surprise. But what almost knocked the researchers off their feet was the difference in the actual muscle tissue. This might sound like something out of *Star Wars*, but the mitochondrial makeup of the cells in the test group was shockingly changed. These seniors had muscle tissues that looked like those of their younger counterparts. Training as a way to turn back the clock? Sure looks like a great way to reverse the effects of aging.

THE SENSE, TENSE, RELEASE TECHNIQUE

Once you've begun to master the Zone-Tone method, it's time to start multiplying your potential. We've got a simple way to compound your progress. When you go to bed at night and lie down to fall asleep, go through the following steps: start at your feet as you're beginning to relax. Focus on your toes and only your toes. Wiggle them a little bit and feel every tiny sensation. Do you feel some tingling in your toes? It's because you've probably never stopped to pay attention to all the feelings in them.

You might wonder why we're starting with the feet. They're certainly not the first body part that comes to mind when you're visualizing an athletic feat. Including your toes aids you in developing the ability to isolate any muscle at will. It's important not to neglect a single body part from your pinky toe all the way up to the muscles in your eyebrows.

Those are the basics, but there's more you need to do in order to benefit from this technique. Just thinking about your muscle doesn't call to mind the way it actually feels when it's in motion. Follow these steps to really zone in and get a feel for each individual muscle:

• As you reach each individual body part, stop and contract that muscle the best way you know how. Contract the muscle three to five times, then relax. Hold the contraction for three to five seconds. Relax for five seconds before you begin the next cycle.

• Recall the exact area where you felt that muscle contract. Now, focus all of your attention on relaxing that exact same area. When you do so, you're teaching yourself how to be in complete control of each muscle in your body. With a bit of practice, you'll be able to call upon any given muscle to perform with maximum efficiency.

Here's another technique for enhancing the overall effects of the Zone-Tone method. This technique is one you'll use at the gym or when working out at home if you've got a full-length mirror nearby.

After you complete a set of an exercise, stand in front of the mirror and contract (flex) the muscles you were just exercising. Contract them as hard as you can and hold it for three to five seconds. Doing this will strengthen your mind-to-muscle connection. It will also help you accurately identify the muscles you're using during an exercise. The result will be an increase in your body to immediately call upon those muscles prior to performing that exercise. Last, it will also help more blood and nutrients flow to those muscles, which will enhance your results.

Remember, the Zone-Tone method isn't just for when you're working out. You should also utilize the Zone-Tone techniques when you're resting. The more you practice the Zone-Tone method, the more powerful it will become.

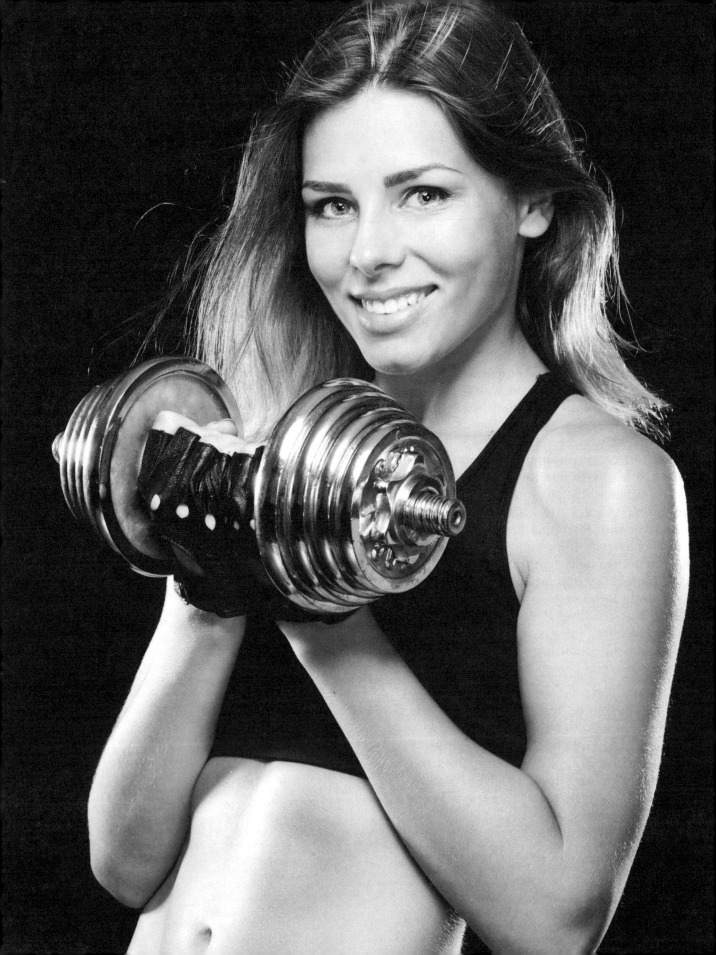

Addendum

Exercise Technique and Why Some Exercises Give You Better Results

THE BODY SCULPTING BIBLE FOR WOMEN

PROPER EXERCISE TECHNIQUE

Learning proper exercise technique is the backbone of every fitness program. If you train improperly you will not stimulate the intended muscle, and will risk major injury as well as receiving little or no results. When you learn to use proper exercise technique you will receive twice the results in half the time, guaranteed! We see people in the gym day in and day out who have no idea how to properly train their muscles. Some of them are professional bodybuilders, some are professional athletes, and some are even certified fitness trainers. Unfortunately, the ones who really suffer the most are people like you who rely on these role models for wisdom and guidance. We will show you the proper exercise technique to use for optimal results. Just remember to utilize your newfound knowledge. Like the old saying, "Feed a man a fish and he'll eat for a day, teach a man to fish and he'll eat for a lifetime." We expect the same of you. We don't want you to read this book once and forget everything you've learned. We want you to learn and utilize that knowledge to achieve astounding results.

Applying proper exercise form and technique is without doubt the most important component of any fitness program. Without it, many setbacks will occur. First, the musculature you intend to exercise will not be stimulated as efficiently as possible. Exercise should not be focused around just lifting barbells and weights. It shouldn't just be about how much you can lift. Optimum fitness is about the quality of exercise, the quality of your form and how you maintain that form, especially during heavier lifting. Proper exercise technique coupled with the Zone-Tone principle that we presented in **Chapter 1** will bring you the most astonishing results with the minimum amount of sets. Why? Because as we

have already discussed, one properly executed set is equivalent to five sets of "just going through the motions" type of exercise. *It comes down to this; if you want to get the most out of your workout, keep the intensity high without sacrificing proper form.* Neglecting to focus on proper form quickly leads to no results, while practicing perfect proper form equals incredible results quickly!

WHICH EXERCISES ARE THE BEST FOR FAST RESULTS?

In weight training, there are a variety of exercises that one can choose from to sculpt the body of your dreams. Results in bodybuilding or body sculpting are generally measured in body composition changes; increased muscle mass or tone, depending on the goal, along with decreases in body fat. The speed at which such changes are acquired depends on the training protocol used, the nutrition plan followed and the amount of rest that the trainee gets. In order for a training protocol to work at peak efficiency, not only must it be periodized or cycled but it also must include exercises that give you the most stimulation in the minimum amount of time.

Different exercises provide different levels of stimulation. Exercises like leg extensions, while excellent for sculpting the lower part of the quadriceps, produce less of a stimulating effect than an exercise like the squat. The efficacy of an exercise really depends on the exercise's ability to involve the maximum amount of muscle fibers and also on its ability to provide a neuromuscular stimulation (NMS). Neuromuscular stimulation is of crucial importance as it is the nervous system that ultimately sends a signal to the brain requesting to start the muscle growth process. How do we determine what the stimulation factor of each exercise is?

THE NMS CLASSES

In order to rate what the NMS of each exercise is, we borrowed the Class rating system used for classifying the speed of DSL systems (the technology used to achieve high speed connections to the Internet through your phone line) and tailored it to fit our purpose. In this system a Class 1 technology has lower speeds than a Class 2 technology. Therefore, in our exercise rating system composed of four classes, a Class 1 exercise yields the lowest NMS (this class is composed of variable resistance machine type exercises) while a Class 4 exercise yields the highest NMS and is therefore the hardest but most stimulating one. In each class we may also have subclasses such as Class 1a and Class 1b. A Class 1a exercise will yield less NMS than a Class 1b.

Class 1a exercises are composed of isolation (one joint) exercises performed in variable resistance machines (such as Nautilus) where the whole movement of the exercise is controlled. These type of exercises provide the least amount of stimulation as stabilizer muscles do not need to get involved since the machine takes care of the stabilization process. An example of such an exercise would be the machine curl.

Class 1b exercises are compound (multi-joint) movements performed in a variable resistance machine. An example of such movement would be the incline bench press performed in a Hammer Strength machine. Since the movement is a compound one, more muscles get involved and therefore the neuromuscular stimulation is higher than that offered by a machine curl. However, the fact that the machine takes care of the stabilization issues limits the growth offered by the exercise.

Class 2a exercises are composed of isolation (one joint) exercises performed with non-variable resistance machines. An example of such exercise would be the leg extension exercise performed in one of those leg extensions attachments that come with the benches that are sold for home gyms. These attachments lack the pulleys and the cams that would make the exercise a variable resistance exercise. Therefore, the muscles need to get more involved in the movement, providing better stimulation.

Class 2b exercises are composed of basic (multi-joint) exercises performed with non-variable resistance machines. An example of such would be the bench press unit that is attached to the Universal type of machines or a leg press machine that contains no pulleys or cams that would make the exercise easier. Since there are no pulleys or cams to make the exercise easier as you lift the weight, the NMS is higher.

Class 3a exercises are isolation (one joint) exercises performed with free weights. An example of such exercise would be a concentration curl performed with a dumbbell. It is still not very clear whether a multi joint exercise performed on a machine offers the same amount or better NMS than the one offered by a free weight isolation exercise. However, for the purposes of this discussion, we will assume that the free weight isolation exercise provides more stimulation as stabilizer muscles come into play (especially if you do the exercise standing up).

Class 3b exercises are multi-jointed basic exercises performed with barbell free weights.

Class 3c exercises are multi-jointed basic exercises performed with dumbbell free weights. The barbell exercises provide less NMS as the movement is more restrained as opposed to dumbbells where the weights can go in all directions unless all of your stabilizer muscles jump in and constrain the movement. Because of this, dumbbells provide the highest NMS in this category.

Finally, Class 4 exercises are free weight exercises where your body moves through space. In other words, any exercise where your torso is the one moving, such as squats, deadlifts, pull-ups, close grip chins, pushups, lunges, and dips, will provide the most stimulation possible and therefore, the fastest results. Haven't you seen at the gym how many people do great amounts of weights in a pulldown machine but have trouble doing pull-ups? The reason for this is that in order for you to perform these type of exercises you need to be capable of not only carrying the added resistance but also involving your bodyweight as well. Therefore, many muscles are called into play in order to perform this feat. Performing dips, chinups, squats and deadlifts you are really hitting every single muscle in your body! These exercises not only give you fast results, but they also create functional strength; in other words strength that can be used for your daily activities. If you are great at performing pull-ups and you go to perform a pulldown you'll see how easy the task of performing a pulldown is. As a matter of fact, depending on your pull-up strength, you might be able to lift the whole stack in most pulldown machines. However, the reverse is not true. While you may be very good at performing pulldowns you may not be able to perform many pull-ups as the strength gained in the pulldown exercise is not as transferable as the one gained in a pull-up. Again, the reason for this phenomenon is NMS.

CONCLUSION

Now that you know what exercises are the ones that give you the most bang for your buck, my recommendations are as follows:

*   If you follow the normal *14 Day Body Sculpting Workout* stick to Class 3 and 4 region exercises.

*   If you follow the *Advanced 14 Day Body Sculpting Workout* you can get away with having 1/3 of your routine composed of lower class (Classes 2 and below) exercises.

Remember that convincing your body to shape up is not an easy task. However, it becomes an impossible one if you choose exercises that do not provide a significant NMS effect. Therefore, always choose exercises from the higher classes in order to show your body that you mean business.

Resources

THE**BODY**
SCULPTING
BIBLE
FOR**WOMEN**

www.bodysculptingbibles.com
The official page of the Body Sculpting Bibles. Pass through here and have access to tons of free resources!

www.facebook.com/bodysculptingbibles
The official Facebook page of the Body Sculpting Bibles. Come and interact with the Body Sculpting Bible online Facebook community and motivate each other.

www.FitWhips.com
James Villepigue's personal website to whip you fit!

www.HugoRivera.net
Hugo Rivera's personal site. Great information on all aspects of bodybuilding, body sculpting & how to live a healthy lifestyle

www.losefatandgainmuscle.com
If you're looking for a companion resource that will truly help you lose fat and gain muscle, this is the website that people visit to achieve it!

TRAINING REFERENCES

Bompa, T.O. (1983). Theory and Methodology of Training—The Key to Athletic Performance. Kendall/Hunt Publishing; Dubuque, Ia.

Bompa, Tudor O., Cornacchia, Lorenzo J., (1998). Serious Strength Training, Human Kinetics Publishers.

Bompa, Tudor O., (1990). Periodization of strength: the most effective methodology of strength training, National Strength and Conditioning Association Journal, 12(5), 49-52. Bompa, Tudor O. Periodization of strength: the new wave in strength training. Toronto, ON: Veritas Publishing Inc., pg. 28, 1993.

Chernyak, A.V. Karimov, E.S. Butinchinov, Z.T. (1979). Distribution of Load Volume and Intensity Throughout the Year (Weightlifting). Soviet Sports Review. 14(2): 98-101

Ebbing, C. and P. Clarkson, (1989). Exercise-induced muscle damage and adaptation. Sports Medicine. Vol 7: 207-234

Edgerton, R.V. (1976), "Neuromuscular adaptation to power and endurance work." Canadian Journal of Applied Sports Sciences, 1:49-58.

Fleck, S.J. Periodized Strength Training: A Critical Review. The Journal of Strength and Conditioning Research, 13 (1) 82-89, 1999

Fry AC, Kreamer WJ, Stone MH, Koziris LP, Thrush JT, Fleck SJ, (2000). Relationship between serum testosterone, cortisol, and weightlifting performance. Journal of Strength and Conditioning Research, 14(13): 338-343.

Fry, R.W., R Morton, and D. Keast (1991), "Overtraining in athletics." Sports Medicine, 2(1): 32-65.

Gilliam, G.M. (1981). Effects of Frequency of Weight Training on Muscle Strength Training. Journal of Sports Medicine. 21: 432-436.

Goldberg, A.L., J.D.Etlinger, D.F.Goldspink, and C.Jablecki.(1975), "Mechanism of work-induced hypertrophy of skeletal muscles." Medicine and Science in Sports and Exercise, 7:185-198.

Hakkinen, K. (1989), "Neuromuscular and hormonal adaptations during strength and power training." A Review of Sports Medicine Physical Fitness, 29(1):9-26.

Hakkinen KA, Pskarinen A, Alen M, Kau hanen H, Komi PV (1987). Relationships between training volume, physical performance capacity, and serum hormone concentrations during prolonged training in elite weight lifters. Internaional Journal of Sports Medicine, 8 (suppli): 61-65.

Kuipers, H. and H.A. Keizer. (1988), "Overtraining in Elite Athletes: Review and directions for the future." Sports Medicine, 6:79-92.

McDonagh, M.J.N. and C.T.M. Davis. (1984). Adaptive response of mammalian skeletal muscle to exercise with high loads. European Journal of Applied Physiology. 52: 139-155.

Minchenko, V.G. (1989). The Distribution of Training Load Throughout the Yearly Training Cycles of Athletes. Soviet Sports Review. 24(1):1-6.

Rhea MR, Ball SD, Phillips WT, Burkett LN., A comparison of linear and daily undulating periodized programs with equated volume and intensity for strength. J Strength Cond Res. 2002 May; 16(2):250-5.

Starkey, D.B., Pollock, M.L., Ishida, Y., Welsch, M.A., Brechue, W.F., Graves, J.E., Feigenbaum, M.S. (1996). Effect of resistance training volume on strength and muscle thickness, Medicine and Science in Sports and Exercise, 1311-1320.

Terjung R.L. and D.A. Hood. (1986). Biochemical adaptation in skeletal muscle induced by exercise training.

NUTRITION REFERENCES

Dragan GI, Vasiliu A, Georgescu E. "Effects of increased supply of protein on elite weightlifters." In Milk Proteins 1984: Galesloot TE, Tinbergen BJ, (Eds). Pudoc, Wageningen, The Netherlands Pudoc, 99-103.

Ivy, J.L. (1991), "Muscle glycogen synthesis before and after exercise." Sports Medicine, 11:6-19.

Lemon, Peter W.R. (1991), "Protein and amino acid needs of the strength athlete." International Journal of Sports Nutrition, 1:127-390.

Munro, H.N. (1951), "Carbohydrate and fat as factors in protein utilization and metabolism." Physiol. Rev., 31:449-488.

STEROID REFERENCES

Bahrke, M.S., Yesalis, C.E. 3rd, Wright, J.E. (1996) Psychological and behavioural effects of endogenous testosterone and anabolic-androgenic steroids. An update. Sports Medicine, 22, 367-90

DiPasquale, M.G. (1990), Anabolic Steroid Side-Effects-Fact, Fiction, and Treatment. Warkworth Ontario: MGD Press.

Gruber, A.J., Pope, H.G. Jr. (1999) Compulsive weight lifting and anabolic drug abuse among women rape victims. Comprehensive Psychiatry, 40, 273-277.

Hickson, R.C., Ball, K.L. Falduto M.T. (1989)

Adverse effects of anabolic steroids. Med Toxicol Adverse Drug Exp, 4, 254-271

Hughes, T.K. Jr., Rady, P.L., Smith, E.M. (1998) Potential for the effects of steroid abuse in the immune and neuroendocrine axis. Journal of Neuroimmunol, 83, 162-167

Lamb, D. (1984). Anabolic steroids in athletics: how do they work and how dangerous are they? American Journal of Sports Medicine. 12(1):31-37.

Malarkey, W.B. Strauss, R.H., Leizman, D.J., Liggett, M., Demers, L.M. (1991) Endocrine effects in female weight lifters who self-administer testosterone and anabolic steroids. American Journal of Obstetrics and Gynecology, 175- 1385-1390

Strauss, R.H., Liggett, M.T., Lanese, R.R. (1985). Anabolic steroids use and perceived effects in ten weight-trained women athletes. JAMA, 253, 2871-2873

Wu, F.C. (1997) Endocrine aspects of anabolic steroids. Clinical Chemistry, 43, 1289-1292

WHEY PROTEIN REFERENCES

Bounouse, G. "Dietary whey protein inhibits the development of dimethylhydrazine induced malignancy." Clin. Invest. Medic. (1988), p. 213-217.

Bounous, G., P., Konshaven and P.Gold. "The immune-enhancing properties of dietary whey protein concentrates," Clin. Invest. Med. 11 (1988), p. 271-278.

Burke, D.G. and P.D. Chilibeck, et al. "The effect of whey protein supplementation with and without creatne monohydrate combined with resistance training on lean tissue mass and muscle strength," Int. Jour. Sport Nutr. Exerc. Metab. 11/3 (2001), p. 349-64.

FINAL THOUGHTS

The techniques presented in the sections above combined with the 14-Day Body Sculpting Training and Nutrition Principles, along with the knowledge presented on how to use your mind to improve your results at the gym are what separate the 14-Day Body Sculpting Workout from anything you have ever read.

After reading this book you should have the knowledge necessary to control the way your body looks. Knowledge is power and the power to change the way your body looks will give you a sense of control that will spill over into other areas of your life. Soon you will discover that the discipline you use to re-sculpt your body can be used to accomplish any other goal that you want to reach in life. Now stop wishing and start doing! Go for it!

About the Authors

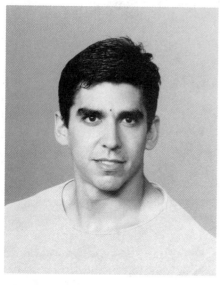

Hugo A. Rivera graduated from the University of South Florida with a Bachelor of Science in Engineering and also holds two certifications from ISSA, as a trainer and a specialist in nutrition. Born on December 5, 1974 in Bayamon, Puerto Rico, he was an overweight child and experienced at an early age the insecurity that comes with obesity and the ridicule of those around him. After going anorexic at the age of 13 and losing a total of 70 pounds in less than a year, his concerned parents took him to a nutritionist in an effort to stop the anorexic cycle. This nutritionist mentioned one thing that would change Hugo's outlook on dieting forever: "Eating food will not make you fat; only abusing the quantities of the bad foods will." Hugo decided to kick his anorexia and instead dedicate his life to studying the effects of foods on the human physiology.

By the age of fifteen, Hugo's interest in how food affects the shape and the form of your body naturally led to an interest in exercise, something that led him to become an avid natural bodybuilder.

He discovered early on that there wasn't much realistic or practical bodybuilding/fitness advice and went on to record what did and didn't work for him. After much trial and error, he started finding principles that he noticed worked on any healthy human being. The best part of it all was his discovery of the fact that there was no necessity to stay all day at the gym in order to get results! Upset at the fact that not many people in the industry cared about trainees actually reaching their goals, he decided to create a web site and start conducting personal training during his college years in an effort to spread all of the knowledge that he had acquired.

Twenty years later Hugo holds a Statewide Natural Bodybuilding Title (Mr. Typhoon Bay) and also a 4th Place in the Nationwide NPC Team Universe (the natural bodybuilder's highest and most competitive contest). Hugo is now considered an expert in the industry and he has dedicated much of his time to helping normal people achieve their dream figures by sharing sensible and practical knowledge that he has found over the years to work ever on the most stubborn metabolisms. Hugo has shared his knowledge on his website www.hrfit.net, through various radio interviews and speaking engagements, as well as on several articles published in the numerous magazines and websites all over the world, such as:

- *Muscular Development en Español* Magazine
- *Maximum Fitness* Magazine
- *Physique* Magazine
- *Be Healthy and Beautiful* Magazine
- *Muscle*
- *Natural Muscle* Magazine
- *Olympian Muscle News*
- *SuperOnda*
- Bodybuilding.About.com
- Bodybuilding.com
- DaveDraper.com
- Dolfzine.com
- MidwestChristianBodybuilding.com
- MSNBC.com
- StrengthPlanet.com

Hugo authored and self-published an online bodybuilding manual called *Body Re-Engineering*. In 2001 he commercially published two books called *The Body Sculpting Bible for Men* and *The Body Sculpting Bible for Women* with co-author James Villepigue, an authority in exercise form and the connection between the mind and the muscle. In these books, both authors apply the periodization principles used by pro athletes to workouts geared for people whose main goal is to lose weight and firm up. Both books soon became bestsellers and now there are over eight book extensions on that franchise.

Hugo was selected from thousands of applicants from all over the world to become the new www.Bodybuilding.About.com guide, an About.com website owned by the *New York Times* Company whose goal is to help beginners start a safe and healthy weight-lifting program, choose the right gear for their needs, and offer motivation to help users meet their personal goals.

Finally, Hugo has co-authored nutrition and training programs along with actress, fitness icon, and six-time Ms. Olympia Cory Everson. He has also served as consultant to high schools helping to put together bodybuilding shows and educating the students on the several aspects of bodybuilding competition and the dangers of steroids. Hugo also visits elementary schools and talks to kids about the importance of a solid education coupled with fitness and exercise. Hugo serves as a consultant to nutrition companies designing nutritional formulas and does seminars all over the world on the subjects of training, nutrition and supplementation.

Hugo's knowledge of the human physiology and anatomy (something that he was exposed to from an early age as his grandfather was a medical doctor), combined with his analytical skills developed through his engineering profession, enable him to produce extremely efficient programs that anyone can fit into their schedule. Because he was overweight and then extremely underweight, he can easily identify with many different groups of people-and his history of juggling several jobs allows him to offer practical advice that people who live a hectic lifestyle can follow.

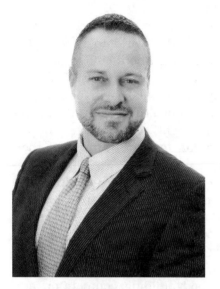

James Villepigue has over 28 years of quality certified experience in the health and fitness industry as a nationally certified personal trainer with The American Council on Exercise and The International Sports Science Association. He has received a degree from the New York College of Health Professions and is a massage therapist. James has also attended the accredited and highly acclaimed training school, the Institute for Professional Empowerment Coaching.

The success of the Body Sculpting Bible system and his extensive training, coaching, and entrepreneurial experience, have propelled James to many exciting career endeavors, including a business partnership with former Governor and A-list fitness powerhouse, Arnold Schwarzenegger, and have resulted in many appearances on national television programs and publication in nationally recognized health and fitness magazines such as:

- *Live with Regis and Kelly*
- *Maury*
- CBS, NBC, FOX, ABC, The WB, and many others
- *Fitness*
- *Women's World*
- *Oxygen*
- *Marie Claire*
- *Cosmopolitan*
- *Muscle-Mag International*

In his own words:

"Fitness training has allowed me to help hundreds of thousands of people throughout the world, of all ages and from all walks of life, to achieve extraordinary results. Besides seeing great changes to their bodies, my clients have additionally received profound changes to all aspects of their lives. This includes being happier, having better relationships, making more money, finding their dream jobs, and achieving all their dreams.

"I've overcome many obstacles in my own life and even most recently, have been dealing with the most challenging obstacle of my life—the tragic death of my beloved father, James Robsam Villepigue. This has been the greatest test for me and my family's very courageous ability to move forward in the wake of chaos. The love that I hold for my dad has empowered me to continue on my wonderful journey of success. I honor my dad and am able to keep to the path I set for myself.

"For those of you who are new to the *Body Sculpting Bible* series, I grew up a skinny kid, who suddenly became very overweight around the age of 14. I was bullied and teased, all the while dreaming for a slim, muscled physique. Unfortunately, in an attempt to lose weight quickly, I became bulimic. I managed to get very thin, but very sick. One's not worth the other, trust me!

"I soon discovered the importance of a clean and healthy lifestyle, comprised of healthy eating, fitness, meditation, and major self-discovery. Fitness gave me the confidence I needed to stand-up for myself and conquer all obstacles in my way. I am so thankful for my discovery of a healthy and fit lifestyle and nly wish that everyone could experience it for themselves."

Believe and achieve!
James Villepigue

getfitnow

GOT QUESTIONS?
NEED ANSWERS?
GO TO:

GETFITNOW.COM

IT'S FITNESS 24/7

Videos, Workouts, Nutrition,

Recipes, Community Tips, and more!